ROADBLOCKS IN COGNITIVE-BEHAVIORAL THERAPY

Roadblocks in Cognitive-Behavioral Therapy

Transforming Challenges into Opportunities for Change

Edited by
Robert L. Leahy

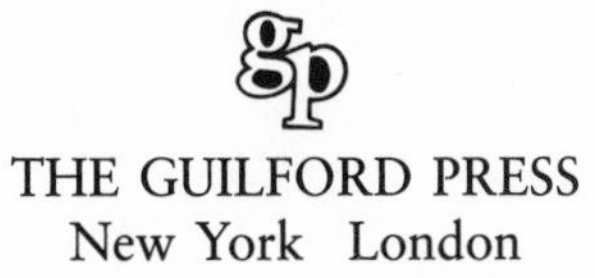

THE GUILFORD PRESS
New York London

A Division of Guilford Publications, Inc.
72 Spring Street, New York, NY 10012
www.guilford.com

Printed in the United States of America

This book is printed on acid-free paper.

Last digit is print number: 9 8 7 6 5 4 3 2 1

Library of Congress Cataloging-in-Publication Data

Roadblocks in cognitive-behavioral therapy : transforming challenges into opportunities for change / edited by Robert L. Leahy.
p. cm.
Includes bibliographical references and index.
ISBN 1-57230-920-2
1. Cognitive therapy. I. Leahy, Robert L.
RC489.C63R635 2003
616.89′142—dc21

2003010581

To Paul Gilbert

About the Editor

Robert L. Leahy, PhD, is President of the International Association for Cognitive Psychotherapy, Founder and Director of the American Institute for Cognitive Therapy in New York City (*www.CognitiveTherapyNYC.com*), Professor of Psychology in Psychiatry at Weill–Cornell University Medical School, and former Editor of the *Journal of Cognitive Psychotherapy.* Dr. Leahy's recent books include *Cognitive Therapy: Basic Principles and Applications, Practicing Cognitive Therapy, Treatment Plans and Interventions for Depression and Anxiety Disorders* (with Stephen J. Holland), *Overcoming Resistance in Cognitive Therapy, Bipolar Disorder: A Cognitive Therapy Approach* (with Cory F. Newman, Aaron T. Beck, Noreen A. Reilly-Harrington, and Laslo Gyulai), *Clinical Applications of Cognitive Psychotherapy* (edited with E. Thomas Dowd), *Psychology and the Economic Mind, Cognitive Therapy Techniques: A Practitioner's Guide,* and the forthcoming *Psychological Treatment of Bipolar Disorder* (edited with Sheri L. Johnson).

Contributors

Donald H. Baucom, PhD, Department of Psychology, University of North Carolina–Chapel Hill, Chapel Hill, North Carolina

Frank M. Dattilio, PhD, ABPP, Department of Psychiatry, Massachusetts Mental Health Center, Harvard Medical School, Boston, Massachusetts

Linda Dimeff, PhD, Behavioral Technology Transfer Group, Seattle, Washington

Norman B. Epstein, PhD, Department of Family Studies, University of Maryland–College Park, College Park, Maryland

Christine Foertsch, PhD, Department of Psychiatry, St. Luke's–Roosevelt Hospital, New York, New York

Arthur Freeman, EdD, Department of Clinical Psychology, Philadelphia College of Osteopathic Medicine, Philadelphia, Pennsylvania

Brad K. Grunert, PhD, Department of Plastic Surgery, Medical College of Wisconsin, Milwaukee, Wisconsin

Gillian Haddock, PhD, Academic Division of Clinical Psychology, School of Psychiatry and Behavioural Sciences, University of Manchester, Education and Research Centre, Wythenshawe Hospital, Manchester, United Kingdom

Stephen J. Holland, PsyD, private practice, Washington, DC

Howard Kassinove, PhD, ABPP, Department of Psychology, Hofstra University, Hempstead, New York

Robert L. Leahy, PhD, American Institute for Cognitive Therapy, and Department of Psychiatry, Weill–Cornell University Medical School, New York, New York

Sharon Y. Manning, PhD, South Carolina Center for Dialectical Behavior Therapy, Columbia, South Carolina

Lynn Marcinko, PhD, Cognitive Behavioral Therapy Clinic, Department of Psychiatry, Harbor–UCLA Medical Center, Torrance, California

Roya Djalali McCloskey, PsyD, Department of Clinical Psychology, Philadelphia College of Osteopathic Medicine, Philadelphia, Pennsylvania

J. Christopher Muran, PhD, Brief Psychotherapy Research Program, Beth Israel Medical Center, New York, New York

Lawrence D. Needleman, PhD, Department of Psychiatry, Ohio State University, Columbus, Ohio

Cory F. Newman, PhD, Center for Cognitive Therapy, University of Pennsylvania School of Medicine, Philadelphia, Pennsylvania

Jeremy D. Safran, PhD, Clinical Psychology Program, New School for Social Research, and Beth Israel Medical Center, New York, New York

Nicole A. Schaffer, PhD, Manhattan Cognitive Behavioral Associates PLLC, New York, New York

Ronald Siddle, PhD, Department of Clinical Psychology, North Manchester General Hospital, Manchester, United Kingdom

Mervin R. Smucker, PhD, Department of Psychiatry and Behavioral Medicine, Medical College of Wisconsin, Milwaukee, Wisconsin

Christopher L. Stevens, PhD, Beth Israel Medical Center, New York, New York

Raymond Chip Tafrate, PhD, Department of Criminology, Central Connecticut State University, New Britain, Connecticut

Michael A. Tompkins, PhD, San Francisco Bay Area Center for Cognitive Therapy, Oakland, California

Adrian Wells, PhD, Academic Division of Clinical Psychology, School of Psychiatry and Behavioural Sciences, University of Manchester, Manchester Royal Infirmary, Manchester, United Kingdom

Jo M. Weis, PhD, Department of Psychiatry and Behavioral Medicine, Medical College of Wisconsin, Milwaukee, Wisconsin

Preface

After I finished writing *Overcoming Resistance in Cognitive Therapy* (Leahy, 2001), I realized that the issue of resistance, noncompliance, therapy-interfering behaviors, roadblocks, and impasses (as it is variously called) was certainly not comprehensively covered in my book. Indeed, over the years, having had the privilege of knowing many experienced and talented cognitive-behavioral therapists, it has become clear to me that there are many patients in therapy who seem to struggle with the process of change. When my colleagues and I put together a number of clinical symposia for the Association for Advancement of Behavior Therapy, I recognized that these panels were a terrific opportunity for me to learn more about impasses in therapy from the world's experts. Several of the contributors to the current volume were participants in those panels.

Indeed, my interest in resistance is a self-interest. I found myself continually frustrated with patients who would not follow my benign guidance and my "powerful" cognitive therapy techniques. My own personal schema of demanding standards and goal setting was being frustrated. I was initially reluctant to utilize empathy for very long because it conflicted with my compulsive tendency to "get the job done." I decided to use cognitive therapy on my own neurotic and anger-provoking thoughts, and I realized that patient resistance and other impasses in the process of therapy provided a window into a world of depth, complexity, challenge, and change that eluded my simple-minded bag of tricks. These impasses, or "roadblocks," I now saw, provide great opportunities to learn more about the patient and my relationship with him or her. Resistance became less of a roadblock and more of a window.

Metaphors—such as the "window" in the previous sentence—help us look at things in a new way. If resistance is a window into the patient's schemas, thoughts, interpersonal history, self-protection, self-limitation, and validation needs, then therapy could become far more interesting and effective. After all, we are so fond of thinking of our patients as poor irrational creatures beset by their neurotic characters and imbalanced biochemical systems that it is refreshing to think of them as individuals who are attempting to construct a world and preserve a reality that affords them some modicum of individuality and respect. It seemed to me that roadblocks could lead to new and deeper levels of cognitive therapy. To paraphrase Freud, we can and ought to view resistance as the "royal road to the psyche."

As I began to examine the meaning of validation and change for a particular resistant patient—who had described himself as the most difficult patient I would ever have—I felt a new freedom for myself. I told this man, "I have been trying to get you to change, but I think, in the process, you have felt that I did not fully understand you. I think I will set aside the pressure to change and simply try to hear you and understand what you are feeling and what it is like for you." As the therapy became more collaborative with this shift on my part, I suggested to him, at the end of each session, that he might think of whatever techniques we had talked about as things that he may or may not want to use for himself. I abandoned, with him, the role of taskmaster and became more the collaborative understanding ear that helped him puzzle out his thoughts and feelings. We examined other failures in validation in his other relationships and his belief that his feelings made no sense to anyone. This focus on exploring the meaning of validation and the risks this patient faced in taking interpersonal chances helped him eventually choose to make the changes. His change was gradual and eventually quite dramatic as my role of taskmaster receded. Understanding his resistance through his eyes opened up my mind immensely. Most important, he found that he had the autonomy and understanding to make the changes he needed to make.

The current volume represents the work of some of the leading cognitive-behavioral therapists in the field. As I put together this collection of contributors, I realized that, indeed, many more outstanding contributors could have been included. This realization made me even more hopeful, because I understood that therapeutic impasses and resistance are the stuff of the real world of the clinician—a world that is experienced daily in clinical practice.

The volume is divided into five parts. Part I (Needleman, Chapter 1; Freeman & McCloskey, Chapter 2; and Tompkins, Chapter 3) includes fundamental examples of roadblocks and the use of case conceptualization. The more complicated the patient, the more important case conceptualization is. My experience may be idiosyncratic, but I seem to be finding my patients to be more complicated than I thought they were when I first began doing therapy. I believe the reason is that, with experience and inevitable frustration and failure, we come to recognize the complexity in individuals that we did not initially see. The newer therapist will find some comfort and irony in recognizing that those of us who have been out here doing this for some time are more aware of how difficult this is—how much there is to learn. Each year I am more impressed with how much I still need to learn and how much that gap dwarfs whatever knowledge I have accumulated. So, if case conceptualization is something used with the more complicated cases, we may find that almost all cases are complicated.

In Part II, Wells, Leahy, and Holland each review some of the potential roadblocks in treatment that are consequences of metacognitive beliefs about anxiety, metaemotional beliefs that impede emotional processing, and experiential and defensive processes that result in avoidance of emotion. Wells, in Chapter 4, has developed a sophisticated model of metacognition that not only has direct relevance for conceptualizing each anxiety disorder but also has treatment implications as well. In Chapter 5, I attempt to develop a model of emotional schemas that can assist the therapist and patient in understanding how roadblocks can arise on the most fundamental level of accessing and experiencing emotions. In Chapter 6, Holland indicates the importance of emotional avoidance as a factor that often escapes cognitive-behavioral therapists. In his analysis of this process, Holland indicates how the skilled therapist can identify this defensive process and utilize it to engage the patient in examining the meaning and fear of negative feelings, thereby accessing underlying assumptions and interpersonal schemas.

Part III covers specific populations—patients with psychosis (Haddock & Siddle, Chapter 7), bipolar disorder (Newman, Chapter 8), posttraumatic stress disorder (Smucker, Grunert, & Weis, Chapter 9), or binge-eating disorder (Schaffer, Chapter 10). Obviously, every diagnostic group or cultural group could be considered here, but we had to limit ourselves in our coverage. In these chapters, the authors examine how specific roadblocks arise for these patient populations and how these roadblocks can be addressed. Part IV addresses couples and families among whom the individual issues are complicated by the systemic issues in families and the underlying agendas within couples. The authors of these chapters, Epstein and Baucom (Chapter 11) and Dattilio (Chapter 12), provide sophisticated analyses of how specific areas can be addressed. Finally, in Part V, various psychotherapy processes are examined. The dialectical behavior therapy approach is presented by Foertsch, Manning, and Dimeff in Chapter 13 as a general model for addressing therapy-interfering behaviors. The chapter on medication compliance by Marcinko (Chapter 16) integrates standard cognitive therapy with motivational interviewing and dialectical behavior therapy. Stevens, Muran, and Safran, in Chapter 14, explicate the interpersonal nature of therapy in evaluating the use of therapeutic ruptures to enhancing progress. In Chapter 15, Tafrate and Kassinove offer specific—and very valuable—ideas of how to address angry patients. This final part should be especially helpful in providing the reader with an integrative approach to dealing with roadblocks.

In sum, I hope that the reader will find these contributions valuable in the following ways:

1. Recognizing roadblocks when they exist.
2. Developing case conceptualization as a strategy in understanding and dealing with these problems.
3. Viewing emotional schemas and emotional processing as important components in activating meaningful emotional experience.
4. Understanding how specific pathology can be an inevitable part of noncompliance with therapy.
5. Expanding therapy to include larger systems in the individual patient's life.
6. Using the transference relationship (and the therapist's own experience) as therapeutic opportunities.

Therapists who are reading this book understand the following experience to be valid in their own lives: A patient does not comply with treatment in various ways and blames the therapist for the failure of the treatment. The therapist may vacillate among anger, guilt, shame, and anxiety. The impasse is viewed as another frustration in the professional life of the therapist. What to do? First, recognizing that all of us have had similar experiences is to recognize that this "comes with the territory." You are not alone. Perhaps, I might add, you are in good company. Second, the impasse may now be an opportunity. Just as pain may tell us the location of the injury, resistance and roadblocks tell us more about the patient's personal experience and the therapeutic relationship we are establishing with him or her. The avenue to change may be through the impasse.

REFERENCE

Leahy, L. (2001). *Overcoming resistance in cognitive therapy.* New York: Guilford Press.

Acknowledgments

Many of my colleagues over the years have influenced my thinking and awareness of the importance of case conceptualization and the potential for resistance to change in therapy, and I am pleased that many of them are represented in this current volume. I have had the good fortune to be surrounded at the American Institute for Cognitive Therapy with the active and energetic minds of clinicians who are dealing daily with roadblocks in therapy. Past or present members of this group include Stephen J. Holland, Lynn Marcinko, Laura Oliff, and Elizabeth Winkelman. Thanks to Randye Semple and David Fazzari from Columbia University for their tireless efforts as editorial assistants on this project and many other projects.

Contents

PART I. CASE CONCEPTUALIZATION

PART II. METACOGNITION AND EMOTION

PART III. SPECIFIC POPULATIONS

PART IV. COUPLES AND FAMILIES

PART V. PSYCHOTHERAPY PROCESSES

Part I

CASE CONCEPTUALIZATION

1

Case Conceptualization in Preventing and Responding to Therapeutic Difficulties

Lawrence D. Needleman

Cognitive case conceptualization plays an essential role in cognitive therapy. This chapter describes the various ways case conceptualizations help prevent and respond to therapeutic roadblocks. Cognitive case conceptualization refers to the process of developing an explicit parsimonious understanding of clients and their problems that effectively guides treatment (Needleman, 1999; Persons, 1989; Sacco & Beck, 1995). When developing an initial case conceptualization, the therapist integrates a thorough intake evaluation with the contemporary cognitive model. Cognitive therapists modify and refine their conceptualizations as a result of new data emerging from ongoing assessment and clients' responses to interventions (selected from the case conceptualization). The case conceptualization is best considered a working model consisting of various testable, interrelated hypotheses (Beck et al., 1990; Carey, Flasher, Maisto, & Turkat, 1984). To decrease the likelihood of confirmatory bias, therapists should search for evidence that refutes their model and honestly consider alternate hypotheses to explain clients' behaviors (Meier, 1999). (For a step-by-step guide to developing effective cognitive case conceptualizations, see Needleman, 1999.)

COGNITIVE MODEL

Stated simply, Beck's cognitive model asserts that cognitive content and processes are central to individuals' emotional and behavioral responses to situations, as well as to individuals' long-standing patterns of adaptive and maladaptive responding (e.g., Beck et al., 1990). When developing case conceptualizations, therapists should incorporate the various elements of the cognitive model discussed in this section.

For therapy to be effective, therapists should have a complete understanding of their clients' belief systems and thought processes. According to Beck et al. (1990), cognitive content is categorically and hierarchically organized. The least durable and least central category of cognition is the *automatic thought*. These are thoughts or images that influence how a person feels and behaves in a particular situation (e.g., "They're trying to get me fired"). As part of the conceptualization, it is important for therapists to identify typical situations that trigger maladaptive automatic thoughts and resulting emotional and behavioral responses.

Core Beliefs

At the other end of the continuum are core beliefs, the deepest or most central category of cognition (e.g., "I am the most brilliant artist alive"). Core beliefs are beliefs that people have held for much of their lives and that are activated across a wide range of situations. These beliefs have a profound influence on how people feel, appraise situations, and see themselves and the world.

To prevent roadblocks in therapy, therapists should identify and address the salient core beliefs that are causing clients distress, that are contributing to their maladaptive behaviors, or that are likely to directly influence their responses to therapy. When attempting to identify core beliefs, cognitive therapists benefit from knowledge of various core-belief themes identified in the literature. Some of these themes include (1) Beck's cognitive triad—beliefs about the self (e.g., "I'll never be enough to satisfy the people I care about"), the world ("Danger lurks around every corner"), and the future ("Nothing will ever work out for me"); (2) disorder-specific core beliefs (e.g., in panic disorder: "I am experiencing a ___________ [medical or mental health] catastrophe"); (3) culturally shared core beliefs (e.g., in Asian cultures: "Having emotional problems is a disgrace"); (4) Erikson's psychosocial stages of development (e.g., in industry vs. inferiority: "I'm incompetent"; Erikson, 1950); and (5) self-handicapping strategies, which serve the purpose of avoiding disappointment or negative self-evaluation (e.g., "If I don't try hard and do poorly, it doesn't really reflect my abilities"; see Leahy, 1999).

Some examples of core beliefs that may directly influence clients' responses to therapy include mistrust beliefs ("People in general will hurt me"), hopelessness beliefs (e.g., "Nothing will ever help me"), and low self-efficacy beliefs (e.g., "I can't do anything that will make my life better"). In addition, beliefs that contribute to *psychological reactance* can be roadblocks to effective therapeutic work if not handled skillfully. Psychological reactance—first described by Brehm (1966)—occurs when individuals perceive that their freedom is lost or threatened and consists of motivation to restore their freedom. Some examples of psychological reactance beliefs are, "No one has the right to tell me what to do" and "Most authority figures are full of it."

Intermediate Beliefs

A third category of cognition is referred to as intermediate beliefs, because they are neither as central and enduring as core beliefs nor as situationally specific as automatic thoughts. Examples of intermediate beliefs are conditional assumptions (e.g., "If I don't succeed at my work, I'm a total failure"), life values (e.g., to be a good person; to dominate others), and implicit rules (e.g., "I shouldn't ever show unpleasant emotions to people").

Other important types of intermediate beliefs are those related to changing problematic responses. Identifying intermediate beliefs based on Prochaska and DiClemente's (1992) influential transtheoretical stages of change model can be particularly helpful. The transtheoretical model suggests that individuals undergo a predictable sequence of stages when changing (Prochaska & DiClemente, 1992; Velicer, Hughes, Fava, Prochaska, & DiClemente, 1995). A growing body of research suggests that, for a wide variety of mental health problems, therapeutic effectiveness increases when therapists match interventions to clients' stage of change (e.g., Prochaska et al., 1994).

According to the transtheoretical model, individuals in the *precontemplation* stage do not intend to change. They may simply be unaware of their problem and are not thinking of it. Freeman and Dolan (2001) called these individuals *noncontemplators*. Alternatively, precontemplators may be actively resisting information that suggests that they have a problem (e.g., "I don't gamble too much; my problem is that my wife nags me all the time, and my boss doesn't pay me enough").

Those in the *contemplation* stage are aware that they have a problem and are seriously thinking about resolving it in the foreseeable future. However, they have not yet made a commitment to take action. Often, the reason is that they continue to have ambivalence about giving up the old (problematic) behavior or replacing it with new behaviors (e.g., "I know my drinking is causing fights with my husband and is creating health problems, but I really need it to relax, and I'm afraid my friends won't accept me if I don't drink"). Another potential roadblock to making a commitment to and planning for change is low self-efficacy.

Individuals in the *preparation* stage intend to take action in the near future and have committed to doing so. They are developing specific plans for changing their problematic behavior. In the *action* stage, individuals have recently begun to make overt changes in behavior and often have restructured their environments to support their new behavior. Finally, individuals in the *maintenance* stage have sustained overt changes over time and are working to stabilize their behavior and avoid relapsing. To increase the likelihood of maintenance, Freeman and Dolan (2001) suggest adding *prelapse*, *lapse*, and *relapse* stages to the transtheoretical model; they describe characteristics of the proposed stages and suggest relevant interventions.

Compensatory Strategies

Another essential element of the cognitive model—and cognitive case conceptualization—is compensatory strategies. Strategies are internal or external coping responses performed to manage distress or challenging circumstances. Some examples of common compensatory strategies include traditional ego defenses (see Vaillant, 2000), experiential avoidance (see Hayes, Strosahl, & Wilson, 1999), social withdrawal, maintaining a façade, self-sacrifice, people pleasing, inactivity, exploitation and manipulation, addictive behaviors, and workaholism. Obviously, strategies can cause difficulties in clients' lives and, if not handled skillfully in therapy, can become roadblocks.

Whether a strategy is adaptive or maladaptive depends on its maturity, appropriateness to the situation, and the flexibility of its use (Vaillant, 2000). Beck et al. (1990) suggest that people with personality disorders underdevelop some strategies and overdevelop others. For instance, individuals with schizoid personality disorder overdevelop their ability to act autonomously and live in isolation but underdevelop their ability to be intimate and reciprocal.

Maintaining Factors

Maladaptive strategies often maintain individuals' distress and dysfunction. Therapists' inattention to maintaining factors often contributes to treatment failure. Therefore, maintaining factors represent another essential component of the cognitive model that should be included in individualized case conceptualizations.

According to Young and colleagues (McGinn & Young, 1996; Young, 1990), individuals with personality disorders take one of three general types of rigid strategies, which help maintain their maladaptive behaviors.

Some individuals with personality disorders acquiesce to their schemas (e.g., dependent individuals selecting dominating partners). Others avoid anything associated with their schemas (e.g., via dissociating, avoiding triggers, abusing substances). Still others overcompensate for their schemas (e.g., a defectiveness schema may lead to acting superior). These different types of strategies might explain why individuals with similar core beliefs can behave in vastly different ways.

Therapists should consider a variety of other factors that may maintain clients' problems. The most important maintaining factors include: (1) schema-consistent appraisal of situations and schema-consistent recall; (2) lack of awareness of more adaptive strategies; (3) high levels of physiological arousal, which interfere with effective problem solving; (4) robustness of behaviors that are intermittently reinforced; (5) immediate reinforcement, which outweighs delayed punishment; (6) avoidance, which prevents disconfirmation of catastrophic beliefs and habituation to triggering situations; (7) self-handicapping, which can bolster one's self-concept (e.g., "If I weren't drinking, I might have given an outstanding talk"); (8) self-fulfilling prophecies; (9) anxiety about change (e.g., "I'll become a completely different person"); (10) feelings of hopelessness; (11) social environments that reinforce maladaptive behaviors, and (12) vicious cycles.

THE ROLE OF CASE CONCEPTUALIZATIONS IN PREVENTING TREATMENT DIFFICULTIES

This section discusses the role of cognitive case conceptualization in selecting effective interventions, predicting and circumventing roadblocks, and using moment-by-moment awareness of clients' in-session experiences to full advantage.

Selecting Effective Interventions

A major purpose of the cognitive case conceptualization is to help therapists select effective interventions. Evidence suggests that matching interventions to particular client characteristics can increase therapeutic success (see Beutler, Clarkin, & Bongar, 2000).

Stage of Change

As mentioned earlier, an important consideration when developing a case conceptualization is clients' stage of change with respect to the problem behavior. Taking this into account helps therapists select effective interventions. For example, when clients are in the contemplation stage, they often benefit from interventions that help tip the balance toward change, such as interventions that evoke from clients concerns about their behavior and reasons for changing; that strengthen self-efficacy; that increase their arousal (e.g., grieving over losses resulting from the problematic behavior) or that help them reevaluate themselves (e.g., value exploration and clarification, imagery).

Single Disorder

When selecting interventions for individuals with a single disorder for which there exists an empirically validated treatment approach, therapists should provide the relevant manualized treatment. Empirically validated cognitive therapy treatment manuals have been developed for a variety of disorders (e.g., depression, Beck, Rush, & Emery, 1979; bipolar disorder, Newman, Leahy, Beck, Reilly-Harrington, & Gyulai, 2002; personality disorders, Beck et al., 1990; substance misuse disorders, Beck, Wright, Newman, & Liese, 1993; social phobia, Chambless & Hope, 1996; and inpatients, Wright, Thase, Beck, & Ludgate, 1993). Within the broad structure of the treatment manual, a cognitive case conceptualization remains important because the client's idiosyncratic beliefs and maladaptive strategies are targets of interventions.

For example, Jeff and Janie both had panic disorder and had a similar core belief, namely that an internal catastrophe could occur instantly and unexpectedly. During panic attacks, Jeff focused on feeling lightheaded and unreal and had the catastrophic cognition that he was "going crazy." Janie focused on chest pain during attacks and believed she was having a heart attack. Although both received the same treatment components (following Barlow & Cerny, 1988; Beck, Sokol, Clark, Berchick, & Wright, 1992), their treatment was individualized based on idiosyncratic features of their conceptualizations. Briefly, cognitive restructuring targeted their specific catastrophic beliefs. In addition, their therapists used different methods to induce panic. During panic inductions, Jeff was exposed to feeling lightheaded by spinning around in a swivel chair while hyperventilating. The purpose was to show him that even when pushed to the limit, he would not go crazy. To expose Janie to sensations of panic, her therapist had her exercise vigorously during the therapy session, beyond the point at which she felt she must stop. This convincingly demonstrated to her that her heart was strong.

Multiproblem Clients

For multiproblem clients or clients for whom no empirically validated cognitive therapy approach yet exists, cognitive therapists must first decide whether it is ethical to treat them. If so, case conceptualization is crucial for selecting targets and selecting and prioritizing interventions. When making these decisions, the therapist should consider several factors, including (1) the relative importance of potential targets (e.g., risks to safety, impaired functioning), (2) the primacy of relevant factors with respect to the client's problems, (3) the relative malleability of various potential targets, and (4) the client's preferences. For example, Jan was an emaciated, 25-year-old client with a 2-year history of a food and eating phobia with associated weight loss, as well as a lifelong history of debilitating anxiety, depression, and social dysfunction. She presented for treatment as a "last hope" effort after failing to gain weight in an inpatient eating-disorder program at a well-known, university-affiliated hospital. Clearly, the priority when she sought treatment was weight gain because of her medical risk.

Although Jan was emaciated and food phobic, she had a normal body image and wanted very much to gain weight. Her eating symptoms were intertwined with obsessive–compulsive, panic, and depressive processes. Figure 1.1 illustrates the working model Jan's therapist developed as a part of Jan's case conceptualization. According to the therapist's working model, when Jan attempted to eat, she had the intrusive automatic thought that

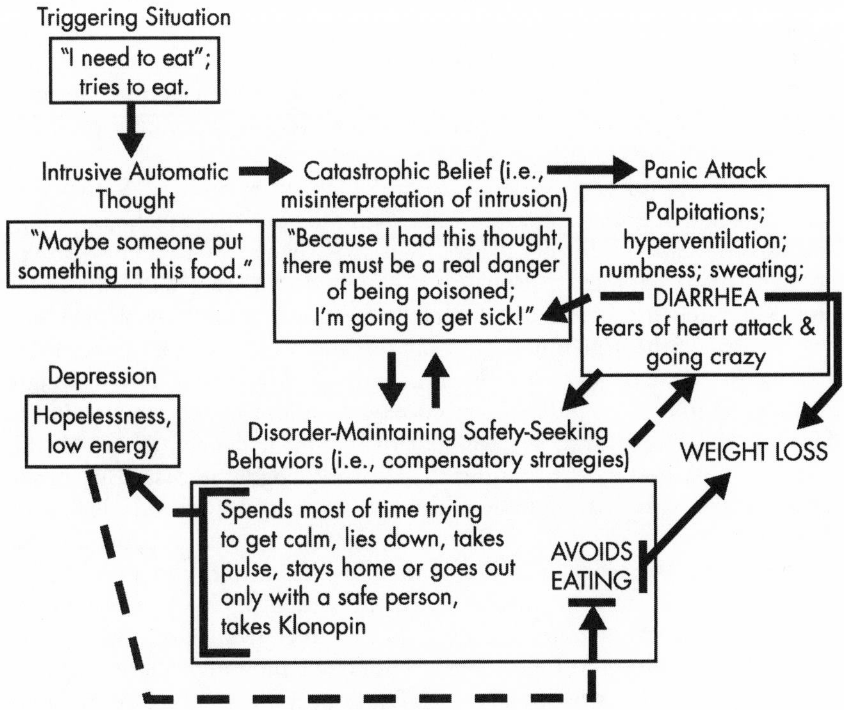

FIGURE 1.1. Working model for Jan.

someone put something in her food. She catastrophically misinterpreted the occurrence of this thought as meaning that the thought reflected reality. Specifically, she believed that someone poisoned her food and that if she ate it, she would get very sick and possibly die. Food and the cognitions associated with food triggered panic attacks consisting of palpitations; hyperventilation; diarrhea (which contributed to her weight loss); and fears of going crazy, becoming deathly ill by food poisoning, and having a heart attack. She typically had many full-blown panic attacks per day. In response to her fears and her intense anxiety symptoms, she engaged in a variety of disorder-maintaining, safety-seeking behaviors (i.e., compensatory strategies). She isolated herself in a quiet, dark room most of each day, lay down, took her pulse, focused on deep breathing, and often avoided eating. When she did eat, she ate very slowly and was hypervigilant to any signs of gastrointestinal symptoms. She rarely left her parents' home and did so only when accompanied by a parent. According to the cognitive model, safety-seeking behaviors such as these prevent individuals from disconfirming their catastrophic interpretations (e.g., Salkovskis, 1996). In addition, by prematurely terminating anxiety, they prevent the natural occurrence of habituation to triggering situations.

The absence of potentially fulfilling activities, social isolation, and failure to progress with respect to developmental tasks contributed to Jan's depression. She was severely depressed and felt hopeless about her life. Feelings of hopelessness, lethargy, resignation, and anger at herself also seemed to contribute to her difficulty with eating. Conversely, starvation probably contributed directly to her depression.

For the sake of brevity, details of Jan's history are omitted. Suffice it to say that beginning very early in life she exhibited extreme psychopathology and was in treatment for her problems at an early age. Her parents showed no signs of psychological problems themselves and were basically caring and moderately protective, although they were understandably burned out.

Because of the urgent nature of Jan's eating problem, therapy began on a twice-per-week basis. Her therapist informed Jan that if her weight dropped another 2 pounds, he would have to admit her to the hospital to have a feeding tube until she was out of imminent danger. Although this was a complicated case, a graphically depicted cognitive case conceptualization made selection of interventions fairly straightforward. The early therapeutic targets for facilitating Jan's weight gain were her panic attacks, her belief that someone was attempting to poison her, and food-related anxiety cues. In therapy, Jan's therapist presented her with the cognitive model of panic. After obtaining medical clearance from Jan's internist, he used hyperventilation to induce panic symptoms and taught her panic coping strategies (à la Barlow & Cerny, 1988; Beck et al., 1992). Over the next few weeks, the frequency and intensity of Jan's panic attacks diminished by approximately 40%. Also, early on in treatment, Jan and her therapist worked on Jan's belief that her food was poisoned (for cognitive restructuring in obsessive–compulsive disorder, see Freeston, Rhéaume, & Ladouceur, 1996; van Oppen & Arntz, 1993). To help Jan desensitize to food cues, she and her therapist constructed an exposure hierarchy for various foods and began graded, *in vivo* exposure to hierarchy items. Initially, Jan did not gain weight, but her weight plateaued and the frequency of diarrhea decreased. After approximately 8 weeks, Jan slowly began to gain weight. Over the next 5 months, she gained on average ½ pound per week. Once she had gained this weight, her psychiatrist put her on a low dose of Luvox; this was the first time in several years that she was able to tolerate a selective serotonin reuptake inhibitor.

After a year in cognitive therapy, Jan had made substantial progress. She was on the low end of normal weight and out of medical danger, had occasional panic attacks but felt confident in her ability to manage or at least live through the attacks, rarely engaged in safety-seeking behaviors, had completely stopped engaging in compulsions, was euthymic, lived by herself in an apartment near her parents, and had begun taking courses at a local community college.

Predicting and Circumventing Therapeutic Roadblocks

Besides helping develop a parsimonious understanding of the client for selecting interventions, a thorough assessment and a thoughtful cognitive case conceptualization help the therapist anticipate potential therapeutic roadblocks. There are many client response patterns (i.e., core beliefs and related compensatory strategies) that, if anticipated, could avoid therapeutic impasses. What follows are several typical examples.

Wilma had the core belief, "I can't tolerate unpleasant feelings." When asked to discuss upsetting issues, she felt overwhelmed with shame and anxiety, and her mind went blank. Mary Ellen believed, "I don't deserve to be happy because there is so much suffering in the world; I should save the world." She felt angry with herself and guilty when she was not feeling depressed or overwhelmed. Because of this belief, she engaged in extreme self-sacrifice to help anyone who was in pain or who had unfortunate circumstances. Her extreme self-sacrifice resulted in mental and physical exhaustion and failed relationships. Steve was severely depressed and lethargic. He believed, "Nothing will ever work out for me; what's the point of trying?". Muhammad clung desperately to people and was hypervigilant to signs that people might want to leave him, a belief that often became self-fulfilling. His terror-provoking belief was, "People will abandon me." Leroy believed, "People are to be used to get what I want." His primary, problematic strategies were externalization of blame, exploitation, and manipulation. He experienced rage when he could not get people to do what he wanted and became verbally or physically threatening to them.

This section focuses on how therapists' conceptualizations can help predict and circumvent three types of potential roadblocks: perfectionism, mistrust, and psychological reactance. Case examples illustrate how therapists address perfectionism and mistrust. In addition, guidelines for helping clients who exhibit psychological reactance are provided.

Perfectionism

Rosita was a client who had the core belief, "If I make a mistake, I'm a complete failure." As a result, she habitually avoided challenging tasks (compensatory strategy). Her avoidance prevented her from progressing in her career and her personal life. Based on the case conceptualization, her therapist predicted that perfectionism put Rosita at risk for not completing self-help work and for feeling discouraged with therapy if she attempted a task and did not complete it perfectly.

Early in therapy, Rosita's therapist addressed her perfectionist beliefs and avoidance behavior with a variety of approaches. He predicted for Rosita that her perfectionistic belief would likely make self-help assignments anxiety provoking and that she might have strong urges to avoid them. (Predictions of this kind illustrate for clients that their therapists understand their problems and can generate hope that the therapists can help with their problems.) The therapist informed Rosita that therapy is a learning process, that mistakes are inevitable, and that, indeed, mistakes are often beneficial and contribute to learning. During tasks performed in sessions, he prescribed making mistakes. As a rationale, he suggested to Rosita that she would benefit from learning to feel more comfortable making mistakes in order to progress in life. He used Socratic questioning to help her realize that it is inevitable for people to make mistakes and, furthermore, that doing some tasks imperfectly could have important benefits (i.e., saving time for more important or enjoyable activities). Rosita benefited from a cost–benefit analysis of her perfectionistic belief. This helped her clearly see the strong, long-term disadvantages of avoidance in various life domains as compared with the weak, short-term advantages.

The therapist used several additional strategies to decrease the risk that perfectionism would impede therapeutic progress. He taught Rosita to monitor her distress and to recognize perfectionistic automatic thoughts and simply label them as such. The therapist began self-help assignments in session. In addition, he attempted to set up self-help assignments that Rosita could not fail. For example, he gave her the following instructions for an early assignment: "If you find yourself avoiding writing down your responses, try to take mental note of the thoughts and feelings that were interfering and describe them to me next time."

Despite these efforts, there were occasions in treatment in which Rosita avoided tasks and felt ashamed and discouraged. The therapist framed these occasions as helpful because they paralleled her behavior in real-life situations and provided opportunities to work with the behavior in session. Also, to decrease her shame and normalize mistakes, the therapist disclosed to Rosita various recent, minor mistakes that he had made, which resulted in no significant difficulties. This therapeutic work lessened Rosita's perfectionism, which improved her mood, decreased her anxiety, and allowed therapy to proceed to other issues.

Mistrust

A second example of a therapist using a cognitive case conceptualization to predict and circumvent difficulties involved the case of John Henry. In the second therapy session during the presentation of the cognitive model, the therapist identified the following core belief: "I shouldn't open up to people or show any weakness; if I do, I will become powerless and at the mercy of people who will judge or mistreat me." (Although many individuals with a mistrust schema are guarded in therapy, many others—especially those seeking treatment voluntarily—disclose their vulnerable thoughts and feelings.) Because of this belief, John Henry often felt anxious in social situations and presented a façade to people. The therapist expected that if John Henry's mistrust belief and his corresponding compensatory strategies were not addressed, they would likely impede progress in therapy.

As a result of this prediction, John Henry's therapist addressed the issue of trust immediately. She assured him that given his life experiences and the resulting mistrust belief, it would be perfectly normal for him to have doubts about her trustworthiness. She conveyed to him that although she hoped he would eventually trust her, she realized that she would have to earn his trust. John Henry's therapist assured him that although she would probably suggest various cognitive-behavioral skills for them to work on, he could always decide what they worked on and what he would share with her. She cautioned him not to tell her "too much too soon," suggesting that doing so might elicit feelings of shame and vulnerability. The therapist also indicated that even if John Henry never fully trusted her, she hoped he could learn useful skills for managing his mood and improving his circumstances.

John Henry's therapist indicated that she would value his collaboration in the therapy process. She proposed that mistrust reactions toward her could provide an excellent opportunity to therapeutically address his mistrust belief in a relatively safe place. She encouraged him to express any doubts he had about her motives or sincerity in order for him to test out his belief. In addition, she strongly encouraged him to let her know if he were planning to drop out of treatment. Telling her would give her a chance to clarify any misunderstandings, be a sounding board for his decision, and, if necessary, make referrals to other clinicians.

Early in therapy, when John Henry was about to tell his therapist a major secret, she stopped him. She provided him with an opportunity to carefully consider whether to share this secret. She asked, "Are you sure you feel ready to tell me this?" and "Are you going too fast?" John Henry decided that he was ready. After John Henry disclosed his secret, the therapist probed his thoughts and feelings. She expressed much empathy, normalized the content of his disclosure, and complimented his courage. Over time, John Henry increasingly revealed more personal information to her. In addition, he eventually shared some personal information with select people in his life and gradually felt more comfortable with self-disclosure.

Psychological Reactance

Identifying the presence of psychological reactance early in therapy and incorporating it into the case conceptualization also can help therapists predict and circumvent later difficulties in therapy (e.g., Therapy Reactance Scale; Dowd, Milne, & Wise, 1991). With respect to therapy, Seibel and Dowd (1999) found that clients' self-rated reactance was negatively associated with global improvement, as rated by the clients and therapists. Reactance also was positively associated with a set of interpersonal distancing behaviors and with premature termination.

Power struggles with reactant clients are almost always counterproductive. For example, when reactant clients are ambivalent about change and the therapist pushes a change agenda, clients immediately take the opposite side and talk themselves out of changing. As part of motivational interviewing, Miller and Rollnick (1991) attempt to have clients convince themselves to change. Therapists summarize clients' ambivalence, emphasizing clients' self-motivational statements. In addition, therapists ask evocative, open-ended questions to (1) help clients recognize their problems (e.g., "What makes you think you have a problem?"), (2) elicit clients' concern (e.g., "In what ways does that concern you?"), (3) elicit intentions to change (e.g., "What's the next step?"), and (4) elicit optimism for making a change (e.g., "What encourages you that you can change in this way if you want to?").

Beutler, Harwood, and Caldwell (2001) provide general guidelines for treating highly reactant clients. According to these guidelines, therapists should take a nonauthoritarian stance and primarily use nondirective interventions. For example, therapists should gently ask open-ended questions; reflect clients' feelings, thoughts, and underlying meanings; allow clients to either generate their own self-help tasks or select self-help tasks from a menu of options; and refrain from reviewing self-help work unless the client requests doing so. If all else fails, therapists might consider carefully using the paradoxical intervention of prescribing the symptom. To avoid client suspicion when doing so, therapists should provide a convincing rationale for paradoxical directives (e.g., "I'd like you to *not* treat each other [spouses] any differently for now, because without a whole lot more clarity on what's going on, it would be a mistake to do anything differently and have more failure experiences"). In contrast to high-reactant clients, those exhibiting low reactance often respond well to directive interventions (e.g., direct suggestions, therapist-assigned self-help tasks, careful review of self-help tasks, structured sessions).

Moment-by-Moment Awareness of Clients' In-Session Experiences

Making ongoing efforts to understand their clients' moment-by-moment experiences are a third way that therapists can prevent roadblocks in cognitive therapy. Understanding clients' moment-by-moment experience is both influenced by and helps modify the case conceptualization. Exquisite attunement to clients' moment-by-moment cognitions and emotions *is* empathy, and it fosters the clients' sense of being deeply understood (Greenberg, Rice, & Elliott, 1993). Mindful awareness of clients' experiences confers several additional advantages, described in this section.

Therapy-Related Cognitions

Awareness of clients' moment-by-moment experience during sessions allows therapists to understand clients' cognitions and emotions about therapy and the therapist. Therapy-related cognitions play an important role in clients' willingness to participate fully in treatment. Moreover, mindfulness of clients' therapy-related responses as they arise helps therapists prevent momentary upsets and misunderstandings from becoming major roadblocks to therapy.

For example, during a therapy session, Abby, a premed student, was discussing her anxiety about her performance on a recent exam. As part of evaluating the relevant thoughts, her therapist asked her the following series of questions: "What's the worst that could happen given the situation? If the worst happened, could you live through it? What would happen over time? What's your estimate of the probability of the worst happening? What's the best that could happen? What's the most likely to happen?".

Abby's therapist noticed her stiffen slightly as they were exploring these questions. He asked her what was going through her mind and how she was feeling. She admitted that she thought the therapist assumed that she had failed the exam and would not be accepted by any medical school. After clarifying his rationale for asking these questions and disclosing his honest belief that she had a good chance of getting into medical school, Abby appeared to relax. Then she and her therapist were able to effectively work through the anxiety-provoking automatic thoughts triggered by the exam.

Microconceptualizations

A related advantage of being attuned to clients' moment-by-moment experiences is that doing so provides a microconceptualization—an understanding of the client in the moment. The new information can contribute to an overall understanding of how clients experience and react to the world. For example, clients' reactions to therapists can reveal clients' automatic thoughts and associated situational triggers, interpersonal core beliefs, and compensatory strategies. A client's in-session, interpersonal responses provide opportunities to directly observe the client's interpersonal behavior, which can be invaluable in refining the case conceptualization. Conversely, mindfulness of the therapist's own reactions to the client can provide invaluable information about reactions the client elicits from others (Layden, Newman, Freeman, & Morse, 1993). (On the other hand, reactions to clients may sometimes represent therapists' own unresolved issues. When in doubt, therapists should consult with colleagues for guidance or seek their own therapy.)

If an observed client reaction is consistent with the case conceptualization, the new information provides more support for the relevant parts of the conceptualization. If an observation conflicts with parts of the initial conceptualization, the therapist should consider changing or modifying the conceptualization to better account for the observation.

For example, a therapist was scheduled to evaluate a new client, Danielle. When he went to the waiting room to meet her, he found Danielle cowering in the corner on the floor. Although she was difficult to interview because of her intense fear and because she regressed in sessions, over several visits the therapist learned that she had been severely abused from early childhood and was afraid that people would hurt or kill her. The therapist's conceptualization of Danielle reflected her chronically activated fear mode. She was hypervigilant to being attacked, and she avoided many situations in which she might be in contact with people.

After working with Danielle for several months and making little progress, the therapist called her at work about scheduling. On the phone, Danielle sounded self-assured. During the next session, the therapist brought up his surprise at her demeanor on the phone. She indicated that in her work setting, she felt confident in her abilities and comfortable. She described her academic and work history. Beginning in high school, some teachers recognized her above-average aptitude in logic and computer programming. Danielle found a series of mentors while in college and in the large company where she worked. Over 10 years at the company, she managed to find a niche for herself and was a valued resource. She consistently received above-average evaluations and felt safe and protected in her work environment.

Danielle's therapist incorporated this new information into his conceptualization of her. This new understanding helped the therapist work with Danielle's strengths. Danielle then made more rapid progress in therapy than might have been possible had he not discovered and incorporated this new information.

Modulation of Clients' Arousal

Attunement to clients' moment-by-moment psychological state also can prevent difficulties in therapy by helping therapists modulate their clients' distress level. Clients' level of distress during sessions is extremely important to therapy outcomes. As a result, therapists should attempt to monitor clients' distress at all times.

Frank and Frank (1991) found that clients benefited most from therapy sessions when they were moderately distressed. Moderate arousal is associated with optimal learning. A sustained, high level of distress is usually counterproductive because it can further sensitize clients to experiences they find aversive (through classical conditioning). Clients might begin to associate the therapist and therapy with aversive feelings and drop out of treatment. Even if they continue with treatment, clients' trust in their therapists might diminish. The reason for this is that they are likely to think and feel that their therapists are not adequately caring for them.

In contrast, sustained low levels of distress in therapy sessions might be counterproductive for two reasons. First, therapy might not be focusing on the most salient cognitions, emotions, behaviors, or issues. Second, clients might be using compensatory strategies to avoid fully contacting important issues (e.g., intellectualizing, dissociating, talking about trivial issues).

When clients are experiencing low levels of distress, it is often necessary for the therapist to increase distress by activating relevant schemas. "Hot cognitions" are typically more responsive to modification than are dormant ones (Beutler et al., 2001). Therapists can help clients activate core schemas using imagery, role plays, or *in vivo* exposure.

For example, Ron sought therapy for feeling extremely anxious at work and for not advancing in his career. These problems resulted from feeling intimidated by male authority figures. In sessions, he dispassionately discussed his relationship with his current male supervisor. Although, during sessions, Ron could calmly and effectively role-play interactions with his supervisor, this work did not generalize to actual interactions with his supervisor. He continued to feel anxious and to act unassertively at work. As a result, Ron's therapist activated relevant schemas by having Ron imagine vividly his current supervisor yelling at him. Ron became intensely anxious (crying, shaking) during the exercise. The imagery triggered memories of his father abusing him. While Ron's schemas were activated, the therapist helped him rationally respond to relevant cognitions and generate coping strategies. After repetitions of imagery exercises over several sessions, Ron experienced markedly less anxiety during the exercises and increasingly believed the adaptive self-statements that he and his therapist generated even in the face of vivid, threatening imagery. These sessions helped Ron feel markedly less anxious around his supervisor and ultimately approach him about redesigning his job. This resulted in an improvement in Ron's work situation and increased his self-efficacy for interacting effectively with supervisors.

Increasing Therapists' Moment-by-Moment Awareness

To heighten their moment-by-moment awareness of clients' experiences, therapists should frequently explore clients' cognitions, opinions, feelings, subjective ratings of distress, and reactions to interventions. Shifts in verbal and nonverbal behavior can signal important reactions that warrant probing. For example, when working collaboratively to identify distorted automatic thoughts, a client, Norman, exhibited a momentary look of disgust. His therapist asked, "What just happened there? What were you thinking and feeling?". Norman admitted thinking, "I'm really screwed up for thinking this way" and feeling very angry with himself. The therapist used this disclosure as an opportunity to normalize cognitive distortions as being very human, to point out the important role of metacognition in distress, and to identify another distortion (i.e., labeling himself). A socially phobic client, Silvia, looked away after awkwardly responding to her therapist's inquiry about a vacation. Knowing Silvia's core beliefs ("I'm defective, and people will think I'm a loser"), he asked her, "I'm wondering if—at this moment—you're making an assumption about what I'm thinking or feeling about you."

Therapists should also inquire about clients' understanding of interventions and ask clients to periodically summarize discussed topics. At the end of each session, therapists should ask clients for verbal or written feedback. Feedback questions can include the following: "What was helpful in today's session?"; "What was upsetting or confusing?"; "How open were you and how hard did you work in today's session?"; "How much time and effort did you spend on self-help work since our last session?"; "What are your thoughts and feelings about the overall direction of therapy so far?"; "Is there anything about your therapist's behavior or style that is particularly bothersome or helpful? If so, what?"; and "In what ways would you like therapy to be modified to be more helpful for you?".

In addition to asking clients for their reactions, therapists should frequently ask themselves questions to help them attune to their clients' experiences. Questions can include: "Does the client understand the cognitive model and the rationale for this intervention?"; "How confident is the client that this can be an effective approach for her?"; "What is she feeling and thinking now?"; "Why is she responding this way?"; "How am I feeling and what am I thinking about this client?"; "How might this be similar to and different from the ways people in her life respond to her?"; "Based on my case conceptualization of this client, what might this mean to her?"; "Based on her belief X, how might she respond to Y?". These questions illustrate that it is useful for therapists to ask themselves both "bottom up" questions (beginning with observations and attempting to abstract more general patterns of responses) and "top down" questions (beginning with the conceptualization and attempting to make sense of a response to a particular situation).

RESPONDING TO THERAPEUTIC ROADBLOCKS

Thus far, it has been suggested that careful selection of interventions, using the cognitive case conceptualization to predict and circumvent difficulties, and moment-by-moment attunement to clients can prevent problems in cognitive therapy. Nonetheless, therapeutic roadblocks—large and small—inevitably arise. This section describes the important role that case conceptualizations play in effectively responding to therapeutic difficulties.

Hostile Clients

A therapeutic difficulty that can be particularly challenging for therapists is clients' directing hostility toward them. Therapists can easily fall into the trap of responding to clients similarly to how others respond to them—that is, with anger, defensiveness, blaming, labeling, discounting, rejecting, and avoiding. These very human, untherapeutic reactions can powerfully strengthen clients' maladaptive beliefs (e.g., "People will try to hurt me if I don't fiercely stand up for myself").

To effectively work with hostile clients, therapists often must first work on their own cognitions and emotions (e.g., Layden et al., 1993). When therapists are attempting to restructure their own thoughts, the case conceptualization of the client can be particularly helpful. It can help the therapist understand possible origins of the client's aversive behavior and how the aversive behavior may have been a reasonable adaptation to extreme childhood circumstances. Also, the case conceptualization might increase therapists' awareness that underlying clients' hostility is deep pain, hurt, shame, fear, embarrassment, or reasonable desires and needs. Therapists should also attempt to be open to the partial truth behind clients' criticism. Many clients, especially those with severe personality disorders, are hypervigilant to subtle or not so subtle signs of rejection or judgment. Therefore, they sometimes detect these therapists' reactions before the therapists do. In short, cognitive restructuring can contribute to therapists feeling empathy for clients who are angry and hostile.

Ideally, therapists then can capitalize on opportunities to work in sessions on behavioral patterns that cause clients much difficulty in their daily lives. An essential ingredient for helping clients who are exhibiting hostility is good listening skills. Therapists should genuinely encourage angry clients to elaborate on their angry thoughts, empathize with their intense underlying feelings (e.g., hurt, shame, anxiety, sadness), accurately reflect the clients' cognitions, and take responsibility for any elements of truth in clients' criticism. As a result of nondefensive, empathic listening, clients' anger usually dissipates, and the therapeutic relationship is strengthened. Clients feel accepted and cared for.

After anger subsides, therapists can use a variety of interventions that can improve clients' interpersonal functioning. For example, therapists can (1) teach clients to restructure distorted, anger-provoking thoughts, (2) set appropriate limits, (3) provide videotaped feedback, (4) examine whether clients' behavior is serving the intended purpose, and (5) teach clients more appropriate ways of getting their needs met (e.g., assertiveness training).

Nonresponse to Interventions

The other situation in which cognitive case conceptualizations can help therapists respond to difficulties involves cooperative clients who are not improving. Kendall, Kipnis, and Otto-Salaj (1992) found that when their clients were not improving, only a minority of therapists developed alternative treatment plans. An important principle in problem solving is, "If it ain't working, try something else."

Because the case conceptualization is a process of organizing, simplifying, and prioritizing a large amount of clinical information, therapists sometimes may overlook or deemphasize relevant issues. For cooperative nonresponders, it is important to look back over the cognitive case conceptualization to see if there are any beliefs (e.g., "I'm incapable of doing anything to improve my lot"), strategies (e.g., avoiding unpleasant emotions), or maintaining factors (e.g., obstructive social environment; reinforcing contingencies) that might account for the current roadblock. For example, Nona was not responding to treatment for her severe depression, despite being diligent about her self-help work, punctual to all sessions, and cooperative in sessions. When reviewing the case conceptualization, her therapist recognized that Nona's belief, "I need a strong person to take care of me," warranted further attention. When the therapist broached this issue with her, Nona admitted to being very worried about terminating treatment because then she would be completely on her own. After working on this issue over the next few sessions, Nona was able to work effectively on her depression.

When treatment nonresponse cannot be readily understood based on the initial case conceptualization, further assessment is needed. For example, Julio's presenting problem was panic attacks and associated avoidance. He initially did not admit to much depression and described himself and his life in fairly positive terms. After eight sessions of standard cognitive therapy for panic disorder, the frequency and intensity of his panic attacks remained the same. When his therapist was attempting to discover factors that may have contributed to Julio's nonresponse, Julio sheepishly admitted to feeling extremely guilty about past promiscuity. He believed that he deserved punishment for his past behavior and that God was in fact punishing him through panic attacks. Initially, his shame prevented him from disclosing this information to his therapist (or even endorsing relevant items on questionnaires). Working through this issue allowed him to work effectively on his panic symptoms. As this case shows, important information may be missing during the initial assessment because clients may be unwilling at first to admit to particular problems (e.g., substance abuse, affairs).

SUMMARY

This chapter described the essential role cognitive case conceptualization plays in preventing and responding to therapeutic roadblocks. First, case conceptualizations help therapists select effective interventions and maximally tailor interventions to client characteristics. Within an empirically validated, manualized treatment for particular disorders (e.g., major depression, panic), the case conceptualization ensures that therapy targets key beliefs, compensatory strategies, and maintaining factors. Awareness of clients' stage of change can also be important in selecting effective interventions. For multiproblem clients, case conceptualizations enable therapists to see the interrelatedness of problems and select and prioritize interventions accordingly.

A second way that case conceptualizations help prevent therapeutic difficulties is by helping predict and circumvent roadblocks. Examples were provided of therapists' detecting potentially derailing beliefs (i.e., perfectionism, mistrust) early in therapy and successfully addressing these issues. Psychological reactance—the perception that one's freedom is threatened and the associated motivation to restore freedom—is another client dimension that can interfere with treatment. Reactance can be detected early, enabling therapists to modify their approach. Guidelines were provided for successfully treating highly reactant clients. Moment-by-moment attunement to clients' in-session experiences is important for predicting and circumventing problems because it helps therapists detect clients' therapy-related cognitions and emotions, refine the conceptualization, and modulate clients' arousal.

In addition to preventing difficulties, case conceptualizations can help therapists effectively respond to roadblocks that arise. Descriptions of ways therapists can use conceptualizations to successfully treat hostile clients and modify interventions for cooperative nonresponders were provided.

REFERENCES

Barlow, D. H., & Cerny, J.A. (1988). *Psychological treatment of panic.* New York: Guilford Press.

Beck, A. T., Freeman, A., & Associates. (1990). *Cognitive therapy of personality disorders.* New York: Guilford Press.

Beck, A. T., Rush, A. J., & Emery, G. (1979). *Cognitive therapy of depression.* New York: Guilford Press.

Beck, A. T., Sokol, L., Clark, D. A., Berchick, R., & Wright, F. (1992). Focused cognitive therapy of panic disorder: A crossover design and one year follow-up. *American Journal of Psychiatry, 149,* 778–783.

Beck, A. T., Wright, F. D., Newman, C. F., & Liese, B. S. (1993). *Cognitive therapy of substance abuse.* New York: Guilford Press.

Beutler, L. D., Clarkin, J. F., & Bongar, B. (2000). *Guidelines for the systematic treatment of the depressed patient.* New York: Oxford University Press.

Beutler, L. D., Harwood, T. M., & Caldwell, R. (2001). Cognitive-behavioral therapy and psychotherapy intergration. In K.S. Dobson (Ed.), *Handbook of cognitive-behavioral therapies* (2nd ed., pp. 138–170). New York: Guilford Press.

Brehm, J.W. (1966). *A theory of psychological reactance.* New York: Academic Press.

Carey, M. P., Flasher, L.V., Maisto, S. A., & Turkat, I. D. (1984). The a priori approach to psychological assessment. *Professional Psychology: Research and Practice, 15,* 515–527.

Chambless, D. L., & Hope, D. A. (1996). Cognitive approaches to the psychopathology and treatment of social phobia. In P.M. Salkovskis (Ed.), *Frontiers of cognitive therapy* (pp. 345–382). New York: Guilford Press.

Dowd, E. T., Milne, C. R., & Wise, S. L. (1991). The Therapeutic Reactance Scale: A measure of psychological reactance. *Journal of Counseling and Development, 69,* 541–545.

Erikson, E. (1950). *Childhood and society* (2nd ed.). New York: Norton.

Frank, J. D., & Frank, J. B. (1991). *Persuasion and healing: A comparative study of psychotherapy* (3rd ed.). Baltimore: Johns Hopkins University Press.

Freeman, A., & Dolan, M. (2001). Revisiting Prochaska and DiClemente's stages of change theory: An expansion and specification to aid in treatment planning and outcome evaluation. *Cognitive and Behavioral Practice, 8,* 224–234.

Freeston, M. H., Rhéaume, J., & Ladouceur, R. (1996). Correcting faulty appraisals of obsessional thoughts. *Behaviour Research and Therapy, 34,* 433–446.

Greenberg, L.S., Rice, L.N., & Elliott, R. (1993). *Facilitating emotional change.* New York: Guilford Press.

Hayes, S. C., Strosahl, K. D., & Wilson, K. G. (1999). *Acceptance and commitment therapy: An experiential approach to behavior change.* New York: Guilford Press.

Kendall, P. C., Kipnis, D., & Otto-Salaj, L. (1992). When clients don't progress: Influences on and explanations for lack of therapeutic progress. *Cognitive Therapy and Research, 16,* 269–281.

Layden, M. A., Newman, C. F., Freeman, A., & Morse, S. B. (1993). *Cognitive therapy of borderline personality disorder.* Needham Heights, MA: Allyn & Bacon.

Leahy, R. L. (1999). Strategic self-limitation. *Journal of Cognitive Psychotherapy: An International Quarterly, 13,* 275–293.

McGinn, L. K., & Young, J. E. (1996). Schema-focused therapy. In P. M. Salkovskis (Ed.), *Frontiers of cognitive therapy* (pp. 182–207). New York: Guilford Press.

Meier, S. T. (1999). Training the practitioner-scientist: Bridging case conceptualization, assessment, and intervention. *Counseling Psychologist, 27,* 846–869.

Miller, W. R., & Rollnick, S. (1991). *Motivational interviewing: Preparing people to change addictive behavior.* New York: Guilford Press.

Needleman, L. D. (1999). *Cognitive case conceptualization: A guidebook for practitioners.* Mawmah, NJ: Erlbaum.

Newman, C. F., Leahy, R. L., Beck, A. T., Reilly-Harrington, N. A., & Gyulai, L. (2002). *Bipolar disorder: A cognitive therapy approach.* Washington, DC: American Psychological Association.

Persons, J. B. (1989). *Cognitive therapy in practice: A case formulation approach.* New York: Norton.

Prochaska, J. O., & DiClemente, C. C. (1992). *Stages of change in the modification of problem behaviors.* Newbury Park, CA: Sage.

Prochaska, J. O., Velicer, W. F., Rossi, J. S., Goldstein, M. G., Marcus, B. H., Rakowski, W., et al. (1994). Stages of change and decisional balance for 12 problem behaviors. *Health Psychology, 13,* 39–46.

Sacco, W. P., & Beck, A. T. (1995). Cognitive theory and therapy. In E. E. Beckham & W. R. Leber (Eds.), *Handbook of depression* (2nd ed., pp. 329–351). New York: Guilford Press.

Salkovskis, P. M. (1996). The cognitive approach to anxiety: Threat beliefs, safety-seeking behavior, and the special case of health anxiety and obsessions. In P. M. Salkovskis (Ed.), *Frontiers of cognitive therapy* (pp. 48–74). New York: Guilford Press.

Seibel, C. A., & Dowd, E. T. (1999). Reactance and therapeutic noncompliance. *Cognitive Therapy and Research, 23,* 373–379.

Vaillant, G. (2000). Adaptive mental mechanisms: Their role in a positive psychology. *American Psychologist, 55,* 89–98.

van Oppen, P., & Arntz, A. (1993). Cognitive therapy for obsessive-compulsive disorder. *Behaviour Research and Therapy, 32,* 79–87.

Velicer, W. F., Hughes, S. L., Fava, J. L., Prochaska, J. O., & DiClemente, C. C. (1995). An empirical typology of subjects within stage of change. *Addictive Behavior, 20,* 299–320.

Wright, J. H., Thase, M. E., Beck, A. T., & Ludgate, J. W. (Eds.). (1993). *Cognitive therapy with inpatients: Developing a cognitive milieu.* New York: Guilford Press.

Young, J. E. (1990). *Cognitive therapy of personality disorders: A schema approach.* Sarasota, FL: Professional Resource Exchange.

2

Impediments to Effective Psychotherapy

Arthur Freeman
Roya Djalali McCloskey

It is significant that Campbell's (1996) *Psychiatric Dictionary* lists nine references related to the concept of resistance. These include "resistance," "character resistance," "conscious resistance," "ego resistance," "id resistance," "state of resistance," "superego resistance," "transference resistance," and "treatment resistance." The common element to all forms of resistance, from the psychoanalytic perspective, is produced by the ego, "which clings tenaciously to its anticathexis [where] the ego finds it difficult to turn its attention to perceptions and ideas the avoidance of which it had until then made a rule, or to acknowledge as belonging to it impulses which constitute the most complete antithesis to those familiar to it as its own" (Freud, 1936, as quoted in Campbell, 1996, p. 626). More simply stated, there are ideas, images, beliefs, and impulses that are uncomfortable for the individual because of the anxiety that they create.

Freud introduced the concept of resistance in the 1890s (Breuer & Freud, 1893–1895/1955). He believed that resistance was the patient's way of coping against unbearable ideas that signaled danger. The opposition to such unbearable thoughts was the cause of the patient's symptoms, and the ego defended against these ideas by filing them in the unconscious and suppressing them from the memory. Typical of anxiogenic thoughts, these cognitions are then avoided.

Resistance had primarily been conceptualized as a negative patient variable and a form of pathology embedded in a narcissistic, false, and pathological character that strove to maintain the status quo at any cost (Menninger, 1958; Stark, 1994). Over time, the view of resistance has changed. Resistance is no longer being viewed as entirely negative and as a patient variable alone. Several authors (Deaton, 1985; Gerber & Nehemkis, 1986; Adelman & Taylor, 1986; Ellis, 1985; Meichenbaum & Gilmore, 1982) have considered the adaptive nature of resistance. A patient may resist treatment as an attempt to gain control over a part of his or her life (Adelman & Taylor, 1986). Or, by not complying with the role that the therapist defines for him or her, the patient experiences a sense a control (Leahy, 2001). Other examples of healthy resistance include the patient reasonably resisting the authority of a therapist who has a poor conceptualization of the patient's problem (Ellis, 1985), or a patient feeling not understood or emotionally validated because a therapist maintains an illusion of competence by throwing a series of techniques at the patient (Leahy, 2001).

The emphasis, however, on patient variables as the sole or major cause of resistance continued both in psychology and in medicine. Essentially, the idea that patients do not "get well" because they are resistant has become common. Until the 1980s, despite the lack of consistent research evidence supporting a correlation between patient variables and adherence, the majority of providers attributed lack of treatment progress to patient characteristics and poor attitudes (Davis, 1966; Gordis, 1976; Becker & Rosenstock, 1984). Therapists often expect patient progress after the patient gains insight into his or her problems (Basch, 1982). In the absence of the expected progress, therapists often feel frustrated and label the patient as resistant. Basch (1982) refers to such resistance as "pseudoresistance." Similarly, Lazarus and Fay (1982) take a position generally opposed to the psychoanalytic one, wherein they dispute the concept of resistance. They believe that what the therapists label as resistance may in fact be a rationalization for their treatment failures. They recommend that, rather than overgeneralizing and labeling every negative therapeutic outcome as resistance, the therapist separate resistance of the patient, resistance of the problem, and the situational factors within which the resistance is maintained.

Since the 1980s, research has provided some evidence for specific patient variables, such as patients' beliefs about their problem or illness (Leventhal, Zimmerman, & Gutmann, 1984; Leventhal & Nerenz, 1983) or their perceived control over treatment process (Trostle, Hauser, & Susser, 1983), as variables that can affect resistance and treatment outcome (Rees, 1985; Fontana, Kerns, Rosenberg, Murcus, & Colonese, 1986; Abbott, Dodd, Gee, & Webb, 2001). However, we know today that patient variables are only one of several major variables that have an impact on therapeutic resistance.

Several theorists and therapists have considered other factors, such as therapist variables, relationship variables, and environmental variables, as contributing to the therapeutic resistance. Robert Mendelsohn (1981) was one of the first to conceptualize resistance at the interpersonal rather than seeing it as solely an intrapsychic event. He identified a therapist variable in addressing the issue of countertransference and how the therapist's resistance to fully experiencing the therapeutic interaction could affect and impede the therapeutic progress. Relationship variables have continued to receive considerable research attention over the years, and the importance of therapeutic bond and its impact on therapeutic progress has been emphasized (Bordin, 1979; Keisler & Watkins, 1989; Ciechanoswski, Katon, Russo, & Walker, 2001; Persons & Burns, 1985; Luborsky & Crits-Christoph, 1990; Luborsky et al., 1985; Safran & Segal, 1990; Safran, 1998; Safran & Muran, 1998; Greenberg & Paivio, 1997). In addition to relationship factors, Bordin (1971) has addressed the importance of goals and tasks of therapy that can strengthen the working alliance and minimize patient resistance to overcome problems. Variables such as the therapeutic bond and setting out the goals and tasks of the treatment hold the therapist as equally accountable, if not more so, as the patient for the progress (or lack of it) in treatment.

Ellis (1985) has taken the causes of therapeutic resistance beyond the patient and therapist variables. He acknowledges that therapist–patient relationship variables and patient variables such as severe disturbance, fear of discomfort, shame of disclosure, and fear of success have an impact on therapeutic resistance. He also has identified environmental factors such as those stemming from problems with significant others, disability factors, and addiction as contributing sources to therapeutic resistance.

The cognitive-behavior model has emphasized patient variables such as the role of patient's cognitive distortions and their impact on noncompliance in treatment (Burns, 1989). Beck, Freeman, and Associates (1990) have emphasized avoidance as a coping style to deal with the vulnerability that results from issues discussed in everyday life and in therapy. Leahy (2001) explicates a number of factors in and solutions for resistance.

Uncomfortable with the psychodynamic term of "resistance" and equally uncomfortable with the more behavioral term "noncompliance," we prefer the term "impediment to therapy." This removes the onus from the patient and describes the broad range of sources of difficulty that can potentially emerge in psychotherapy, of whatever the orientation. In this chapter we have identified 41 specific sources of impediments to therapy. These stem almost equally from four sources—the patient, the therapist, the environment, and the patient's problem or pathology. We have not listed the areas of impediment in order of importance, nor is the listing of the manifestations of the impediments in a hierarchy of importance. The patient factors are those impediments that come primarily from the patient. Similarly, the therapist factors are those primarily from the therapist. The environmental impediments come from family, culture, organizations, and institutions. Finally, the patient's pathology is, in and of itself, a source of impediment to the therapy. There can be multiple impediments, thereby increasing the resistance and noncompliance and making the therapy more difficult.

The essential issue for the therapist is to identify the source (or sources) of impediment, to make the impediments manifest for the patient, and to include in the treatment plan an organized approach for lessening or eradicating the impediments so that therapy can proceed more smoothly.

PATIENT FACTORS

Lack of Skill to Comply with Therapeutic Regimen and Expectations

Often, the assumption that is made by therapists and patients is that all patients have the basic skills to comply with therapeutic expectations. We assume that the depressed patient knows how to create pleasure for him- or herself or that the anxious patient has the skills and understanding to self-soothe.

Beck, Freeman, and Associates (1990) make the point that individuals with personality disorders often have never gained the skills necessary for more adaptive functioning.

Negative Cognitions Regarding Previous Treatment Failure

For the patient who is familiar to the mental health system, the negative experiences with agencies and therapists, the money spent on therapy, services not delivered as promised, medication not working as expected to, or maintenance of the problems over time can equal a negative set regarding therapy. Even when gains have been made in therapy or problems ameliorated, the patient may still perceive having failed in therapy or therapy having failed him or her. They may reason that, after all, if therapy had worked, they would not now be seated in the current therapist's office.

Negative Cognitions Regarding Consequences to Others of Altering Behavior Patterns

The systemic perspective holds that the identified patient is often the carrier of the family pathology. This being the case, any change on the part of the patient to reduce his or her pathology will then cause significant problems for others in the patient's system. The patient is concerned that if he or she changes, some catastrophic consequence will occur to significant others or, in cases of severe obsessive–compulsive disorder, to the world at large.

Secondary Gain from Symptoms

Many individuals learn that being impaired, despite the price that they pay for that impairment and consequent decrease in adaptive function, brings about certain rewards or advantages. The secondary gain may be a perception of power over others, a perception of security, or a perception of being loved. The gain may come from significant others, institutions, or a more simple relief of anxiety for the individual.

Fear of Changing One's Actions, Thoughts, or Feelings

This factor is best expressed as, "The devil that you know is better than the devil that you don't know." Some individuals are unhappy, disappointed, or depressed about their circumstance but see any other approach as a black void that might swallow them up. They wonder what it would be like to be different, how being different would feel, how others would view their being different, and what would happen if they did not like the difference. Could they ever go back to their old ways?

Lack of Motivation to Change

The lack of any "force or energy that propels (the individual) to seek a goal and/or to satisfy a need" (Campbell, 1996) will leave the patient in a static state. In some cases there are forces that are "demotivating" to the patient. In other cases, there is simply no motivation to do things differently. The individual has reached a point of homeostasis and continues in what appears to be the most comfortable situation. Freeman and Dolan (2002) describe a clinical revision of the stages of change. They identify 10 stages: noncontemplation, anticontemplation, precontemplation, contemplation, action planning, action, prelapse, lapse, relapse, and maintenance.

The patient must be assessed as to his or her present stage of motivation. The patient who is noncontemplative may not be motivated because he or she has no idea that change is desirable or useful. His or her "resistance" is based on a lack of information. When the need to change is pointed out, this individual will readily try to change. The anticontemplative individual approaches therapy with a "screw you" perspective. He or she does not want to change and will work hard to avoid change. By leading the patient through the stages as described by Freeman and Dolan (2002), a change strategy can be developed.

Negative Set

Related to several of the previously noted impediments is the factor of negative set. The patient demonstrates a readiness or even propensity to respond to almost any therapeutic strategy, intervention, or direction with an overt "no" or a covert "yes . . . but." There is no one reason or rationale that can explain the negative set. It may be protective, it may be challenging, it may be habituated, or it may be stylistic of the individual's pathology.

It may also be seen in the individual's response to specific situations, circumstances, or stimuli. The set may, over time, become generalized so that an initial negative reaction to a therapist can become generalized to all therapists and then to all therapy. Or a negative reaction to a relationship becomes generalized to all relationships and then to the notion of having a relationship. This style can be seen as diagnostic of posttraumatic stress disorder, in which the traumatic incident can then predispose an individual to respond in his or her stereotypic way to situations that have elements of the traumatic event.

Limited or Poor Self-Monitoring or Monitoring of Others

Therapy requires some level of self-examination of thoughts, actions, and emotions. Some individuals have difficulty because their "vocabularies" or repertoires are limited. They might have a limited emotional vocabulary or a limited behavioral repertoire. They may not be able to access their thoughts or not understand why or how to do it.

They may be limited because their self-view is one that does not permit or accept any need to monitor what they say or do. Therapy is negatively affected by this poor, limited, or nonexistent self-monitoring. The insight regarding the source or etiology of a behavior or thought is the initial step in the therapeutic process. The operative step is the ability to use that self-knowledge to produce therapeutic change.

The term "alexithymia" has been used to refer to these individuals who have difficulty recognizing, labeling, or describing their emotions.

These patients seem to go through life with blinders. Their tunnel vision causes them to respond to situations with partial data. They miss the environmental cues that will alert them to potential danger. Unlike the hyperarousal of the individual with negative set, these patients have poor or limited ability to assess sometimes gross and obvious situations.

Frustration with Lack of Treatment Progress over Time and Perceived Lower Status by Being in Therapy

Many patients come to therapy after having been to a number of therapists over many years. They ask the question, "When will I have enough therapy?" They have expected (and therapists have often promised) cures for their emotional distress. They have been taught that if they could attain insight, get in touch with their feelings, change their thinking, take their medication, withdraw from negative interactions, or learn to meditate that their emotional problems will be reduced or ameliorated. To their frustration and the frustration of therapists, the patient's significant others, and the mental health system, the changes have not been forthcoming.

In fact, the patient may be in the same state that he or she was in years earlier. Time has gone by, and life has passed them by. Opportunities have come and gone and may not return. The patient may generalize his or her frustration and take it out on the present therapist, which may be a major source of therapeutic impediment.

The frustration may not all be past. The patient may also be frustrated with what he or she perceives as a lack of progress in the present therapy. He or she may have expected to be able to change or to do things that he or she is still not able to act on. This could lead to anger and frustration.

A part of the picture may also be the idea that if one is in therapy, there is something wrong with him or her. Conversely, not being in therapy or resisting therapy can become a way of viewing oneself as being mentally healthy.

Lack of Personal Resources (Physical, Cognitive, or Intellectual)

As with the skills deficit described previously, patients come into therapy with different physical, cognitive, or intellectual equipment. The individual who is physically challenged is not necessarily limited. He or she can compensate for challenges and use the challenge as a motive to excel. The same is true of any individual, whether the challenge is physical, cognitive, or intellectual. On the other hand, these life challenges can also become real and imagined impediments to success in any realm, including therapy.

The therapist cannot assume that these life challenges will have the same meaning for all individuals. In fact, for some, even the most minimal challenge has the potential to paralyze the individual for life. For other patients, the challenges or limitations must be taken into account in developing therapeutic strategies and interventions. One area that is often overlooked is cognitive deficit—that is, limited cognitive development that renders the individual unable to process information in a sophisticated manner. For example, a therapist could expect an adult individual to process information in accord with formal operations. Abstraction and the abilities to conceptualize and generalize would be expected. However, an adult patient may still be operating at lower than expected levels, more likely concrete operations. The expectation that a patient will be able to generalize one learning or insight to other situations is too often frustrated because the patient simply does not have the formal operational skills. In general, it would be far better to cast interventions at the level of the concrete rather than to expect every patient (or even most) to have the expected level of cognitive ability.

Summary

The patient brings a number of factors to the therapeutic collaboration. Understanding that the collaboration will rarely be 50:50, the aforementioned impediments are only part of the total picture.

PRACTITIONER/THERAPIST FACTORS

Lack of Skill or Experience

Skill and experience are quite different. A novice therapist may have acquired the basic necessary skills for effective therapy, but lack of experience may encourage patient resistance. The unskilled therapist clearly needs skill building. Either situation may interfere with adequate treatment. What is necessary is the ability to collaboratively design a treatment plan that has a synergistic quality and then implement it. A good treatment plan is not just a mechanical introduction of a series of skills but requires collaboration.

Adequate experience provides the therapist with the practice in using his or her skills. The key ingredient for enhancing both skills and experience is supervision.

Congruence of Patient and Practitioner Distortions

Although we do not expect practitioners to be totally free of cognitive distortions, it is essential that therapists build the self-knowledge that will allow them to label their personal distortions. When these distortions are congruent with the distortions of the patient, a significant impediment emerges. There is also the potential that the patient's pathology may in fact be reinforced by the congruence.

Poor Socialization of Patient to Treatment and to a Specific Treatment Model

Patients achieve socialization to psychotherapy through several sources. First can be their previous experience. A second source of socialization and understanding comes from TV and films. Third, patients learn from friends and family what is expected of them in therapy. Fourth, some "education" comes from other patients on an inpatient unit. Fifth, socialization and understanding can come from the therapist.

It is this latter source that is often not well utilized. If the patient is not aware of what the therapy entails, of how it works, of what is expected of him or her, or of the length of the therapy, the patient has insufficient information on which to base his or her informed consent for treatment. Without the patient's informed consent, then treatment cannot ethically proceed.

The patient must be informed of all of the details of therapy. The fact that he or she may have been in therapy previously has no impact on this factor. After all, if the previous therapy had been successful, the patient would likely be seeing his or her previous therapist.

Lack of Collaboration and a Working Alliance

The working alliance is a central feature of all therapies. The therapist and patient work together as a team. The collaboration is not always 50:50, but may be 30:70, 90:10, or 95:5. In the latter case the therapist will be providing most of the energy or work within the session or in the therapy more generally. The more severely depressed the patient, the less energy the patient may have available to use in the therapy. In working with patients who have been adjudicated for therapy or are otherwise there against their will, the collaboration must be built slowly. This is true of almost all therapy with adolescents.

The therapeutic focus would be to help the patient to make maximum use of his or her energy, to build greater energy, and to take a greater proportionate share of the collaboration.

Lack of Data

Sometimes practitioners focus on a label, and once they identify a "disorder," they proceed full force with treatment without any further data. The organized collection of data will give the therapist valuable information about the severity, situational variability, and individual uniqueness of the problem for the given patient. Without the necessary data, practitioners may implement general treatment guidelines that lack specificity, or the goals may be reached after much detour and delay. The question is how long the patient is willing to be dragged through the detours before he or she loses interest and hope and eventually gives up.

Therapeutic Narcissism

Therapeutic narcissism takes many forms. Some practitioners pride themselves in their loyalty and dedication to their patients, because they consider how poorly their patients may do in their absence. They overestimate their importance in their patient's lives and assume that the patients may not be able to survive without their help. On the surface this seems like act of dedication and sincerity, but in fact this is a good example of therapeutic narcissism. In another variant of therapeutic narcissism, the therapist believes that he or she is smarter or more skilled than he or she actually is.

Often these therapists believe that charisma is an adequate substitute for skill and that theoretical grounding in any psychotherapy model is unnecessary.

This problem may play itself out in therapy as offering interpretations to the patient that must be totally accepted by the patient lest the patient's lack of acceptance be interpreted as resistance. When questioned about why they do what they do, these therapists reiterate their model, which cannot or should not be challenged, inasmuch as they believe that their model must be accepted as applicable to all patients without question or modification. Given their "priestly" function, they believe that calls for empirical support of one's therapeutic model must be resisted as unnecessary. The therapy that they practice is the only true religion, and mechanotechnical (skills-based) approaches are to be avoided in favor of the intrinsic beauty of purely theoretical models.

Therapeutic narcissism involves the belief that long-term therapy is the gold standard for therapy and that "less is more." The less you do for or with the patient, the better therapy you do. Finally, therapeutic narcissism may be presented in other ways. The therapist may overestimate his or her effectiveness with the patient and therefore hesitate to refer the patient when referral is necessary. This is often done under the shield of caring so much about the patient that the practitioner cannot trust that others would take as good care of the patient as he or she has done.

In another example of therapeutic narcissism, the practitioner assumes that he or she knows what is best for the patient. Furthermore, the practitioner may expect that the patient in all instances should implement his or her suggestions without ever being challenged. This can easily lead to a sense of powerlessness and resentment on the part of the patient.

Poor Timing of Interventions

Often, the major factor in the success or failure of an intervention is timing and circumstance. An intervention that is properly done but poorly timed may be of little or no value. It is not simply a matter of the therapist's skill at mounting the intervention but also of the patient being ready to "hear" that interpretation. Nor is it a matter of the therapeutic relationship. The therapeutic relationship and working alliance can be superb, but it will not necessarily accommodate a poorly timed intervention.

Problems of timing can be rooted in the therapist's anxiety, therapeutic narcissism, lack of therapist skill, or the therapist's lack of understanding of the patient. Rather than allowing the intervention to "develop" and ripen, the therapist may feel compelled to launch an intervention as soon as he or she thinks of it. If, by chance, the moment is appropriate, the intervention might work quite well. If, however, the patient is not ready, the intervention may be ignored, refused, or become a source of breach in the therapeutic relationship. Alternatively, an intervention that is withheld may not just ripen but rot on the vine and be equally poorly timed and thereby ineffective.

Unstated, Unrealistic, or Vague Therapy Goals or a Lack of Patient Agreement with Goals

One of the most important steps in providing good treatment is clarification of the goals of therapy. Without such clarification, the therapist and the patient may be working on different goals. As a result, the patient and the therapist will not feel connected, as each of them marches to an entirely different drum. Poor agreement on therapy goals may occur if the patient presents a problem that is different from his or her desired goal because he or she fears confronting that issue directly or fears negative evaluation by the therapist and others in his or her life.

The therapist must be clear when working with the patient about setting goals for therapy. The goals must be reasonable, proximal, realistic, and possible. The patient must clearly state his or her agreement with the goals of therapy.

The therapist must be able to inform the patient when the goals set by the patient may be idealistic and not realistic.

Limited Understanding of the Developmental Process

DSM-IV-TR specifically enjoins the diagnostician from making a diagnosis when the behaviors that have been identified can be better explained by developmental factors. For example, the term "rebellious adolescent" may be redundant, as would "dependent toddler." In fact, behavior contrary to these developmental processes would be questionable.

Understanding development in terms of cognitive development, moral development, psychosocial development, or physical development are essential. Without this perspective, the clinician would assume that everyone functions in the same way in every situation. By taking a developmental perspective, the therapist can easily craft interventions that will have a higher likelihood of working.

Generalized Negative Beliefs about Mental Illness or Unrealistic Expectations of Patient

The therapist's negative beliefs about mental illness can have a direct impact on the conceptualization of the patient, as well as the formulation of the treatment. For example, if a practitioner believes that depression or anxiety is untreatable and that it takes over the person and makes him or her useless in day-to-day functioning, not to mention in relationships, then treatment will be limited. Although this seems silly, many other disorders carry with them a hopelessness, so that the therapist who is not conversant with the emerging literature will be likely to give up on a patient before therapy even begins. These disorders include bipolar illness, schizophrenia, substance abuse, or pedophilia. A negative conceptualization will impose unnecessary restrictions on what the patient is capable of doing, what should be required of the patient, how he or she may function in a therapeutic relationship, and what adjunctive therapies may be necessary. This in turn directly influences treatment planning and may in fact reinforce areas of the patient's difficulties.

Lack of Flexibility and Creativity in Treatment Planning

An effective treatment plan requires not only the right skills and experience but also a high degree of flexibility and creativity on the part of the therapist. These qualities allow the treatment plan to be more fluid and individually tailored to the patient's needs. One of the criticisms of treatments is that they are rigid and unyielding and do not allow creativity. Many experienced practitioners may find themselves rigidly using the same protocols without deviations with different patients who share a common condition. What these practitioners seem to focus on is treating the condition alone rather than the condition within a unique patient. They fail to use the manual as a base and to make alterations as needed. What motivates one patient with a certain problem may be quite different from the motivation of another patient with the same problem. Similarly, some patients find certain treatment plans easier to process and to incorporate into their lives than others.

Summary

Inasmuch as therapy is collaborative, the therapist contributes a substantial portion of the interaction. If the therapy is not going well, the therapist has to look at what he or she is doing or not doing that may contribute to the therapeutic problems or impasses.

ENVIRONMENTAL FACTORS

Environmental Stressors That Preclude Change

Maslow's hierarchy of needs posits that when one's basic biological or physiological needs are unmet, it is difficult for the individual to consider issues of self-actualization; he or she may even choose to compromise safety and security to meet these needs. Often, patients have difficulty in therapy in that they need to cope with high levels of environmental stress. When DSM-III (American Psychiatric Association, 1980) was published, it included for the first time a multiaxial system of diagnosis that included Axis IV, an assessment of the individual's psychosocial stressors.

The goal would be to use environmental manipulation, problem-solving techniques, or advocacy to help the patient to reduce the stressors that may serve to preclude change. As one patient commented, "It is hard to think about changing when you are treading water just to keep from sinking and drowning."

Significant Others Who Actively or Passively Sabotage Therapy

The boundaries between individuals and their significant others may range from poor to nonexistent. Patients may be living or working with significant others (SOs) who will enable the negative behavior in any number of ways. They may serve to actively discourage change, may passively discourage the patient from changing, may covertly interfere with change, or may directly fight any different thoughts, feelings, and actions on the patient's part.

With children, legal and therapeutic issues require that the parents be involved. However, parents can easily sabotage therapy by not bringing the child, by not cooperating with medication or behavioral regimens, or by discouraging the child or adolescent from risk taking or trying to change. In couples' work, the families of the individuals may be "helping" by talking negatively about the partner.

The therapeutic goals may include trying to enlist the SOs in the therapy or, if that is not possible, work to disempower the SOs. By establishing "firewalls" against the interference, therapy can proceed in a far more effective manner.

Agency Reinforcement of Pathology and Illness via Compensation or Benefits

Individuals who receive benefits through Social Security Supplementary Income (SSI), veterans' benefits, or worker's compensation often receive payments based on their degree of injury, dysfunction, or impairment. They may receive their pension until they no longer qualify. That might mean that if an individual is no longer impaired, he or she stands to lose this financial support. This is in no way a description of all benefit recipients. Many would prefer to be rid of their disability so that they could function more effectively. However, when a behavior is reinforced by a financial reward, it may lead to fraud or malingering.

Cultural or Family Issues Regarding Help Seeking

In some cultures and in some families, help seeking is encouraged and even rewarded. In other cultures or families, seeking help is an admission of weakness or aberration. There may be concerns about the therapist learning family secrets or about family activities that the family would prefer not to expose.

In many cases, the patient may feel uncomfortable with a therapist of a different cultural group, just as a therapist may be equally uncomfortable with a patient of a different group (Aponte, Rivers, & Wohl, 1995; Dana, 1993).

Significant Family Pathology

Individuals coming from chaotic, dysfunctional, and pathological families can be said to come by their problems honestly. It is no surprise when the therapist discovers, in evaluating a patient, that there is a significant positive family history for a particular symptom or disorder. Disorders that are known to be heritable (e.g., bipolar illness, depression, or schizophrenia) are often diagnosed by the presence of the family history. In other cases, the family pathology results in a physically, mentally, or psychologically abusive environment that requires that the therapist report the abusive setting or behaviors to social welfare or legal offices.

This situation can become an impediment to therapy when the chaos or pathology of the family make it difficult or impossible for the patient to change. Some patients can escape the influence of their families only by physically leaving the home or geographic area. For children this is impossible, though the society may choose to remove the child or adolescent from the home and place him or her in a foster care or institutional setting.

The family pathology may also cause missed appointments, problems in doing homework, difficulty in maintaining gains, or the maintenance of a negative set concerning therapy.

Unrealistic or Conflicting Demands by Family Members or Significant Others

Patients can be confused or even paralyzed by their internal demands. The demands may be accompanied by additional ideas of hopelessness related to inability to challenge their internal dialogue. In this case the patient may end up in a downward spiral. When the external voices of family, friends, and significant others is added to the mix, the patient may be frozen in place or may even take a contrary position and do whatever is opposed to the demands of others. The therapist may be placed in the same role as these demanding "others."

Unrealistic or Conflicting Demands by Institutions

The major demands on patients from institutions and agencies are a two-edged sword. The message is that change is desired but that change must occur within a limited time frame due to reimbursement policies. Insurers and therapists voice the goal that there be services for patients in need. At the same time the patients know that if they do not or cannot change within the limits of reimbursed services, the therapy that they will receive may be insufficient.

Financial Factors That Limit Change

Financial factors can impede therapy in several ways. Related to the aforementioned point, once reimbursed services run out, therapy will end unless the patient has the financial resources to continue (or if the therapist is willing to see the patient for a substantially reduced or no fee). The financial issue can also be a factor in abusive relationships in which a partner is frightened of leaving because she fears that she will not have the financial resources to support herself and her family. She may then choose to stay in an abusive situation against the best interests of her personal safety or the safety of her family.

System Homeostasis

The system perspective posits that family systems, like physical systems, reach a balance or state of homeostasis. This implies that when any action in any way disrupts or unbalances the system, the system will act to restore the balance. If, for example, the issue for a patient is being in a position of power, any event or interaction that places him or her in a less than powerful position will be seen as threatening and he or she will take immediate action to restore the perception of power.

In many interactions (especially in family and couples work) the participants know when the actions will reach the homeostatic point. If any member crosses that line, the system will be unbalanced. To avoid that, the members will withdraw from the interaction, thereby using a homeostatic cutoff to keep things balanced even when they are dysfunctional.

Inefficient or Limited Support Network

Patients may come to see the therapist as their principal support person. Patients may experience few people in the world as accepting, understanding, caring, and thoughtful as the therapist. They may then place all of their eggs in the therapist's basket. One of the goals of therapy with all patients is to help them build a broader, more useful, more accepting, more available, more generous, and more appropriate support network. Sometimes this can be done through the use of recognized support groups, such as Alcoholics Anonymous, parenting groups, or disability-oriented groups.

Summary

Living as we do in a number of overlapping social systems, the environment, both proximal and distal, will influence the changes that an individual will make. Although the environment can be a strong support and offer encouragement, it can also curtail the individual's motivation and ability to change.

PATHOLOGY FACTORS

Patient Rigidity

Most individuals prefer a balance in their lives. They work hard to maintain control and to keep a certain level of stability in their daily lives. The therapy process is often about creating a change in thoughts, feelings, and behaviors that have not particularly served the patient well. Most patients are, at best, ambivalent about the treatment process and the changes to come. This ambivalence is stronger for those who fear change and having to confront new situations.

Some patients rigidly hold on to what is familiar. They prefer predictable patterns as a way to cope, even though at some level they acknowledge that their ways of handling life issues are problematic and can become painful. A chronically depressed patient with an additional Axis II diagnosis is a good example of someone who holds on to the same beliefs, feelings, and behaviors, even though he or she may be suffering. Cognitive and emotional rigidity prevents him or her from alternative thinking and more diverse problem-solving patterns. Therefore, these patients resist learning in therapy, and, no matter what kind of therapy is offered, they may not develop healthier coping styles.

Difficulty Establishing Trust

The therapeutic relationship is an important framework through which the therapeutic tools to recovery are delivered. Trust is one of the most important ingredients in the therapeutic relationship. There are several reasons that patients may have difficulty trusting their therapists. Attachment history, client–therapist mismatch, unrealistic expectations of the therapist, and therapist qualifications are among the variables that impede the establishment of a trusting therapeutic relationship.

First, the quality of the patient's relationship with his or her primary caregiver often serves as a blueprint for future relationships, and the therapeutic relationship is no exception. Previously established core beliefs about self and others will activate related negative thoughts that can prevent the patient from experiencing the therapist accurately.

Second, sometimes just as the match between the temperament of a child and the parent may not be ideal, the match between the patient and therapist is not satisfactory. Therefore, the patient and therapist start the relationship with some fundamental differences that make it more difficult to build an adequate trusting relationship. Consequently, the therapist does not have a fair chance to therapeutically influence the patient.

Third, some clients enter treatment with preconceived notions about the qualities of their therapist, from the age, sex, and the ethnicity of the therapist to his or her political views. These patients find it difficult to adjust their expectations and ways of thinking, therefore resisting treatment.

Finally, sometimes the therapist is obviously poorly qualified, and the patient correctly resists trusting the therapist and the suggested treatment plan.

Self-Devaluation

The patient's negative view of him- or herself can be a contributing factor to therapeutic resistance. These patients attribute negative outcomes to themselves rather than to a variety of potential factors. Such negative self-attributions affect the patient's self-esteem, leaving the patient questioning whether he or she is good enough, is not healthy enough, or has achieved enough. In turn, the self-devaluation will impair the patient's performance (Arkin & Oleson, 1998), reinforcing that he or she is not good enough and is not capable of change. This in turn creates a sense of despair and hopelessness, which then fuels the ongoing pattern of self-defeating behaviors and ultimately self-punishment.

The patient may fear disclosure to the therapist about his or her "shortcomings." He or she apologizes for his or her needs, and any discussions about needs lead to negative outcomes of depression and anxiety (Leahy, 2001). The patient may have bad feelings about the way he or she is. Add to this the idea that sharing such dark secrets with someone else, in this case, the therapist, will make things better. The patient will resist disclosure, while frantically covering up his or her flaws.

Limited Energy

After identifying the patient's problems or destructive beliefs, the therapist needs to assess the cognitive strength of the patient's beliefs and the force and energy that maintain them (Ellis, 1985). The patient must gain both intellectual and emotional insight into his or her problems, because intellectual insight alone does not lead to major powerful changes for the patient (Ellis, 1985). When patients are depressed, they often do not have the energy to act, or even think. They report a sluggishness of mind. The frequent goal of the depressed patient is to wait until his or her energy level returns.

The goal in this case is to help the patient to develop a plan to get the ball rolling, not simply wait for the return of energy. Once the patient has an action plan, the therapist can guide him or her by providing the necessary steps toward change.

Impulsivity

Impulsivity is characterized by poor decision making and by *re*acting to rather than acting in given situations. Furthermore, impulsivity involves a sense of time. An impulsive individual simply considers the moment and event, while ignoring the history and the context of time within which the moment is to be considered. Adequate learning and decision making involves interruption of what is going on in the moment to evaluate one's action against the experience of the past, which will then help the person move forward. This is how hindsight is developed and then used to create forethought (Barkley, 1998). Impulsive patients often live a life of chaos, as they do not anticipate the consequences of their actions prior to reacting to situations. Further, due to their poor incorporation of past life experiences, they are poor learners. When engaged in treatment, they acknowledge and understand the presented therapeutic tools. However, in their daily lives, they are often unable or unwilling to delay immediate gratification long enough to access the learned therapeutic tools. This is the reason impulsive patients resist treatment and often do not learn from their experiences. Furthermore, their impulsivity and lack of therapeutic progress often activates the therapist's own negative cognitions, creating frustration for the therapist, which then in turn affects the therapeutic relationship and progress.

Autonomy Press

Some patients have a difficult time accepting help. They portray themselves as having an autonomous style, and they have difficulty allowing others into their emotional inner circle. Further, they often fear failure if they rely on someone else, whether family members or the therapist, to help them feel better. They fear loss of self-esteem if they allow themselves to engage in a therapeutic relationship. Their fear is that they may lose control of their feelings and their lives.

This need for autonomy will play itself out in problems in collaboration and difficulties in establishing a working alliance and cooperation with therapeutic planning and interventions.

Dependence

Dependent patients seek solutions to their problems from others. Unlike the autonomous individual, they adopt a submissive position in relationships with the hope of gaining approval and nurturance. There are several variables that can negatively affect the outcome of the therapeutic relationship and treatment with a dependent patient. First, a dependent patient expects the therapist to take over his or her life and to lead him or her toward nurturance and protection. Therefore, engaging a dependent patient in a collaborative treatment plan will be challenging for the therapist.

Second, dependent individuals are very sensitive to criticisms and disapproval, and the therapist may spend considerable time and effort addressing a patient's responses to the feedback given to him or her in therapy.

Third, it is often difficult to create a sense of efficacy in the dependent patient. These individuals mostly seek comfort in what they have obtained through the help of others or the therapist. They avoid self-determination, downgrade their own accomplishments, and do not comfort themselves by what they do for themselves. Therefore, these patients may seek treatment year after year but avoid learning and practicing the essential therapeutic elements in order to recover and to cope.

Symptom Profusion

It is rare that patients come to therapy with a single problem. They are often hesitant about presenting all of their problems to the therapist, either because they find the list of problems overwhelming or because they are embarrassed by it. Therefore, they may present with only one or two problems, such as depression, panic attacks, or marital problems, that are most distressing to them. However, most likely the patient has eight to nine problems (Persons, 1989).

Treatment is only as good as the assessment. After a thorough assessment, some patients may meet criteria for several Axis I and Axis II disorders, in addition to a lengthy list of Axis III and Axis IV difficulties. Imagine a 38-year-old woman with severe depression, severe obsessive–compulsive disorder on Axis I, dependent personality disorder on Axis II, and poorly controlled high blood pressure and seizure disorder on Axis III who has lost her mother, divorced her husband after he left her with two children, ages 2 and 11, and lost her job of 13 years, all within one year (Axis IV).

When encountering patients with multiple serious problems, it is likely that even an experienced clinician may feel overwhelmed, not knowing where to begin. (And if the therapist feels overwhelmed by this problem list, imagine what the patient is experiencing.)

Realistically, progress in such complicated cases will be slower than what the patient is desperately hoping for or demanding. Therefore, as progress is not happening fast enough, the patient may give up or passively resist treatment.

Confusion or Limited Cognitive Ability

The treatment plan has a greater chance of being effective after the patient fully understands the plan and agrees to actively participate in his or her treatment. When the patient has limited cognitive ability and does not understand what the therapist is presenting, the collaboration will be impeded. The plan may not be presented in the simple terms and procedures that the patient can understand. In such cases, the patient not only does not feel relieved by the help that he or she is receiving but also feels further frustrated and may be angered by the complicated, difficult material presented.

These will be deterrents to cooperation, and the patient will often resist engagement in treatment. If the patient suffers from confusion and organically based memory and concentration difficulties, the patient is unable to transfer information from one therapy session to another and to utilize the presented material in his or her daily life. Therefore, minimal progress is made in treatment, and the patient may feel frustrated and resist further treatment.

Significant Medical/Physiological Problems

Significant medical/physiological problems present several variables that may impede treatment progress. First, even though the patient's emotional difficulties are a greater obstacle to successful coping, he or she may perceive medical problems as more "real" in comparison with emotional difficulties. The underlying belief may be that dealing with emotional issues is more of a luxury and will have to be secondary. After all, physiological complications are often visible and tangible and may be more difficult to deny. On the other hand, emotional struggles are not visible and are easier to dismiss, at least for a period of time. Therefore, if psychotherapy is introduced too early or at a time when the patient is preoccupied with medical complications, he or she may resist full participation in treatment.

Second, on some occasions a patient may be suffering from a pressing medical condition. As Maslow has pointed out, urgent physical needs must be met before the patient can attend to higher emotional needs. If the patient is suffering from a medical condition, he or she may instinctively avoid engagement in or proceeding with therapy.

Third, some patients may receive far more support and sympathy from their significant others for their medical problems than for their emotional issues. Patients' significant others may share a similar belief that the medical problems are visible, tangible, and easier to sympathize with than emotional difficulties. Therefore, it is not surprising that some patients with physiological and medical problems may resist psychological treatment and recovery.

SUMMARY

When therapy is not going well, therapists must look to four areas to assess what might be impeding the therapy process and progress. To assist in doing this, we have developed a checklist survey. The therapist or supervisor can review the therapy work and evaluate where the sticking points are in therapy with this patient, at this point in time, at this point in therapy, and related to the goals of the therapy.

Figure 2.1 (pp. 47–48) is an example of an assessment tool that can be used to evaluate the problems and the level of significance of that problem area for the patient. Each of the noted areas of impediment are listed. The therapist can review the list with the patient or supervisor. As the therapy team reviews the therapy progress, they can indicate the level of contribution of each of the impediments. The therapy can then be designed to deal with the problems. The patient must be included in addressing the impediments, as they are the individuals most affected by the therapy or change difficulties.

As the impediments are identified, the treatment plan can be revised to cope with the impediments. The interventions are then tailored to encourage overcoming the roadblocks to therapy.

REFERENCES

Abbott, J., Dodd, M., Gee, L., & Webb, K. (2001). Ways of coping with cystic fibrosis: Implications for treatment adherence. *Disability and Rehabilitation, 23*(8), 315–324.

Adelman, H. S., & Taylor, L. (1986). Children's reluctance regarding treatment: Incompetence, resistance, or an appropriate response? *School Psychology Review, 15,* 91–99.

American Psychiatric Association. (1980). *Diagnostic and statistical manual of mental disorders* (3rd ed.). Washington, DC: Author.

Aponte, J. F., Rivers, R. Y., & Wohl, J. (Eds.). (1995). *Psychological interventions and cultural diversity.* Needham Heights, MA: Allyn & Bacon.

Arkin, R. M., & Oleson, K. C. (1998). Self handicapping. In J. M. Darley & J. Cooper (Eds.), *Attribution in social interaction: The legacy of Edward E. Jones* (pp. 313–347). Washington, DC: American Psychological Association Press.

Barkley, R. A. (1998). *Attention-deficit hyperactivity disorder: A handbook for diagnosis and treatment* (2nd ed.). New York: Guilford Press.

Basch, M. F. (1982). Dynamic psychotherapy and its frustrations. In P. L. Wachtel (Ed.), *Resistance: Psychodynamic and behavioral approaches* (pp. 3–24). New York: Plenum Press.

Beck, A. T., & Freeman, A., & Associates. (1990). *Cognitive therapy of personality disorders.* New York: Guilford Press.

Becker, M. H., & Rosenstock, I. M. (1984). Compliance with medical advice. In A.

Steppe & A. Matthews (Eds.), *Health care and human behavior* (pp. 175–208). New York: Academic Press.

Bordin, E. S. (1979). The generalizability of the psychoanalytic concept of the working alliance. *Psychotherapy: Theory, Research, and Practice, 16*, 252–260.

Breuer, J., & Freud, S. (1955). Studies on hysteria. In J. Strachey (Ed. and Trans.), *Standard edition of the complete psychological works of Sigmund Freud* (Vol. 2, pp. 1–311). London: Hogarth Press. (Original work published 1893–1895)

Burns, D. D. (1989). *The feeling good handbook: Using the new mood therapy in everyday life*. New York: Morrow.

Campbell, R. J. (1996). *Psychiatric dictionary* (7th ed.). New York: Oxford University Press.

Ciechanowski, P. S., Katon, W. J., Russo, J. E., & Walker, E. A. (2001). The patient–provider relationship: Attachment theory and adherence to treatment in diabetes. *American Journal of Psychiatry, 158*(1), 29–35.

Dana, R. H. (1993). *Multicultural assessment perspectives for professional psychology*. Needham Heights, MA: Allyn & Bacon.

Davis, M. S. (1966). Variations in patients' compliance with doctor's advice: Analysis of congruence between survey responses and results of empirical observations. *Journal of Medical Education, 41*, 1037–1048.

Deaton, A. V. (1985). Adaptive non-compliance in pediatric asthma: The parent as expert. *Journal of Pediatric Psychology, 10*(1), 1–14.

Ellis, A. (1985). *Overcoming resistance: Rational-emotive therapy with difficult clients*. New York: Springer.

Fontana, A. F., Kerns, R. D., Rosenberg, R. L., Marcus, J. L., & Colonese, K. L. (1986). Exercise training for cardiac patients: Adherence, fitness and benefits. *Journal of Cardiopulmonary Rehabilitation, 6*, 4–15.

Freeman, A., & Dolan, M. (2002). Revisiting Prochaska and DiClemente's stages of change theory: An expansion and specification to aid in treatment planning and outcome evaluation. *Cognitive and Behavioral Practice, 8*(3), 224–234.

Gerber, K. E., & Nehemkis, A. M. (Eds.) (1986). *Compliance: The dilemma of the chronically ill*. New York: Springer.

Gordis, L. (1976). Methodological issues in the measurement of patient compliance. In D. L. Sackett & R. B. Haynes (Eds.), *Compliance with therapeutic regimens* (pp. 51–68). Baltimore: Johns Hopkins University Press.

Greenberg, L., & Paivio, S. (1997). *Working with emotions in psychotherapy*. New York: Guilford Press.

Keisler, D. J., & Watkins, L. M. (1989). Interpersonal complementarity and the therapeutic alliance: A study of relationship in psychotherapy. *Psychotherapy: Theory, Research and Practice, 26*, 183–194.

Lazarus, A. A., & Fay, A. (1982). Resistance or rationalization?: A cognitive-behavioral perspective. In P. L. Wachtel (Ed.), *Resistance: Psychodynamic and behavioral approaches* (pp. 115–132). New York: Plenum Press.

Leahy, R. L. (2001). *Overcoming resistance in cognitive therapy*. New York: Guilford Press.

Leventhal, H., & Nerenz, D. R. (1983). A model of stress research with some implications for the control of stress disorders. In D. Meichenbaum & M. Jaremko (Eds.), *Stress reduction and prevention* (pp. 5–38). New York: Plenum Press.

Leventhal, H., Zimmerman, R., & Gutmann, M. (1984). Compliance: A self-regulation perspective. In W. D. Gentry (Ed.), *Handbook of behavioral medicine* (pp. 369–436). New York: Guilford Press.

Luborsky, L., & Crits-Christoph, P. (1990). *Understanding transference: The core conflictual relationship theme method.* New York: Basic Books.

Luborsky, L., McLellan, A. T., Woody, G. E., O'Brien, C. P., & Auerbach, A. (1985). Therapist success and its determinants. *Archives of General Psychiatry, 42*(6), 602–611.

Meichenbaum, D., & Gilmore, J. B. (1982). Resistance from a cognitive-behavioral perspective. In P. L. Wachtel (Ed.), *Resistance: Psychodynamic and behavioral approaches* (pp. 133–156). New York: Plenum Press.

Mendelsohn, R. (1981). Active attention and focusing on the transference/countertransference in the psychotherapy of borderline patient. *Psychotherapy: Theory, Research, and Practice, 18*(3), 386–393.

Menninger, K. (1958). *Theory of psychoanalytic technique.* New York: Basic Books.

Persons, J. B. (1989). *Cognitive therapy in practice: A case formulation approach.* New York: Norton.

Persons, J. B., & Burns, D. D. (1985). Mechanisms of action of cognitive therapy: The relative contributions of technical and interpersonal interventions. *Cognitive Therapy and Research, 9*, 539–551.

Rees, D. W. (1985). Health beliefs and compliance with alcoholism treatment. *Journal of studies on Alcohol, 46*, 517–524.

Safran, J. D. (1998). *Widening the scope of cognitive therapy: The therapeutic relationship, emotion and the process of change.* Northvale, NJ: Jason Aronson.

Safran, J. D., & Muran, J. C. (Eds.). (1998). *The therapeutic alliance in brief psychotherapy.* Washington, DC: American Psychological Association.

Safran, J. D., & Segal, Z. V. (1990). *Interpersonal process in cognitive therapy.* New York: Basic Books.

Stark, M. (1994). *Working with resistance.* Northvale, NJ: Jason Aronson.

Trostle, J. A., Hauser, W. A., & Susser, I. S. (1983). The logic of noncompliance: Management of epilepsy from the patient's point of view. *Culture, Medicine, and Psychiatry, 7*, 35–56.

FIGURE 2.1. Freeman Impediments to Change Scale—Individual (Arthur Freeman and Roya Djalali McCloskey)

Instructions: For each of the following impediments, identify the contribution of that issue to the problems being encountered in therapy. It will be essential for the therapist to review all areas with the patient.

0 = no importance; 1 = some importance; 2 = moderate importance; 3 = great importance; 4 = major impediment.

Patient Factors	**Significance**
1. Lack of skill to comply with therapeutic regimen and expectations	0 1 2 3 4
2. Negative cognitions regarding previous treatment failure	0 1 2 3 4
3. Negative cognitions regarding consequences to others of altering behavior patterns	0 1 2 3 4
4. Secondary gain from symptoms	0 1 2 3 4
5. Fear of changing one's actions, thoughts, or feelings	0 1 2 3 4
6. Lack of motivation to change	0 1 2 3 4
7. Negative set	0 1 2 3 4
8. Limited or poor self-monitoring or monitoring of others	0 1 2 3 4
9. Frustration with lack of treatment progress over time and perceived lower status by being in therapy	0 1 2 3 4
10. Lack of personal resources (physical, cognitive, or intellectual)	0 1 2 3 4
Practitioner/Therapist Factors	
1. Lack of skill or experience	0 1 2 3 4
2. Congruence of patient and practitioner distortions	0 1 2 3 4
3. Poor socialization of patient to treatment and to a specific treatment model	0 1 2 3 4
4. Lack of collaboration and a working alliance	0 1 2 3 4
5. Lack of data	0 1 2 3 4
6. Therapeutic narcissism	0 1 2 3 4
7. Poor timing of interventions	0 1 2 3 4
8. Unstated, unrealistic, or vague therapy goals or a lack of patient agreement with goals	0 1 2 3 4
9. Limited understanding of the developmental process	0 1 2 3 4
10. Generalized negative beliefs about mental illness or unrealistic expectations of patient	0 1 2 3 4
11. Lack of flexibility and creativity in treatment planning	0 1 2 3 4

(continued)

FIGURE 2.1. *(continued)*

Environmental Factors	
1. Environmental stressors that preclude change	0 1 2 3 4
2. Significant others who actively or passively sabotage therapy	0 1 2 3 4
3. Agency reinforcement of pathology and illness via compensation or benefits	0 1 2 3 4
4. Cultural or family issues regarding help seeking	0 1 2 3 4
5. Significant family pathology	0 1 2 3 4
6. Unrealistic or conflicting demands by family members or significant others	0 1 2 3 4
7. Unrealistic or conflicting demands by institutions	0 1 2 3 4
8. Financial factors that limit change	0 1 2 3 4
9. System homeostasis	0 1 2 3 4
10. Inefficient or limited support network	0 1 2 3 4
Pathology Factors	
1. Patient rigidity	0 1 2 3 4
2. Difficulty establishing trust	0 1 2 3 4
3. Self-devaluation	0 1 2 3 4
4. Limited energy	0 1 2 3 4
5. Impulsivity	0 1 2 3 4
6. Autonomy press	0 1 2 3 4
7. Dependence	0 1 2 3 4
8. Symptom profusion	0 1 2 3 4
9. Confusion or limited cognitive ability	0 1 2 3 4
10. Significant medical/physiological problems	0 1 2 3 4

3

Effective Homework

Michael A. Tompkins

Homework has been an important component of cognitive therapy from its conception (Beck, Rush, Shaw, & Emery, 1979). Empirical evidence suggests that homework may assist clients to become well faster and remain well longer and that homework compliance may be an important predictor of a positive treatment outcome (Detweiler & Whisman, 1999; Kazantizis, Deane, & Ronan, 2000). Nonetheless, clinicians who assign homework know that clients do not always do it or do it well and that much of the clinical work with some clients centers on improving their compliance with structured tasks such as homework.

Three general factors can impede the successful use of homework in cognitive therapy: task factors, therapist factors, and client factors (Detweiler & Whisman, 1999). *Task factors* are particular features of the homework assignment that increase the likelihood that clients *can* carry them out, such as the clarity and concreteness of homework assignments. *Therapist factors* are aspects of the therapist's manner that increase the likelihood that clients *will* carry out a homework assignment, such as whether the therapist is able to develop and maintain a positive therapeutic alliance and effectively reinforce homework compliance. *Client factors* are psychological or dispositional variables within the client, such as perfectionism or rejection sensitivity, that decrease the likelihood that clients *will* follow through with structured tasks such as homework.

Whereas one or all of these factors may cause many of the homework roadblocks that cognitive therapists typically encounter, I recommend that therapists attend to the first two (task and therapist factors) before assuming that homework noncompliance is due to the psychopathology of their clients. There are several reasons for this recommendation.

First, this approach may lead to more efficient treatment. Seeing homework noncompliance only in terms of client psychopathology overlooks the real and often significant improvements in homework compliance that can be achieved by a slight change in the homework assignment or in the therapist's manner when setting up and reviewing it. For example, consider a socially anxious client who is highly motivated to begin dating women but cannot begin or maintain a conversation because he lacks the necessary conversational skills. If a therapist instructs the client to begin a conversation with a woman and carry on that conversation for 15 minutes, who is to blame when the client fails? True, the client has a skill deficit, but does that deficit necessarily need to lead to homework failure? The therapist can make small adjustments in the homework so that the assignment better matches the client's current skill level, such as asking the client to smile and say hello to a woman he passes in the street.

Second, this approach can help secure and reinforce homework compliance early in treatment, thereby getting the therapy off to a good start. Seldom are therapists aware in the first session or two of the full extent and form of the client's maladaptive beliefs that may contribute to homework noncompliance. Making certain that we have controlled what we can control (task and therapist factors), regardless of the client's particular maladaptive beliefs, enables therapists to move ahead with homework early.

Third, this approach can help maintain a positive therapeutic alliance. When therapists tend to what they have the most control over, they are less likely to perceive themselves as incompetent or to become hopeless about the treatment or frustrated with their clients. In addition, therapists are less likely to blame their clients ("He doesn't really want to get better") when they fail to complete homework assignments. When therapists blame their clients for their homework failures without considering that the failure may be due to some problem with the homework task itself, they are no longer working to solve their client's problems, including their homework noncompliance. Instead, they are contributing to a process that can further aggravate homework noncompliance, as well as erode the therapeutic alliance.

However, even after therapists have carefully considered the structure of homework assignments and their manner when setting up and reviewing them, certain clients consistently fail to complete the homework they have agreed to do. In these instances, client factors come to the fore, and therapists must manage homework noncompliance as they might manage any other client behavior that interferes with progress toward the client's treatment goals (Persons, 1989; Tompkins, 1999).

In summary, I propose that many homework roadblocks are due to inattention to features of the homework task and to the therapist's manner and that, with straightforward adjustments to each, many roadblocks can be prevented or overcome. This chapter begins with a discussion of strategies for evaluating a client's potential for homework noncompliance, as many homework roadblocks can be prevented if therapists anticipate and plan for them when designing and implementing homework. I then present five common homework roadblocks and strategies for preventing or overcoming them.

EVALUATING THE POTENTIAL FOR HOMEWORK NONCOMPLIANCE

Many factors can influence whether a client can or will complete therapy homework. Many are client factors, such as a client's level of hopelessness, and often are the same factors that are responsible for problems in the client's life (e.g., perfectionism, anger). Other client factors, such as poor hearing or eyesight or physical limitations, although not psychopathological, can still influence a client's ability to complete homework assignments.

I recommend that therapists evaluate a client's potential for homework noncompliance by attending to five areas (Tompkins, 2003): (1) the client's beliefs about illness and treatment; (2) the client's level of skill and knowledge; (3) the client's history of noncompliance; (4) environmental factors (e.g., unsupportive spouse, no transportation); and (5) the function of noncompliance in the client's life.

The Client's Beliefs about Illness and Treatment

A number of studies have underscored the importance of addressing clients' cultural expectations about the nature of their illness, as well as the appropriateness of an intervention strategy (Marsella & Pedersen, 1981; Pedersen, Draguns, Lonner, & Trimble, 1981). Therapists who understand their client's explanatory model of illness can develop and implement treatment interventions that match this explanatory model, thereby increasing the likelihood of treatment compliance (Kleinman, 1977; Sue & Zane, 1987). In other words, if clients do not believe that a homework assignment addresses their problem because it does not consider their unique sociocultural makeup, they are not likely to try it. For example, a single Latino woman who wants to meet eligible men is not likely to complete a homework assignment that instructs her to go to a party alone and introduce herself to several men.

I encourage therapists to sample their client's beliefs and cognitions about their problems, about therapy in general, and about therapy homework in particular. Therapists can ask directly, "Why do you want help with your problems now?" "What do you think will happen in therapy?"

"What do you think would help you the most and the least?" "What do you think is my role and your role in therapy?"

The answers to these questions can provide therapists with hypotheses about the likelihood and form of homework noncompliance. Does the client lack information about treatment and what it consists of? Has the client been forced by someone to come to therapy? Is the client afraid of the therapist or some aspect of the treatment? For example, Beth, who was agoraphobic and had not driven in 2 years, became very anxious when her therapist suggested that she would be expected to drive on a nearby freeway as part of future homework assignments. When the therapist asked what was going through her head, she blurted out, "You want me to drive on a freeway now. I can't do that. I can't even drive to this office." To address Beth's fears, the therapist corrected Beth's assumptions about how treatment would proceed. He explained to her that driving homework would begin with small and easy driving assignments and work up to driving on the freeway and, furthermore, that this part of the treatment would begin after she had learned tools to help her manage her driving fears. This information reassured Beth and helped her to move ahead with treatment. Had the therapist not noted Beth's anxiety about homework and not inquired about her thoughts, the treatment might have ended then and there.

The Client's Skill and Knowledge Level

At times, therapists will develop a homework assignment with a client only to discover that the client lacks the skills and knowledge necessary to effectively carry it out. Many clients lack common life skills that therapists may take for granted, including the ability to identify, prioritize, and solve everyday problems; to manage time effectively; to be appropriately assertive; to communicate clearly and effectively; to interact appropriately with others; and to anticipate and navigate social and interpersonal difficulties (e.g., social problem solving). It is a good idea for therapists to note not only the limitations in their clients' skill repertoire but also the flexibility with which they apply certain skills to certain problems in certain situations. For example, a client who has learned to be cool and business-like when asserting himself with his boss at work may find that this approach creates more problems than it solves if he tries it with his wife.

Perhaps the best indication that clients have the skills needed to succeed at a specific homework assignment is whether they use (or have used) the required skills in their everyday lives. For example, a therapist treating a graduate student who is having trouble writing her dissertation might ask her if there have been times when writing was not a problem. If the therapist discovers that the client has been a compulsive letter writer all her life and has published several magazine articles and a short story, the therapist can assume that the client has the necessary writing and composition skills to complete homework assignments designed to increase her writing output, such as writing for a short time each day.

Therapists can assess clients' skill levels by asking them to try a homework task in session while the therapist observes. Role plays can be used for this purpose. For example, Cecil, a socially anxious computer programmer who was quite isolated and depressed, decided with his therapist that spending time with a trusted friend would help lift his mood. Cecil and his therapist agreed that Cecil would call his friend Joe to invite him to his house to watch a movie. However, when Cecil role-played calling Joe, the therapist observed Cecil mumbling an invitation that was cold and off-putting. The therapist realized that Cecil needed training in basic telephone pleasantries, as well as how to appropriately begin and end a telephone conversation.

A client's performance outside the office in natural settings can also provide therapists with useful and accurate information about their client's skill level and repertoire. Therapists can obtain permission from clients to watch them purchase a cup of coffee or ask directions from a stranger. Similarly, therapists can ask clients to speak with a confederate in the waiting room or outside the office while they observe the interactions.

Environmental Factors

At times, a client's failure to follow through with homework reflects an environment that does not reward (and sometimes punishes) change. A depressed woman is not likely to try more pleasurable activities if her husband berates her when she calls a friend to chat or when she asks him to accompany her to a movie. Clients who have been depressed for many years or who have grappled with long-standing life problems may live in environments that are devoid of positive reinforcement for attempting something new or for working at something until it is done. Other clients who may have suffered a panic attack or a major depressive episode for the first time may experience well-intentioned but counterproductive responses from caring family members who are just trying to help. Family members may ignore a client's fears rather than encouraging him or her to face them, thereby contributing to his or her avoidance, or they might harangue a depressed client to try to drive him or her out of the depression. Other clients may experience cultural, social, or physical restraints to homework compliance. For example, a single mother who feels anxious and panicky and who lives with her three children in a one-bedroom apartment may have trouble complying with homework that instructs her to practice progressive muscle relaxation for 30 minutes each day because she cannot find the time or the space to be alone.

Therapists can begin by asking a general question, such as, "Can you think of anything that might interfere with the progress you would like to make with your therapy?" Other probe questions that are sometimes helpful include, "Who in your life now is the most supportive and the least supportive of your therapy?" "Who could I call on for help if we run into a problem?" "What have you tried in the past to solve your problem and what has gotten in the way?"

The Client's History of Noncompliance

Clients who are resistant to trying homework assignments or who work at homework halfheartedly often have histories that reflect long-standing difficulties in following through with other assignments or activities they agreed to complete. Clients with a pattern of homework noncompliance may report similar problems with school homework. They may have received poor performance evaluations because they failed to follow through with what they agreed to do or were chronically late in turning in work assignments. These clients may also report that they have had trouble following the recommendations of their physicians or therapists and may tell you that they have been prescribed a medication but seldom take it or were not able to attend past therapy appointments although they wanted to.

In general, when inquiring about a client's history of noncompliance, it is a good idea for therapists to be respectful but direct. The therapist might ask, "How do you typically respond to people when they give you advice or suggest you change something you're doing?" or "Was homework a problem for you in school?"

The Function of Homework Noncompliance

Newman (1994) noted that it is useful to explore the factors that make it in the client's "best interest" to oppose the therapist and the goals and tasks of therapy. A client's maladaptive beliefs appear to be the starting point for much of homework noncompliance (Russo, 1987). For example, some clients will not try a homework assignment because they believe they are "fundamentally flawed or incompetent." They fear that if they try it and fail, the therapist or others will rebuke or criticize them. Bill sought treatment because he was unhappy in his marriage but could not discuss this with his wife nor accept a referral for couple therapy. His therapist was puzzled because Bill had learned assertiveness skills and had practiced them dutifully in session, but on numerous occasions he had not tried even the mildest of assertive statements with his wife or anyone else. When questioned, Bill told his therapist that he was not going to try something unless his therapist could guarantee he would succeed.

Perfectionistic clients typically have unrealistic expectations about how a homework assignment is to be done, which may cause them not to do the homework, to delay beginning the assignment until the last minute, or to bail out prematurely because they view the homework as "spoiled" or a failure. These clients typically have beliefs such as "If I don't do it perfectly, I'm a failure," or "People are critical and rejecting." Julianne, a 24-year-old writer who was anxious about the difficulty she was having writing her first book, was given a homework assignment to practice progressive muscle relaxation daily. Julianne tried the relaxation practice only once because she worried that she was not doing it correctly. She wrote four pages of questions to ask her therapist at the next session so that she could learn to do it correctly in the future.

Other clients fear control or loss of autonomy (Dowd & Sanders, 1994) or suffer affective instability or emotional and interpersonal dysregulation (Linehan & Kehrer, 1993). Therapists who treat these clients believe that they are walking on eggshells, and they may not assign or review homework for fear the client will become angry.

A case formulation offers therapists a way of understanding how a client's particular maladaptive beliefs and interpersonal and behavioral problems may contribute to homework noncompliance, as well as to other problematic behaviors (Eells, 1997; Persons, 1989; Tompkins, 1999). Furthermore, understanding the function of a maladaptive behavior, such as homework noncompliance, may help therapists to feel greater empathy for their client's distress and to better tolerate their maladaptive ways of managing it (including homework noncompliance).

COMMON ROADBLOCKS TO EFFECTIVE HOMEWORK

I now discuss five common homework roadblocks and strategies for overcoming them. These strategies focus on adjusting the homework *task* or the therapist's *manner* to improve homework compliance rather than on strategies to change client factors, such as maladaptive beliefs, that may contribute to homework noncompliance (Tompkins, 2002).

"I Didn't Do the Homework Because I Didn't Think It Would Help."

Clients are more likely to comply with a homework assignment if they believe it will help them solve the problems for which they have sought treatment. Goldfried and Davison (1976) noted that presenting clients with a general rationale for treatment, as well as explaining its link to the client's treatment goals, heightens the client's view that therapeutic tasks, such as homework, are valid and credible. In addition, a number of studies suggest that clients who agree with the rationale for a treatment improve more rapidly and are more likely to have successful outcomes (Addis & Jacobson, 1996; Fennell & Teasdale, 1987).

When presenting a rationale for homework assignments, it is important that therapists link the homework to the client's goals:

"Sue, I think getting out of the house some this week would be a good homework assignment for you, and we'll talk about the specifics of that in a minute. Right now I want to remind you that over the last few sessions we've learned that you tend to be most depressed when you're home alone. Since your goal at the beginning of therapy was to be less depressed in general, I see this homework assignment as an opportunity to practice a strategy that not only helps you now but also can help you in the future improve your mood when you're feeling down. What do you think?"

In this way, the therapist underscores for Sue that the homework assignment is consistent with her overarching goal of managing her depression.

I recommend that therapists never assign a homework assignment if the client has not understood and accepted its rationale (Persons, Davidson, & Tompkins, 2001). Clients who reject a homework rationale may be less open to change (Addis & Jacobson, 2000), perhaps because they feel hopeless that anything will help. Others may have clear beliefs about what will and will not help them solve their problems that the therapist has not explored, or they do not understand the reason for doing it. Therapists can ask, "Does the reason I'm recommending the homework assignment make sense to you?" Or "To what degree does the homework match with your ideas about what needs to change to solve your problem on a scale of 0 to 10, where 10 means the homework completely matches with your ideas about what needs to change?"

"I Didn't Do the Homework Because I Wasn't Sure What I Was Supposed to Do."

Clients may have trouble completing homework assignments that are too vague. If the homework is not described in concrete and specific terms, clients may not understand exactly what they are to do. A concrete and specific homework assignment includes details about when, where, with whom, for how long, and using what materials. A concrete and specific homework assignment would be, "Call Julia tonight at 7:00 P.M. and invite her to dinner this Saturday night." A vague assignment would be, "Call a friend this week and invite him or her to do something with you."

"I Forgot to Do the Homework."

Prompts are cues, instructions, or gestures that facilitate the client beginning a desired response, such as a homework assignment. Because prompts alert clients that a homework assignment is to be done, they increase the likelihood that the homework will be attempted.

Prompts are particularly useful for clients who have memory problems or are easily distracted or who live in chaotic, loud, or disorganized environments. Also, prompts may be needed if a homework assignment involves an action that is often repeated, as when clients are asked to write down the intensity, time, and place of their anxious episodes or what they are doing each time they feel depressed.

Prompts can take many forms—written instructions, reminders from significant others, or visual or audible cues. A distressed couple who agree to take turns over dinner listening to each other speak without interrupting for 10 minutes can be prompted to begin the homework assignment by having them place the written instructions for the assignment in the center of the dining table. A socially avoidant child can be prompted by his mother to begin a therapy homework assignment, such as saying "hello" to his teacher, as his mother escorts him into the classroom. Therapists who want to remind anxious clients to take calming breaths throughout the day can have them place brightly colored dots on objects they see frequently during the day (computer monitors, watch faces, telephone receivers) or in environments that are potentially stressful or anxiety evoking (on the wall across from where they sit in a conference room, on the rearview mirrors of their cars). In addition, therapists have numerous technological gadgets, such as pagers, voice mail, or e-mail, that they can use to cue their clients to initiate homework assignments.

Written instructions can prompt clients to begin the assigned homework, and they have been shown to increase homework compliance (Cox, Tisdelle, & Culbert, 1988). Written instructions represent a public statement of the client's intention to comply with the homework, much like a written contract. They also serve as a record of what the client has agreed to do (see the previous section) that can circumvent misunderstandings and disagreements that erode the therapeutic alliance. A concrete and explicit format for written homework instructions leads both client and therapist through the main elements of a successful homework assignment and provides a check that all elements have been considered and included.

To organize this task, I recommend that therapists follow the ABCDE's of written homework instructions, which is a modification of the format proposed by Shelton and Ackerman (1974).

Action

This statement describes exactly what clients (and others involved in the homework assignment) *will do* (read, practice, say, observe) to complete the homework assignment and *how often* they will do it: "Call Joyce once this week and invite her to the movies on Saturday," "Say hello to three strangers this week on your walk to work in the morning."

Bring

This statement describes what clients will bring to the next session: "a completed activity schedule," "a written list of four situations that make you anxious," "the want ads from the Wednesday morning newspaper." A therapist can ask a client to bring anything to a session, such as his or her spouse, the self-help book he or she agreed to purchase, or the telephone number of his or her physician.

Chart

This statement describes how clients will record the results of the homework assignment, which can include a record of what happened or what was learned. For example, therapists can provide clients with activity schedules, checklists, or graphs that they complete and bring to the next session: "Complete the Beck Depression Inventory and enter the total on your mood graph," "Count the number of times each day you think or use the word 'should' and record it on this piece of graph paper."

Do/Do Not

This statement describes what will happen when clients *do* (reward) or *do not* do (consequence) the homework assignment. Therapists are encouraged to document what clients have agreed to do when they complete (or fail to complete) the homework assignment. "Do/Do not" statements can include praise—"Tell yourself you did a good job"—or more tangible rewards, such as "Put $25 in your vacation fund." Consequences might include: "If the homework is not completed, we will focus exclusively in our next session on what went wrong."

Extra

This statement describes what clients will do if they encounter problems completing the homework assignment. Because potential problems cannot always be anticipated, it is helpful to specify what clients will do if they are unable to complete the homework assignment. Backup plans can be an alteration in the homework assignment, such as: "If you call Julie and she's not home or cannot go to the movies with you, call Cheryl, then Kathy, and then Monica." Or they can involve an alternative homework task that has been discussed and agreed on: "If you call Julie and she does not want to go to the movies on Saturday, ask her if she would like to go to dinner or to lunch the next day."

"I Didn't Do the Homework Because It Was Too Difficult."

Typically, when clients report that a homework assignment was too difficult, they mean either that it was beyond what they could try at this time or that they encountered some problem when trying to execute the homework that they could not overcome.

It is always better to start with small homework assignments and then shape approximations to the desired final outcome than it is to insist that clients try homework tasks they doubt they can complete. Such graded tasks play a central role in cognitive therapy for depression, as well as exposure-based treatments for anxiety disorders (Beck et al., 1979; Goldfried & Davison, 1994). For example, asking a socially anxious client to nod and smile at coworkers might open the door for the client to consider other, more challenging homework assignments, such as asking a coworker how she spent her weekend. A less demanding homework assignment that the client completes enhances the client's confidence in the therapist and therapy, thereby strengthening the therapeutic alliance and motivating the client to try more.

As a rule, it is best when beginning treatment to start with homework assignments that ask clients to do what they are already doing 30% of the time or more. For example, Cheryl, a nurse who sought treatment to help her become more assertive, agreed that homework designed to help her practice her newly learned assertiveness skills made sense. She and her therapist identified several types of people with whom she had trouble being assertive and ranked them in order of the percentage of time she was assertive with them. She and her therapist decided that at first she would try being assertive with Phyllis, a coworker whom she liked and with whom she was able to be assertive 40% of the time.

Many clients will begin a homework assignment as agreed on only to stop when the going gets a bit tough. Two strategies are useful in such situations. The first is to anticipate possible difficulties clients may encounter and develop backup plans. The second is to have clients practice homework assignments in session prior to implementing the assignments on their own outside of session.

Anticipating obstacles and planning for them increases the likelihood that clients will complete homework assignments. For example, Jason, a depressed auto mechanic, agreed to call George, a friend, later in the day to invite him to go to a movie. At the agreed-on time, Jason dutifully called George but, when he heard a busy signal, hung up the telephone and did not try again. Had Jason and his therapist developed a list of other people

Jason might have called if he could not reach George, Jason might have completed his homework assignment.

There are a number of ways to uncover potential homework obstacles. Therapists can ask their clients directly, "Do you see any obstacles that would make it hard for you to carry out the assignment?" Therapists can ask clients whether they have tried similar homework assignments in the past and, if so, how they turned out. What problems did they encounter? Watch for clients who qualify their answers—"I think that I can handle that if it happens"—or who quickly dismiss the therapist's concerns—"No, there won't be any problem." Ask these clients how they would handle a typical homework problem and see whether the solution is appropriate and can be done given the client's current level of functioning. Or ask clients to rate the likelihood (0–100%, where 100% is definitely) that they will do the homework as agreed. Low numbers can alert therapists to potential homework obstacles. Therapists can then explore with clients why they believe they may not do the homework and alter the homework assignment or plan a different assignment altogether, such as monitoring the problem the client is not ready to tackle.

Therapists can use covert rehearsal (Beck, 1995) to identify obstacles to completing homework assignments. In covert rehearsal, the client is asked to imagine going through all the steps involved in completing the homework assignment, talking aloud to the therapist, who listens for potential obstacles. For example, Betsy, a depressed unemployed teacher who spent her days in bed, agreed to give herself a manicure as a pleasurable activity to improve her mood and hygiene. During covert rehearsal, Betsy imagined, out loud, each step of the process. As she imagined reaching for the nail polish, she remembered that she had run out of polish several weeks ago. Betsy and her therapist then discussed how and when she would go to the store to buy polish, and this task became her homework assignment. Had Betsy not rehearsed her homework assignment beforehand, she might have thrown up her hands and gone back to bed when she could not find any nail polish. In addition to identifying what is needed but unavailable, covert rehearsal can be used to identify environmental factors, such as critical relatives, that may decrease homework compliance and to develop a plan to help the client overcome them.

In-session practice is particularly helpful when therapists anticipate that clients will have to perform homework assignments in the presence of intense negative affect, such as fear, anger, guilt, or shame. For example, Ginny, a depressed young attorney who sought help because she had little social life, agreed that she needed to become more comfortable setting limits with the managing partner who insisted she work long hours every weekend. As homework, Ginny agreed to say "no" to the managing partner when he asked her to work that weekend. Ginny practiced the homework assignment, while the therapist played the role of the managing partner. Ginny did well until her therapist began to turn up the heat. He repeatedly asked her to work and would not take no for an answer. Eventually, Ginny succumbed to her feelings of guilt and gave in to the partner's demands. The therapist stopped the role play, praised Ginny for hanging in there as long she did, and reviewed with her the rationale for the homework. The therapist and Ginny then developed a set of adaptive responses that she was to read through to help her better tolerate her feelings of guilt. With more practice, Ginny was able to hold her ground in the role plays with her therapist and later with the managing partner.

"I Didn't Do the Homework Because It Didn't Seem Important."

Frequently, clients do not complete homework assignments because they believe that it is not really important. Usually they believe this for a reason. In fact, their therapists, when setting up the homework, may give them the impression that it will be OK if they do not try the homework, much less complete it. Or their therapists may fail to review the homework or, when they do, give the clients the impression that it is OK that they did not do the homework this time and will be OK if they do not do it the next time, either. Therapists can prevent or overcome this roadblock by recognizing that they are important reinforcers of client behavior and that their manner when speaking with clients can increase or decrease the likelihood that homework will be tried and completed. To help, therapists can attend to the four C's of setting up and reviewing homework: be *Consistent,* be *Curious,* be *Collaborative,* and be *Careful.*

Be Consistent

It is imperative that therapists review the homework every session. If homework is not reviewed, therapists do not have the opportunity to praise clients who have completed it or discuss with clients the reasons why they failed to do it. Clients may think that homework is not important if their therapists do not take an active interest in it or that the therapists really did not think they could do it, thereby reinforcing clients' hopelessness about changing their situations.

I recommend that therapists review the previous week's homework before moving to any other significant piece of work in the session. In this way, therapists emphasize the importance of homework over everything else in a session and make certain that they will have adequate time to review homework. For some clients, an indirect question may be enough: "Shall we take a look at your homework assignment from last week?" or "What stands out in your mind from this homework assignment?" For clients who need more direct prompting, therapists can ask, "We agreed last week that you would call Bonnie to invite her to go to a movie with you.

How did it go?" For clients who tend to wander, therapists can gently summarize what was said and then redirect them to a review of the homework assignment

> "Kathy, I hear you saying that it's been a rough week. Your husband has been out of town and you've had to take care of the kids all by yourself, which made you feel more depressed than usual. This sounds important and I want to hear more about it. But first I'd like to review the homework from last week and then we'll come back to this. Would that be OK?"

During the review, it is a good idea for therapists to ask clients whether they modified the homework assignment in any way, and if so, how and why. Often, clients will change homework assignments to accommodate some unanticipated obstacle. Perhaps a client needed to modify a homework assignment to better match his or her skill level (he or she tried the assignment and was not as good at it as he or she thought) or to accommodate to a change in situation (he called someone else because the person he called was not home) or to work around an unanticipated external factor (she practiced the homework assignment with her sister rather than her father, who was unsupportive). For example, Peggy—who had trouble with assertiveness—agreed to a homework assignment to discuss with her supervisor a salary raise during her performance review that week. However, when her supervisor rescheduled Peggy's review because he had to attend an unexpected off-site meeting, Peggy changed the homework assignment and assertively negotiated with him a time the following day for her performance review. This was an excellent outcome, and Peggy's therapist praised her resourcefulness. Changes clients make to their homework assignments may say something about the difficulty of an assignment, about the client's level of motivation, or about the quality of the therapeutic alliance. Information such as this may be useful to therapists when designing future homework assignments and may increase the likelihood that homework will be tried and completed.

Be Curious

A stance of curiosity rather than firm certainty avoids assumptions that may lead to misunderstandings that derail attempts to set up or review homework and that may leave clients feeling criticized or put down. Clients always have more information about what contributed to an unsuccessful homework assignment than their therapists do, and a curious stance recognizes and takes advantage of this fact. A curious stance encourages clients to become curious about the homework themselves, including the obstacles they encounter or may encounter and their role in homework noncompliance. Last, and perhaps most important, curious therapists shift the responsibility for solving homework compliance problems to clients. Overresponsible therapists suggest, "Try this next time," where curious therapists probe, "Tell me what you might try next time."

Be Collaborative

Make certain that the client—not just the therapist—has contributed to developing the homework assignment. There are clear advantages to the therapist and client working collaboratively to design homework assignments. First, clients who have input into homework may perceive themselves as having greater control of the assignment itself. This may lessen their anxiety and thereby increase the likelihood that the assignment will be tried. Second, each time the therapist and client successfully work through misunderstandings and disagreements to set up homework, the therapeutic relationship is enhanced. Third, clients usually understand more fully than their therapists do what is or is not a useful homework assignment and what difficulties may arise. Therapists who consult with their clients about potential obstacles to homework increase the likelihood that the homework will be completed. Initially, the therapist assumes the responsibility for suggesting relevant homework assignments. As the therapy proceeds, however, the client is encouraged to share and then assume the responsibility for developing homework assignments. I recommend that therapists start any discussion of potential homework assignments by asking the client, "Perhaps you have an idea for a homework assignment that would help you with this problem?" At times, clients may suggest a homework assignment that seems tangential to the focus of the therapy session. Rather than dismissing the assignment out of hand, therapists can explore the client's rationale for the assignment (be curious), perhaps soliciting the advantages and disadvantages of this homework assignment over another one the therapist might suggest. Often, client and therapist must briefly negotiate a mutually agreeable homework assignment. Successful negotiations can strengthen the therapeutic alliance and thereby foster greater motivation to try this and future homework assignments.

Be Careful

Be careful when responding to the client during discussions of past or future homework assignments. When clients say, "I thought about what I learned from the homework on my drive here today," or "Perhaps I could try a little tougher exposure assignment this week," nod, smile, and praise them. Similarly, avoid reinforcing homework noncompliance. Avoid saying, "That's OK," "No problem," "No big deal," or "Better luck next time," when luck had nothing to do with it. When clients complete homework assignments, congratulate them and chat (if this is reinforcing to them) for a few minutes to reinforce homework compliance. Take care that the praise is appropriate to the effort and is not overblown.

When clients fail to do homework, respond in a neutral, curious manner and focus on identifying problems that may have contributed to homework noncompliance. If the homework was not completed (or attempted), set aside some time—even the entire session—to review why the homework was not done. Did we make the homework too difficult? Were the homework instructions unclear? Did some unanticipated problem arise?

At times, therapists may need to use the telephone to prompt clients to begin a homework assignment or to answer questions they may have about it. When speaking to clients via telephone about homework, focus only on the homework. Do not discuss other issues that may come up. Many clients find telephone contact with their therapists rewarding and will use it to that end. If this appears to be happening, get this issue out on the table to discuss at the next session (not during a telephone contact). If the client has not completed the homework assignment, either speak to him or her about repeating the assignment and calling the therapist when it is completed or about repeating the assignment with a change that the client and therapist work out over the telephone or end the conversation by recommending that the client discuss the assignment at the next scheduled session.

When clients attempt the homework and were successful at some part of it, focus on that part and praise their efforts: "Although we agreed that you would walk 5 minutes three times this week, you walked 5 minutes one day. Congratulations for walking 5 minutes that one day." Then negotiate with the client modifications to the homework assignment so that he or she can do a bit more next time and reassign: "Now, let's take a look at how we can help you meet your goal of 5 minutes each day. What do you say?" However, if a client continues to fail to complete homework assignments, consider breaking future assignments into smaller, easier-to-do pieces. In that way, the client can be reinforced for completing the entire homework assignment, even if it is smaller. Take care that clients do not interpret their therapists' efforts to shape approximations to the desired homework to mean that their therapists accept incomplete homework. The goal of rewarding small steps is to have clients *always* complete their homework consistently and as agreed upon. When therapists notice that clients try homework assignments but continue to fail to complete them, they should discuss this issue directly.

SUMMARY

The ability of therapists to increase a client's compliance with therapy homework may be one of the crucial therapeutic skills that determine the success of psychosocial interventions in real-world clinical settings (Addis

& Jacobson, 2000). To that end, I have presented strategies for evaluating the potential of homework noncompliance and, when encountered, for overcoming the more typical homework problems. For the most part, the strategies focused on how therapists can manage features of the homework task and their manner when setting up and reviewing homework, as therapists have greater influence over these factors than they do over the client factors presented to them. Even when therapists suspect that homework roadblocks are due to client factors, I encourage therapists to first consider whether they have implemented the homework assignment well and whether they are giving clients the clear message that homework is important before assuming that clients fail to do homework because of their psychopathology.

In conclusion, there is perhaps no better index of how well client and therapist are working together than whether homework is done and done well. When clients fail to complete homework, therapists fail, too. Yet many failures can be prevented through thoughtful attention to this important and perhaps essential element of cognitive therapy.

REFERENCES

Addis, M. E., & Jacobson, N. S. (1996). Reasons for depression and the process and outcome of cognitive-behavioral psychotherapies. *Journal of Consulting and Clinical Psychology, 64,* 1417–1424.

Addis, M. E., & Jacobson, N. S. (2000). A closer look at the treatment rationale and homework compliance in cognitive-behavioral therapy for depression. *Cognitive Therapy and Research, 24,* 313–326.

Beck, A. T., Rush, J. A., Shaw, B. F., & Emery, G. (1979). *Cognitive therapy for depression.* New York: Guilford Press.

Beck, J. S. (1995). *Cognitive therapy: Basics and beyond.* New York: Guilford Press.

Cox, D. J., Tisdelle, D. A., & Culbert, J. P. (1988). Increasing adherence to behavioral homework assignments. *Journal of Behavioral Medicine, 11,* 519–522.

Detweiler, J. B., & Whisman, M. A. (1999). The role of homework assignments in cognitive therapy for depression: Potential methods for enhancing adherence. *Clinical Psychology: Science and Practice, 6,* 267–282.

Dowd, E. T., & Sanders, D. (1994). Resistance, reactance, and the difficult client. *Canadian Journal of Counseling, 28,* 13–24.

Eells, T. T. (Ed.). (1997). *Handbook of psychotherapy case formulation.* New York: Guilford Press.

Fennell, M. J. V., & Teasdale, J. D. (1987). Cognitive therapy for depression: Individual differences and the process of change. *Cognitive Therapy and Research, 11,* 253–271.

Goldfried, M. R., & Davison, G. C. (1976). *Clinical behavior therapy.* New York: Holt, Rinehart & Winston.

Goldfried, M. R., & Davison, G. C. (1994). *Clinical behavior therapy.* New York: Wiley.

Kazantizis, N., Deane, F. P., & Ronan, K. R. (2000). Homework assignments in cognitive and behavioral therapy: A meta-analysis. *Clinical Psychology: Science and Practice, 7,* 189–202.

Kleinman, A. M. (1977). Depression, somatization and the "new cross-cultural psychiatry." *Social Science and Medicine, 11,* 3–10.

Linehan, M. M., & Kehrer, C. A. (1993). Borderline personality disorder. In D. H. Barlow (Ed.), *Clinical handbook of psychological disorders: A step-by-step treatment manual* (2nd ed., pp. 396–441). New York: Guilford Press.

Marsella, A. J., & Pedersen, P. B. (Eds.). (1981). *Cross-cultural counseling and psychotherapy.* New York: Pergamon Press.

Newman, C. F. (1994). Understanding client resistance: Methods for enhancing motivation to change. *Cognitive and Behavioral Practice, 1,* 47–69.

Pedersen, P. B., Draguns, J. G., Lonner, W. J., & Trimble, J. E. (Eds.). (1981). *Counseling across cultures.* Honolulu, HI: University Press of Hawaii.

Persons, J. B. (1989). *Cognitive therapy in practice: A case formulation approach.* New York: Norton.

Persons, J. B., Davidson, J., & Tompkins, M. A. (2001). *Essential components of cognitive-behavior therapy for depression.* Washington, DC: American Psychological Association.

Russo, T. (1987). Cognitive counseling for health care compliance. *Journal of Rational-Emotive Therapy, 5,* 125–134.

Shelton, J. L., & Ackerman, J. M. (1974). *Homework in counseling and psychotherapy: Examples of systematic assignments for therapeutic use by mental health professionals.* Springfield, IL: Thomas.

Sue, S., & Zane, N. (1987). The role of culture and cultural techniques in psychotherapy. *American Psychologist, 42,* 37–45.

Tompkins, M. A. (1999). Using a case formulation to manage treatment nonresponse. *Journal of Cognitive Psychotherapy, 13,* 317–330.

Tompkins, M. A. (2002). Guidelines for enhancing homework compliance. *Journal of Clinical Psychology, 58,* 565–576.

Tompkins, M. A. (2003). *Therapy homework: Key steps in creating and implementing successful homework assignments.* Unpublished manuscript.

Part II

METACOGNITION AND EMOTION

4

Anxiety Disorders, Metacognition, and Change

Adrian Wells

Difficulties and roadblocks in cognitive therapy are numerous in typology and have multiple potential causes. Roadblocks can present as forms of resistance (Dowd & Seibel, 1990; Liotti, 1987; Mahoney, 1988), a term that has been used as a general rubric for the different forms of noncompliance or patient opposition to therapists (e.g., Newman, 1994) and that includes behaviors as diverse as avoidance, noncompliance with homework, and lack of motivation. The source of resistance has been conceptualized in terms of internal cognitive processes such as the inherent stability of meaning structures, the functional significance of elements of pathology that confer some advantage for the individual, cognitive and behavioral coping processes that are counterproductive, and elements of personality disturbance (Freeman & Jackson, 1998; Leahy, 1999; Liotti, 1987; Wells, 1997). Freeman and Jackson (1998) suggest that noncompliance or resistance in the context of treating personality disorder can be viewed in terms of four areas of impediments to therapy: patient factors, diagnostic factors, environmental factors, and therapist factors. *Patient factors* are those that are specific to an individual, such as negative cognition concerning previous failed therapy, secondary gain, and poor self-monitoring capabilities. *Disorder-* or *problem-linked factors* include patient rigidity, medical complications, and excessive dependence. *Environmental factors* include significant others who may sabotage therapy through overt or covert interventions and reinforcement of pathology through compensation. Examples of *therapist factors* are lack of therapist skill, of congruency between therapist and patient attitudes, and of collaboration and a good working alliance. Leahy (2001, 2002) has contributed significantly to the analysis of resistance and proposes a multidimensional model in which resistance occurs due to validation demands, self-consistency, schematic processing, emotional processing, moralistic thinking, victim roles, risk aversion, and self-handicapping.

The multiplicity in form of roadblocks and the mechanisms underlying them is compounded further by a consideration of the mechanics and dynamics of cognitive-affective change in cognitive therapy. A theme of this chapter is that roadblocks are often the result of inadequate specification of the internal cognitive and behavioral factors that lead to persistence of psychological dysfunction. On a theoretical information processing level, we know little about how an individual's cognitive system regulates and modifies its own content and organization. This lack of knowledge has a general impact on therapeutic efficiency, as the basic techniques used are not derived from a model of how or what it takes to change cognition. On a more applied level, roadblocks in treatment arise as a function of self-regulation strategies executed by patients. An important subset of self-regulation is coping that is used by anxious patients to avoid or minimize danger to the self.

THE SELF-REGULATORY EXECUTIVE FUNCTION MODEL, METACOGNITION, AND COGNITIVE CHANGE PROCESSES

What are the internal cognitive computations required to establish and maintain cognitive-affective change in psychological disorder? Although this is an important question and although the answer is fundamental to the nature and conduct of cognitive therapy, most of the existing models of disorder do not provide an answer. In order to answer this question, models of psychopathology are required that specify in detail the internal information processing mechanisms and processes that support cognitive modification. For instance, what are the cognitive and behavioral operations that lead to a revision of beliefs? Failure to understand the information processing mechanisms that support cognitive change and failure to modify mechanisms that maintain disorder can lead to roadblocks in treatment.

The Self-Regulatory Executive Function (S-REF) model of emotional disorder (Wells, 2000; Wells & Matthews, 1994, 1996), provides a cognitive framework for understanding how multiple levels and components of cognition and behavior interact dynamically in the persistence and modification of disorder. Psychological disturbance is equated with the activation of a generic cognitive-attentional syndrome, a marker for which is inflexible self-focused attention. This syndrome consists of perseverative forms of processing in the form of worry/rumination, activation of negative self-beliefs, attentional strategies of threat monitoring, and coping behaviors that fail to restructure maladaptive beliefs. This configuration derives predominantly from the person's metacognitive beliefs that specify the use of perseveration, threat monitoring, and certain thought control strategies as predominant modes of coping. These beliefs exist as implicit plans ("programs") that guide processing and as explicit declarative beliefs that are amenable to verbal report (e.g., "Worrying about what might happen means I will be prepared").

Content-specific metacognitions may also be identified in specific disorders, such as generalized anxiety disorder, obsessive–compulsive disorder, and depression. According to the S-REF model, cognitive and behavioral responses of the individual produce a range of consequences in parallel that affect both lower (reflexive) and higher (knowledge, beliefs) levels of cognition. Furthermore, the type of thinking and coping strategies adopted by patients may divert resources away from the cognitive operations required to modify cognition itself. For instance, a distinction has been made between two different *modes* of cognition that have implications for cognitive change processes (Wells, 2000). Blocks to cognitive modification occur when therapy is unable to establish a metacognitive mode of processing. There are also dynamic factors involving coping that perpetuate dysfunction. Some internally directed coping strategies backfire and maintain negative beliefs or disrupt normal self-regulation. For example, coping with anxiety by suppressing disturbing thoughts can lead to a disturbance of mental control (Purdon, 1999; Wegner, 1989), and the use of worry as a coping style appears to incubate intrusive images and posttraumatic stress disorder (PTSD) following stress (Holeva, Tarrier, & Wells, 2001; Wells & Papageorgiou, 1995). Some varieties of coping involve unhelpful patterns of interaction with the external environment. Avoidance of feared situations in anxiety disorders contributes to failure to discover that situations are not dangerous, and more subtle forms of safety behavior, such as avoiding self-disclosure in social phobia, can negatively bias the reactions of others, leading to negative cycles of social interaction.

Because the S-REF model provides an account of the mechanisms and dynamics of cognitive stasis and modification, it provides a framework that augments our understanding of blocks to therapeutic change. The implication for the process of overcoming therapeutic blocks is that metacognitive beliefs should be explored and challenged as a source of maladaptive coping strategies. For instance, patients may be unable to discontinue negative ruminative thinking styles because of beliefs about the dangers of doing so. Coping strategies such as worry/rumination, threat monitoring, thought control, and avoidance should be specifically targeted for modification, and the reduction of these strategies should facilitate cognitive modification. Unrealistic and inflexible standards or goals for self-regulation should be explored as a source of repeated activation of the cognitive-attention syndrome.

The model makes a distinction between two modes of processing that can have an impact on cognitive-affective change: *object mode* and *metacognitive mode*. In object mode, self-regulatory processing is dominated by plans for processing that specify that threat is objective and that the goal is to evaluate threat, to focus attention on danger, and to engage in threat-reducing strategies. The outcome of this mode of processing is the maintenance and strengthening of plans for threat appraisal and strengthening of dysfunctional beliefs. However, an alternative mode of processing is represented by the metacognitive mode, in which the plan for processing specifies that thoughts are events (not realities), that the goal is to evaluate cognition, that attention be focused on disconfirmatory information, and that worry and rumination be suspended. The outcome of this mode is modification of knowledge and the strengthening of plans for adaptive processing. Cognitive therapy can be viewed as shifting patients to a metacognitive processing mode, which is an important resource for cognitive modification. An implication for therapy is that individual differences may exist in the propensity to use and/or establish a metacognitive mode, and generally therapeutic effort should be focused on shifting to this mode early in treatment.

With this theoretical framework in mind, I now turn to a discussion of specific difficulties or blocks in treatment linked to coping strategies, perseveration (i.e., worry/rumination), and attention. Finally, some more general common issues relating to specific anxiety disorders are considered.

COPING STRATEGIES

A typical mode of coping in anxiety disorders is avoidance, which can manifest as avoidance of situations, of behaviors, and of internal events. Avoidance can block therapeutic progress in three predominant ways:

1. It prevents access to "hot cognitions" and activation of symptoms, thereby restricting assessment and case formulation.
2. Some avoidant forms of coping, particularly involving the control or concealment of anxiety symptoms, can backfire and worsen symptoms and negatively affect aspects of the external environment.
3. Avoidance prevents exposure to situations or experiences of symptoms that would provide an opportunity to disconfirm negative appraisals and beliefs.

The patient with panic disorder who avoids strong emotions because of fear of loss of control and the patient with obsessive–compulsive disorder (OCD) who controls his or her stream of consciousness so as to avoid thoughts of harming another are locked into coping strategies that deny them access to experiences that can disconfirm their fears. The very act of disclosing thoughts or discussing emotions can be enough to elicit the experience of the unwanted emotion or thought and the dangers that the patient believes are associated with such an experience. The patient chooses not to discuss these events with the therapist, denying the therapist access to valuable information that is required for eliciting appraisals and devising strategies for testing them.

Avoidant forms of coping are often motivated by fear and are associated with danger-related appraisals. In anxiety disorders avoidance can also be motivated by shame and embarrassment, in cases in which self-appraisals concern the interpretation of symptoms as unacceptable, abnormal, or aberrant in relation to some internalized social rule system. For instance, the ego-dystonic nature of obsessional thoughts and impulses can lead the patient with OCD to censor or sanitize descriptions of these events. The resulting lack of detail interferes with the construction of personally valid strategies of exposure to obsessions. A solution to this problem is the "normalization" and destigmatizing of obsessions at the outset of treatment.

The therapeutic situation can be contaminated by the anxious patient's coping behavior. For instance, patients with OCD may be unwilling to think about and describe obsessional thoughts, as this will lead to inflated risk of catastrophe, and the patient with social phobia will censor his or her speech or say very little so that he or she does not sound foolish to the therapist. Censorship and avoidance of this kind, if they go unchecked, will produce an incomplete formulation of the presenting problem and retard the rate of therapeutic progress.

Coping responses are often more subtle in form than overt avoidance. Patients with anxiety disorders use subtle safety behaviors (Salkovskis, 1991) to prevent feared catastrophes. Both avoidance and safety behaviors may well provide short-term relief of anxiety, but in the long term they interfere with cognitive modification. In particular, patients attribute the nonoccurrence of catastrophe to use of their behavior and fail to learn that their negative thoughts and beliefs are false. In some disorders further problems with safety behaviors exist in that these behaviors intensify negative symptoms and can contaminate situations. For example, a patient with panic disorder who misinterpreted sensations of breathlessness as a sign of suffocation prevented such a catastrophe by taking repeated deep breaths. This made him feel light-headed and, paradoxically, made his breathing seem more difficult. Further deleterious effects of safety behaviors are described in the cognitive model of social phobia (Clark & Wells, 1995). Safety behaviors often consist of saying little, asking questions rather than self-disclosing, and mentally rehearsing sentences before speaking. These behaviors increase self-consciousness, impair concentration, contribute to difficulties in speaking, and make the person with social phobia appear withdrawn or unfriendly. Safety behaviors pose blocks to therapy when they remain unmodified. Irrespective of the amount of exposure an anxious patient receives, the commission of safety behavior during exposure prevents disconfirmation of belief in appraisals because it supports a "near miss" attribution in which the patient believes he or she managed to prevent a catastrophe this time but may not succeed in the future. Moreover, such behaviors reduce anxiety by blocking exposure to feared events, and this is a problem when the events feared are components of the anxious response itself. In behavioral terms, the safety behavior prevents full exposure so that anxiety does not habituate, and, in cognitive terms, exposure fails to provide a true test of belief because the situation is bereft of the source of threat (i.e., anxiety itself).

OVERCOMING BLOCKS TO DISCONFIRMATION

The solution to the blocks in cognitive-emotional change presented by avoidance and safety behaviors is for the therapist to spend time in the detailed analysis of the full range of avoidance and safety behaviors linked to target dysfunctional cognitions. The emphasis here is on identifying which specific behaviors are linked to each dysfunctional appraisal. Behavioral experiments will produce unambiguous disconfirmation of belief in appraisal when the correct safety behaviors are manipulated during exposure. For example, in the treatment of social phobia (Wells, 1997), patients are instructed to drop specific safety behaviors such as hiding their faces (in cases of fear of blushing) while observing the nature of other people's attention to them in feared social situations. Behavioral experiments of this kind follow the P-E-T-S protocol for effective behavioral experiments for maximizing belief change (Wells, 1997). Four stages should be distinguished in designing and implementing experiments, according to the P-E-T-S protocol.

1. In the first stage (P), which signifies *preparation*, the therapist must elicit a key target cognition and belief level, along with a detailed description of the safety behaviors used to prevent or conceal catastrophe linked to the appraisal. A cognitive rationale is then presented in the context of the active case formulation that emphasizes exposing the patient to the feared situation or stimulus while he or she performs actions that allow him or her to discover that the catastrophe predicted (in line with the negative appraisal) does not happen.

2. In the second phase (E), the patient is *exposed* to the feared situation. This situation should resemble as closely as possible the type of situation that activates the patient's fear. Approximations to the situation or stimulus may suffice as a first step, but they are not usually a complete substitute for exposure to typical situations or stimuli. In particular, the situation that activates fear may contain very specific elements, the presence or

absence of which will determine whether anxiety and negative appraisals are activated. The exposure situation must produce anxiety as this is the marker for activation of the negative appraisal and because the anxious feelings themselves are often part of the situation that is interpreted as dangerous. If anxiety is not activated, the patient can simply discount the threat value of the exposure experience, and the experiment then fails to provide a disconfirmatory learning experience.

3. The third phase (T) of the P-E-T-S protocol is the *test*, or disconfirmatory maneuver. Exposure alone is not typically sufficient to provide rapid and direct disconfirmation of negative appraisals. To achieve unambiguous disconfirmation, it is recommended that the patient perform a deliberate action that disconfirms the appraisal (or prediction). This will consist of abandoning safety behaviors and/or paradoxical strategies, such as pushing symptoms or showing feared responses, depending on the stage of treatment and the nature of the presenting problem. For instance, in the treatment of social phobia a patient may be asked to focus externally on the reactions of others while deliberately showing signs of performance failure, such as spilling a drink. In the treatment of panic disorder the disconfirmatory maneuver often consists of pushing symptoms to discover that physical or psychosocial catastrophe does not occur.

4. The final stage of behavioral experiments is the *summarize* (S) phase, in which the results of the experiment are reviewed in terms of the patient's belief or prediction. Belief level is rerated, experimental results are discussed in the context of the case formulation, and the experiment is modified or finely tuned prior to further implementation.

Empirical studies support the usefulness of manipulating in-situation coping behaviors and attention during exposure. In a study of patients with social phobia (Wells et al., 1995), brief exposure and the dropping of safety behavior within the context of a rationale emphasizing disconfirmatory processing were more effective than brief exposure alone with a habituation rationale in reducing in-situation anxiety and negative beliefs. Similar results were obtained in a subsequent study of panic and agoraphobia (Salkovskis, Clark, Hackmann, Wells, & Gelder, 1999). Another study of patients with social phobia also supports the view that disconfirmatory maneuvers that focus attention on belief-incongruent information (external attention focus) appear to produce stronger effects than brief exposure alone (Wells & Papageorgiou, 1998a).

THE PROBLEM OF LOW CONGRUENCE (VALIDITY)

One of the factors that can block the effective implementation of behavioral experiments is lack of congruence between the feared situation and the situation used to test the negative belief. In panic disorder, the symptoms induced in the therapist's office may not resemble closely enough the symptoms that are normally catastrophically misinterpreted. In social phobia, specific features of the feared situation often make the difference between whether or not anxiety is activated. For example, a patient at our clinic reported that reading in front of a group of five or more people always made him feel anxious. However, it was not possible to activate this anxiety by mock-up group reading tasks in therapy. After several failed attempts and further detailed assessment of a recent episode in which he felt anxious in his work situation, the patient realized that he felt anxious only in a confined room when the audience sat close to him. Accordingly, modifications were made to the mock reading task that were successful in eliciting anxiety and activating his belief that he "looked anxious." Video feedback of his performance was used to challenge his erroneous belief.

The importance of precision in determining whether or not disconfirmation occurs is evident in obsessive–compulsive disorder. When challenging beliefs about intrusive thoughts in metacognitive focused therapy (Wells, 1997, 2000), exposure and response prevention experiments are used in which obsessional thoughts are deliberately invoked and patients are asked to refrain from neutralizing behaviors. This procedure is done to test predictions concerning the power and influence of thinking, such as the belief that having mental images of the devil will lead to specific negative events unless these are prevented by engaging in special rituals. Although these experiments are effective in reducing belief in the power of such thoughts, a residual belief level may persist despite further efforts at verbal and behavioral reattribution. A source of this problem is failure to fully induce obsessional experiences that faithfully reproduce the nature of spontaneous experiences outside of therapy sessions. An illustration from our clinic will help in demonstrating this point. A patient troubled by thoughts that she would inadvertently transform her personality by having mental images of a well-known serial killer stated that inducing the thoughts was not the same as having the thoughts spontaneously during her normal routine. Rather than relying on constructing an experiment around the vagaries of the time at which the next spontaneous thought would occur and on her poor ability to ban neutralizing, a detailed analysis of a recent experience of a spontaneous obsessional thought was undertaken. The aim was to determine what was special about a spontaneous thought. This explored the nature of the thought, such as its size, color, shape, vividness, and the nature and bodily location of feelings that accompanied it. It was discovered that it was not only the image of the serial killer but also the co-occurrence of a specific sensation of "weightlessness" in the pit of the stomach that determined whether or not the thought would lead to the feared transformation of personality. Taking account of this discovery, exposure and response prevention experiments were refined and repeated for both deliberate and spontaneous thought occurrences in which the patient was instructed to focus on and enhance the bodily sensation in association with the thought.

PERSEVERATION (WORRY AND RUMINATION)

Perseveration refers to repetitive and often purposeful occurrences of thought and/or behavior. Anxiety disorders are characterized, at least in part, by such activity, which often has a brooding quality. In generalized anxiety disorder (GAD), a predominant feature is excessive and uncontrollable worrying about a number of topics; in OCD it involves repetitive thoughts or actions; PTSD involves preoccupation with traumatic events; and social phobia involves a tendency to worry about forthcoming social encounters and to dwell on memories of one's performance in difficult social situations. Perseveration of this kind can be difficult to bring under control, and if it goes unchecked it can be a source of roadblocks in cognitive therapy.

We saw earlier how perseveration has been viewed as a component of a cognitive-attentional syndrome that underlies vulnerability to emotional disorder and that is involved in disorder maintenance (Wells, 2000; Wells & Matthews, 1994). Evidence suggests that worry can have a negative effect on emotional processing following stress and trauma (Butler, Wells, & Dewick, 1995; Wells & Papageorgiou, 1995). The tendency to use worry to control intrusive thoughts is predictive of PTSD following road traffic accidents in prospective analyses (Holeva, Tarrier, & Wells, 2001). More generally, brief periods of worrying appear to be associated with an increase in thought intrusions (Borkovec, Robinson, Pruzinsky, & DePree, 1983).

Worrying contributes to intrusive thoughts, and perseveration is problematic because it focuses attention on negative information and negates the consolidation of positive information necessary for belief change. As the empirical evidence suggests, it also appears to lead to an amplification of stress responses under some circumstances. Progress in individual treatment sessions can be limited if patients engage in worry processes following sessions. Worry or postmortem processing involving the selective focusing on negative feelings or events has the capacity to change the meaning of experiences such that potentially positive and reconstructive experiences become negative events. This type of thinking style should be identified and targeted early in treatment. The therapist should review with the patient the advantages and disadvantages of worry, reinforce the disadvantages, challenge beliefs about the advantages, and then ask the patient to ban the activity.

Acute worry episodes in which the content of worrying or catastrophizing shifts from session to session are problematic when the patient's agenda becomes dominated by the need to resolve the current worry crisis and/or when the treatment session readily dissolves into a search for reassurances. It is important for the therapist to move away from challenging the content of worries and to intervene at the process and metacognitive level. An effective strategy is the worry postponement technique, a form of which was first introduced by Borkovec and colleagues (Borkovec, Wilkinson, Folensbee, & Lerman, 1983) and later modified and developed as a behavioral experiment (Wells, 1997). Here, patients are instructed to notice themselves worrying the next time a worry episode is activated and to disengage from the worry process by setting aside a time later in the day as a designated worry time, during which he or she will spend 15 minutes worrying with a clear onset and offset time for worrying. The worry time should be used only if the patient feels that it is necessary. Typically patients forget to use the worry time or feel that it is not necessary. This technique can be presented as a behavioral experiment to challenge beliefs about the uncontrollability of worry. The technique also has the advantage of taking maladaptive worry processes off-line, thereby minimizing the negative consequences of worrying. A further technique is training in detached mindfulness (Wells & Matthews, 1994). Not to be confused with mindfulness meditation (e.g., Kabat-Zinn, 1990), detached mindfulness is simply an instruction to be aware of engaging in worry or rumination, with the further instruction to watch such thoughts in a detached way without engaging with them. The aim is to train patents in alternative styles of responding that can be used to override cyclical negative thinking patterns. All of these strategies may fail if the patient is not motivated to give up negative and perseverative forms of thinking. To understand such motivational blocks, it is necessary to turn to analyzing the individual's metacognitive beliefs.

ATTENTIONAL STRATEGIES

The attentional strategies used by patients can block therapeutic change when they focus processing resources on information that is consistent with negative appraisals and beliefs. In the S-REF model, psychopathology is considered to be associated with the preponderance of two attentional styles that either coexist or alternate. These styles are inflexible self-focused attention, and hypervigilance, or monitoring for threat. Self-focus and threat monitoring are often the same strategy, as, for instance, in cases of panic disorder, health anxiety, social phobia, and obsessional disorder in which internal cognitions and somatic events are feared. In PTSD, threat monitoring may take the form of hypervigilance for environmental stimuli that resemble those encountered during the trauma, such as scanning the environment for particular types of people. These attentional strategies may be triggered by lower level reflexive cognitive activity and/or be sustained as a component of active coping. An example of the latter is seen in a patient with health anxiety who believes that it is advantageous to scan the body for symptoms so that untoward symptoms can be detected early and lifesaving help obtained. The problem with attentional strategies of self-focus and threat monitoring is that they fuel negative appraisals and perpetuate the perception of danger and threat. In PTSD, threat monitoring may actually strengthen a cognitive configuration that maintains the perception of danger. and contributes to failed emotional processing (Wells, 2000; Wells & Sembi, 2001).

Attentional strategies can produce mixed effects. Distraction, when used by a patient to prevent catastrophe, is a safety behavior that blocks effective belief change. In the exposure literature, distraction following exposure has been associated with a return of fear following exposure (Grayson, Foa, & Steketee, 1982; Sartory, Rachman, & Grey, 1982). However, external attentional focusing on disconfirmatory information has been shown to enhance the effects of brief exposure in patients with social phobia (Wells & Papageorgiou, 1998b). Difficulties are likely to be encountered in treatment when attentional strategies are used in a way that prevents unambiguous disconfirmation of negative beliefs, such as their use as an anxiety-management or avoidance strategy when anxiety symptoms themselves are a source of fear. Nevertheless, attentional manipulations may be useful if they interrupt perseverative forms of inflexible thinking or self-focus, and for this purpose a specific technique of attention training has been developed (Wells, 1990). It should be noted, however, that this technique is not intended to be practiced as a symptom-control procedure but that it provides a means of restoring executive control over processing. The potential blocks in treatment generated by attentional strategies can be overcome by using strategies that focus attention on disconfirmatory information. The effects of procedures such as distraction may be used as evidence to challenge specific beliefs, but their use as symptom-control strategies when symptoms themselves are feared should be avoided or followed up by techniques that challenge negative appraisals.

COMMON BLOCKS IN SPECIFIC ANXIETY DISORDERS

Panic Disorder

The goal of cognitive therapy for panic disorder is the elimination of belief in catastrophic misinterpretations of symptoms. This goal is achieved through behavioral experiments that utilize symptom induction. An initial block of treatment can be the patient's level of disease conviction in which panic or anxiety symptoms are seen as being due to an organic disease event though no disease is present. In this instance socialization may take longer than usual, and the therapist should aim to shift the patient to a psychological model of the presenting problem. In order to do so, several panic attacks should be reviewed in detail and the vicious-cycle model drawn out in an attempt to find exceptions to the psychological model. The failure to find exceptions is used as preliminary evidence for a psychological model. Behavioral experiments should be used early on as socialization strategies. Typical experiments include body-focusing instructions and reading paired-associate word lists (e.g., breathless–suffocate, chest tight–heart attack, dizziness–fainting, numbness–stroke) to show how specific types of thinking can elicit anxiety and/or affect bodily sensations. Experiments illustrating the model also consist of manipulating safety behaviors. For instance, if the patient copes with fear of suffocation by engaging in deep breathing, the role of such safety behaviors on symptom experiences can be demonstrated by the deliberate intensification of deep breathing in the session.

A damaging block in the conceptualization and treatment of panic disorder is failure to elicit catastrophic misinterpretations. This block often occurs when avoidance is severe, such that the patient rarely experiences anxiety, and therefore access to hot cognitions is diminished. This pattern occurs when patients show moderate to severe levels of long-standing agoraphobic avoidance. The solution is the use of behavioral exposure tests to activate hot cognitions. The therapist should use the nature of avoidance as a marker for situations that will activate hot cognitions. A proportion of early treatment sessions may then be devoted to interoceptive and/or situational exposure in which the therapist probes for the content of misinterpretations. Questioning specifically the *worst consequences* that could happen in a situation when anxiety is activated provides a means of determining the content of catastrophic misinterpretations.

A further factor that can block access to catastrophic misinterpretations that drive panic disorder is the repeated articulation of secondary escape or avoidance-related cognitions. For instance, when asked, "What thought went through your mind when you noticed your heart beating fast and sensations of breathlessness?" a patient replied, "I thought I had to get out of the supermarket." In this type of scenario, it is useful for the therapist to question specifically what the patient believes would be the consequences of failure to escape or to avoid if such failure were accompanied by an intensification of anxious symptoms (e.g., "If you were unable to escape and your anxiety got worse, what is the worst thing that could happen?").

Behavioral experiments aimed at challenging catastrophic misinterpretations often involve exposure to bodily symptoms. The induction of panicogenic symptoms is highly aversive and anxiety provoking for patients and may therefore be resisted. When this situation arises, the therapist can take a graded approach to symptom induction. For example, the therapist can ask the patient to begin by taking three deep breaths, then five, then seven, and so on, in an experiment using hyperventilation provocation. As a further strategy, the therapist can perform the experiment with the patient or start the symptom induction before the patent does so that the patient may witness any catastrophe happening to the therapist first and can decide to discontinue the procedure before a similar thing happens to him or her. Resistance to behavioral experiments should be discussed in terms of the case formulation, and the therapist must emphasize that resistance will contribute to a failure to disconfirm negative misinterpretations that are the engine driving panic.

A final specific type of block that I will mention here is the presence of panic attacks in the apparent absence of catastrophic misinterpretations. Assuming biological mediation has been ruled out, this situation arises during the course of treatment, in cases in which specific misinterpretations—such as belief in collapsing, in having a heart attack, or in going crazy—have been successfully challenged but the patient still finds bodily sensations and anxiety intolerable. Here the catastrophic misinterpretation appears absent, but it is most likely that the misinterpretation exists in a slightly different form. More specifically, the misinterpretation is often the idea that the anxious feelings or symptoms will never end, or the misinterpretation may occur in the form of a mental image or memory of a previous panic attack. In these circumstances, it is necessary to challenge the belief in the permanence of symptoms and anxiety and to use imagery modification strategies and/or techniques focused on reinterpreting memories of anxious experiences. Interoceptive exposure experiments may be used to challenge belief in the permanence of symptoms and to build a greater tolerance of symptom experiences.

Health Anxiety

Engagement difficulties are common in individuals presenting with health anxiety. The patient believes strongly that he or she is physically ill and that psychological processes are not involved in the problem. Treatment can be viewed as extended socialization in which the therapist aims to strengthen an alternative psychological explanation of the patient's problem. The desirable end point is the acquisition by the patient of the belief that the problem is one of worry about health rather than a problem of suffering from a life-threatening disease process. Worry about health should be reduced in its frequency and severity, and general disease conviction should be challenged so that the patient no longer believes that it is likely that he or she is physically ill. Motivation to persist with psychological treatment is low when patients perceive treatment as inappropriate, as in some cases of hypochondriasis in which the patient believes the problem is physical rather than psychological.

Motivation and engagement problems can be tackled with a number of strategies. First, treatment should be presented as a no-lose experiment. This can be done by discussing the length of time the patient has been pursuing a medical explanation for the problem and how well this pursuit has solved the problem. It should be pointed out, when appropriate, that seeking medical treatment has not resolved the problem and that the patient has nothing to lose by engaging in an alternative psychological treatment approach. Moreover, the patient should be told that, if the psychological approach does not work, he or she can then return to the previous strategy as a means of finding the solution. A case formulation that offers an alternative (no-disease) explanation of the patient's symptoms offers a powerful alternative perspective (e.g., Wells, 1997). The role of body checking, body-focused attention, guarded movements, and other maladaptive coping behaviors (e.g., use of alcohol, excessive exercise, avoiding food) in exacerbating symptoms should be illustrated early in socialization.

Motivation may be increased by undertaking an advantages–disadvantage analysis of cognitive therapy. The disadvantages should be challenged and the advantages increased in scope. Gaining evidence for the cognitive formulation early on in treatment is essential. Evidence may be obtained through symptom monitoring, in which patterns in the occurrence of feared symptoms can be observed and an alternative explanation sought. Manipulation of the intensity of body checking and maladaptive coping behaviors should also be used to demonstrate the effect of behaviors on symptom preoccupation and intensity when possible. Early and effective intervention targeted at symptom relief can be used as evidence of the validity of the cognitive approach. For example, with the patient who presents with health anxiety and panic attacks, the intervention may initially focus on the conceptualization and treatment of panic attacks using a panic model before concentrating on remaining disease conviction using a health anxiety formulation.

In some cases health anxiety and associated disease conviction offer a number of advantages for the sufferer. They may influence the nature of personal relationships and provide either a strategy for avoiding intimacy or a vehicle for the expression of dependency. In a case reported by Wells and Dattilio (1992), a patient with health anxiety showed a negative response (strengthening of cognitions) to cognitive restructuring strategies aimed at directly challenging his disease conviction, whereas this response was not shown to a relaxation strategy. Eventually the patient dropped out of treatment, after disclosing that his health anxiety and worry protected him from engaging in exhibitionistic behaviors and that, without these constraints, he feared that he would descend into sexual depravity.

Generalized Anxiety Disorder

Until recently cognitive models of the factors that underlie uncontrollable worry, the characteristic feature of GAD, have not been available. The absence of such has been a conceptual block to developing effective treatment. It has also meant that patients continue to engage in maladaptive worry processes despite the therapist's best effort to challenge the content and validity of individual worries. In some more severe presentations, patients present with patterns of repeated worrying that change in content, and the worrying propensity does not appear to decrease across treatment sessions. It has been argued that this problem emerges from a failure to modify the factors underlying repetitive negative thinking, that is, worry (Wells, 1995, 1999). A case conceptualization needs to specify the individual's beliefs that lead to worrying as a predominant means of dealing with threat. The metacognitive model of GAD (Wells, 1995, 1997) provides a basis for such a conceptualization and treatment.

The metacognitive-focused cognitive model and treatment (Wells, 1995, 1997) emphasizes the role of patients' erroneous negative and positive beliefs about worry in the persistence of the problem. This model is supported by empirical evidence from a range of sources (e.g., Cartwright-Hatton & Wells, 1997; Wells & Carter, 1999, 2001; Wells & Papageorgiou, 1998a).

One of the main blocks for the therapist aiming to implement metacognitive-focused cognitive therapy for the first time is the conceptual shift that is required to deal with beliefs about worry, rather than dealing with the content of individual worries directly. It is easy for the therapist to drift into focusing on individual worries and to challenge their content, even though the focus should initially be on challenging beliefs about the uncontrollability and dangers of worrying and then on challenging positive beliefs about the usefulness of worrying as a coping strategy. It is useful here for the therapist to remind him- or herself of the question, "How much of a problem would my patient have if he or she believed that worrying was normal, controllable, and harmless and did not use worry as a predominant means of coping?" Instruments such as the Generalized Anxiety Disorder scale (GADS; Wells, 1997) may be administered to patients each session and used as a source of focal metacognitions that should be targeted in treatment in order to reduce therapeutic drift.

Social Phobia

Three common blocks in the treatment of social phobia are considered in this section: (1) the contaminating effect of social anxiety on the therapeutic relationship; (2) difficulty in discontinuing worry/rumination-based thinking prior to or after social situations; and (3) inflexible and locked-in self-consciousness.

The therapeutic situation can be contaminated by social anxiety. In particular, patients may avoid eye contact with the therapist, may give short yes/no answers, or may control their speech and behavior in an attempt to avoid feared social responses such as babbling, blushing, or appearing foolish. Although distracting for the therapist, responses of this kind are typically manifestations of dysfunctional avoidance and safety behaviors. The therapist may feel uncomfortable addressing these behaviors, but it is imperative that material from the therapeutic encounter is overtly analyzed and incorporated into the case conceptualization.

A further contaminating mechanism in therapy is the therapist's own level of social anxiety or social-evaluative concerns. If the therapist is high in fear of negative evaluation, he or she may find it difficult to suggest and model behavioral experiments involving the deliberate commission of embarrassing or failed performance in public. This reluctance can generate a significant obstacle to therapeutic progress. In these circumstances the therapist should attempt to isolate and challenge his or her own cognitions and predictions through the personal practice of treatment strategies.

A small number of patients report considerable difficulty in stopping worry in the form of anticipatory processing prior to social situations or postmortem processing afterward, and for some patients the worry is worse than the actual exposure to the feared social situation. Ruminatory responses of this kind can transform the meaning of events and strengthen negative self-processing. The targeting and modification of rumination-based processing early in treatment has contributed to the development of a brief treatment for social phobia (Wells & Papageorgiou, 2001). Rumination tendencies persist when patients continue to believe that worry/rumination is advantageous and allows them to avoid social catastrophe or to "save face." The problem can be addressed by reviewing with the patient the advantages and disadvantages of worry. The disadvantages should be reinforced and, when necessary, an alternative to rumination devised. Alternatives to anticipatory worry include worry postponement, reducing the amount of rehearsal before social encounters, and task focusing instead of self-focusing. Techniques for dealing with postmortem processing include shifting perspective in the memory of the social situation such that patients are asked to recall what other people did in the social situation rather than recalling how they themselves felt and acted. In this way it becomes apparent that information concerning other people's reactions is sketchy and that recall is biased toward the negative sense of self. The therapist can then examine the potentially unhelpful effects of such selective biased processing on the patients' self-concept, and, having established that the postmortem is unhelpful, ask patients to renew efforts to ban it. Alternatives to the postmortem may also be introduced, such as keeping a positive social-data log after events instead of the negative postmortem and postponing the postmortem until the following day, engaging in it then only if they feel they must. When worry persists, the therapist should assess whether specific metacognitive beliefs are driving the process. Such beliefs are usually uncovered while reviewing the advantages of rumination/worry, and they may need to be subjected to a more sustained and broader use of verbal and behavioral reattribution techniques directed at weakening them.

The final block to be considered in this section is that presented by inflexible self-consciousness. A cognitive therapist under my supervision discussed a patient who could give a detailed description of the cognitive model and who clearly understood the importance of dropping safety behaviors and shifting to external-focused attention during exposure to social situations. However, the patient repeatedly failed to achieve this goal. This pattern is apparent in a small number of patients, and I have observed two different factors that appear to account for the problem. The first is a preoccupation with performance and "doing things right," such that dropping safety behaviors becomes an "all or nothing" task, which itself interferes with shifting attention to external disconfirmatory information and reinforces self-focus. Normally, the coupling of external-attention instructions with instructions to drop specific safety behaviors counteracts the problem of self-focus caused by monitoring and changing safety behaviors. This potential block can be resolved by placing more emphasis on shifting patients to external attention than on dropping safety behaviors. The second factor that appears to contribute to failure in reducing self-focus is an inability to formulate specific strategies for anchoring attention on aspects of the external environment. To solve this problem, a range of strategies can be suggested and practiced in session, such as focusing on the number of people in the social environment, evaluating whether other people have a good dress sense, trying to work out whether other people look happy or sad, and focusing on how many people are paying attention to the patient. In brief cognitive therapy (Wells & Papageorgiou, 2001), we introduced the strategy of instructing patients to focus externally on features of the nonsocial environment when not in feared social situations as additional practice in flexible attentional responding. These strategies must be followed by techniques focused on modifying both specific negative predictions about the consequences of failed social performance and the distorted self-image that patients have of themselves when anxious. The strategies are not intended to be used as symptom-control strategies that could serve as additional safety behaviors.

Obsessive–Compulsive Disorder

Cognitive therapy for OCD typically consists of exposure to obsessional thoughts and impulses combined with ritual prevention. This strategy is intended to facilitate habituation and can be configured as a behavioral experiment for challenging negative beliefs about the power and consequences of obsessions, impulses, and feelings.

Failure to Access Obsessional Thoughts

Obsessional thoughts are experienced as repugnant by the patient. Thoughts of committing violent and obscene sexual acts and similar thoughts are associated with feelings of guilt, shame, fear, and embarrassment. As a result patients are often reluctant to disclose the full extent of their obsessional thoughts, images, and impulses. Censorship of this kind retards therapeutic progress and, in extremes, renders impossible the design and implementation of exposure and response prevention experiments and other reattribution procedures. To reduce this complication, the therapist should normalize patient experiences and facilitate disclosure at the outset of treatment. This can be achieved by describing the types of obsessional thoughts that patients often present and introducing the idea that it is normal to feel uncomfortable disclosing full details of obsessional thoughts. It can be stressed that obsessions are commonly occurring phenomena and that more than 80% of people have them. In some cases it may be helpful for the therapist to disclose the nature of his or her own obsessional thoughts and impulses.

A patient may not describe obsessional thoughts because he or she is engaged in chronic cognitive avoidance. In some instances, the very act of disclosure can be perceived as giving the obsessional thought additional power to affect outcomes. Under these circumstances, the therapist should ensure that the patient understands the formulation of the problem in terms of dysfunctional beliefs about the power of thoughts and the role of neutralizing and avoidance in preventing the falsification of such beliefs. Beliefs about thoughts may be elicited without discovering the details of the obsession, and preliminary verbal reattribution strategies should then be implemented to weaken such beliefs as a prerequisite to accessing of obsessions and the implementation of exposure and response prevention experiments.

Inability to Experimentally Falsify Predictions

Difficulties arise in the experimental test of beliefs about obsessions when the time course of any predicted negative outcomes is indeterminate or distant. For example, a patient believed that having thoughts about an unlikable person while performing an action would make him unlikable unless actions were repeated with images of likable people in mind. When questioned about how long this process of personal transformation would take, he replied that it could take many years. To overcome this problem, treatment was shifted to focus on another obsession that had a shorter predicted time course but that was linked to the same belief about the power of thinking. In addition (and when this cannot be achieved), verbal reattribution strategies were used to challenge the belief. These strategies included questioning the evidence for the belief, questioning the mechanism by which thoughts can influence events, and taking a historical perspective and questioning why, after a long period of OCD, the catastrophe had not yet occurred. Behavioral experiments involving the attempted causation of positive outcomes through the power of thought are also useful in challenging beliefs about the power of thinking (e.g., try to win the lottery by thinking about winning).

Beliefs about obsessions and rituals are resistant to modification when they are a part of an extensive and elaborate belief system—for example, social or religious beliefs. Some behaviors and interpretations of cognitive events may be sanctioned and reinforced by members of the patient's family or community. Such attitudes can work against the best therapeutic efforts to challenge beliefs. In these circumstances the therapist may rely more on a habituation model rather than focusing explicitly on challenging beliefs about obsessions. A useful strategy is to question how other people within the community who have similar beliefs deal with obsessional thoughts, with the focus on changing responses to intrusions and on learning that such intrusions do not have to be acted on by sustained neutralizing.

Failure and Resistance in Exposure and Response Prevention

In some cases, habituation, adaptive learning, and modification of negative predictions do not occur because the patient is continuing to engage in subtle avoidance, neutralizing, and safety behaviors. In one case, the belief that having an obsessional thought would lead to loss of control was successfully reduced to 15% through exposure and response prevention experiments, but further reductions seemed untenable. The patient reported that he was not using any neutralizing responses and that he was deliberately holding in mind an image of strangling the therapist. However, detailed questioning revealed that he was not paying full attention to the image because he believed that giving full attention to it would lead to commission of the imagined action. It is necessary to analyze in fine detail the cognitive, attentional, and behavioral strategies that patients use during exposure and response prevention and to guide attention and modify behavior in a way that maximizes cognitive-affective change.

When patients refuse to engage in exposure, the therapist should initially consider less anxiety-provoking exposure sessions in which exposure occurs to a thought or contaminant that provokes modest rather than extreme anxiety. A clearly structured approach to exposure during therapy sessions is required as a prerequisite to exposure work for homework. The responsibility for devising exposure and response prevention experiments should be a shared responsibility, with the emphasis for the design of such experiments gradually shifted onto the patient as treatment progresses. Clear presentation of the case formulation and treatment rationale provides a means of facilitating engagement with exposure tasks, and motivational techniques may be used to increase patient readiness to accept the intervention.

SUMMARY

Many different types of blocks can be encountered in cognitive therapy for anxiety disorders. This chapter has focused on the blocks that emerge from a lack of detailed specification in theory of cognitive change processes, an area that requires greater attention and formulation. Internal dynamic and metacognitive factors that contribute blocks to cognitive modification were discussed in the context of the S-REF model of disorder. This model identifies different modes of processing, metacognitive beliefs, maladaptive coping strategies, perseveration, and attentional factors as an influence on therapeutic change processes. It was suggested that many types of blocks can be viewed as the consequence of particular self-regulation or coping strategies that remain unformulated and/or unmodified during the course of treatment. In addition, progress in the treatment of anxiety depends significantly on the therapist's ability to expose patients to stimuli or situations that resemble those that are the focus of misinterpretation. We saw how a poor level of congruence, therapist anxiety or reticence, and failure to adequately configure exposure as an unambiguous test of specific predictions can contribute blocks to cognitive modification in behavioral experiments. The P-E-T-S protocol for behavioral experiments was described as a means of overcoming these potential difficulties. Finally, some common roadblocks in the treatment of several specific anxiety disorders and a range of solutions were examined.

REFERENCES

Borkovec, T. D., Robinson, E., Pruzinsky, T., & DePree, J. A. (1983). Preliminary exploration of worry: Some characteristics and processes. *Behaviour Research and Therapy, 21*, 9–16.

Borkovec, T. D., Wilkinson, L., Folensbee, R., & Lerman, C. (1983). Stimulus control applications to the treatment of worry. *Behaviour Research and Therapy, 21*, 247–251.

Butler, G., Wells, A., & Dewick, H. (1995). Differential effects of worry and imagery after exposure to a stressful stimulus: A pilot study. *Behavioural and Cognitive Psychotherapy, 23*, 45–56.

Cartwright-Hatton, S., & Wells, A. (1997). Beliefs about worry and intrusions: The Metacognitions Questionnaire. *Journal of Anxiety Disorders*, 11, 279–315.

Clark, D. M., & Wells, A. (1995). A cognitive model of social phobia. In R. Heimberg, M. Liebowitz, D. A. Hope, & F. R. Schneier (Eds.), *Social phobia: Diagnosis, assessment and treatment*. New York: Guilford Press.

Dowd, E. T., & Seibel, C. (1990). A cognitive theory of resistance and reactance: Implications for treatment. *Journal of Mental Health Counselling*, 12, 458–469.

Freeman, A., & Jackson, J. T. (1998). Cognitive behavioural treatment of personality disorders. In N. Tarrier, A. Wells, & G. Haddock (Eds.), *Treating complex cases: The cognitive behavioural therapy approach* (pp. 319–329). Chichester, UK: Wiley.

Grayson, J. B., Foa, E. B., & Steketee, G. J. (1982). Habituation during exposure treatment: Distraction versus attention focusing. *Behaviour Research and Therapy, 20*, 323–328.

Holeva, V., Tarrier, N. T., & Wells, A. (2001). Prevalence and predictors of acute stress disorder and PTSD following road traffic accidents: Thought control strategies and social support. *Behavior Therapy, 32*, 65–83.

Kabat-Zinn, J. (1990). *Full catastrophe living: The program of the stress reduction clinic at the University of Massachusetts Medical Center.* New York: Dell.

Leahy, R. L. (1999). Strategic self-limitation. *Journal of Cognitive Psychotherapy, 13*, 275–293.

Leahy, R. L. (2001). *Overcoming resistance in cognitive therapy.* New York: Guilford Press.

Leahy, R. L. (2002, July). *Cognitive therapy of resistance.* Workshop presented at the British Association for Behavioural and Cognitive Psychotherapies, University of Warwick.

Liotti, G. (1987). The resistance to change of cognitive structures: A counterproposal to psychoanalytic metapsychology. *Journal of Cognitive Psychotherapy, 1*, 87–104.

Mahoney, M. J. (1988). Constructive metatheory: 1. Basic features and historical foundations. *International Journal of Personal Construct Psychology, 1*, 1–35.

Newman, C. F. (1994). Understanding client resistance: Methods for enhancing motivation to change. *Cognitive and Behavioural Practice, 1*, 47–69.

Purdon, C. (1999). Thought suppression and psychopathology. *Behaviour Research and Therapy, 37*, 1029–1054.

Salkovskis, P. M. (1991). The importance of behaviour in the maintenance of anxiety and panic: A cognitive account. *Behavioural Psychotherapy, 19*, 6–19.

Salkovskis, P. M., Clark, D. M., Hackmann, A., Wells, A., & Gelder, M. G. (1999). An experimental investigation of the role of safety-seeking behaviours in the maintenance of panic disorder with agoraphobia. *Behaviour Research and Therapy, 37*, 559–574.

Sartory, G., Rachman, S., & Grey, S. J. (1982). Return of fear: The role of rehearsal. *Behavioural Research and Therapy, 20*, 123–134.

Wegner, D. M. (1989). *White bears and other unwanted thoughts.* New York: Viking.

Wells, A. (1990). Panic disorder in association with relaxation induced anxiety: An attentional training approach to treatment. *Behavior Therapy, 21*, 273–280.

Wells, A. (1995). Meta-cognition and worry: A cognitive model of generalized anxiety disorder. *Behavioural and Cognitive Psychotherapy, 23*, 301–320.

Wells, A. (1997). *Cognitive therapy of anxiety disorders.* Chichester, UK: Wiley.

Wells, A. (1999). A metacognitive model and therapy for generalized anxiety disorder. *Clinical Psychology and Psychotherapy, 6*, 86–95.

Wells, A. (2000). *Emotional disorders and metacognition: Innovative cognitive therapy.* Chichester, UK: Wiley.

Wells, A., & Carter, K. (1999). Preliminary tests of a cognitive model of generalized anxiety disorder. *Behaviour Research and Therapy, 37*, 585–594.

Wells, A., & Carter, K. (2001). Further tests of a cognitive model of generalized anxiety disorder: Metacognitions and worry in GAD, panic disorder, social phobia, depression, and non-patients. *Behavior Therapy, 32*, 85–102.

Wells, A., Clark, D. M., Salkovskis, P., Ludgate, J., Hackmann, A., & Gelder, M. (1995). Social phobia: The role of in-situation safety behaviours in maintaining anxiety and negative beliefs. *Behavior Therapy, 26*, 153–161.

Wells, A., & Dattilio, F. (1992). Negative outcome in cognitive-behaviour therapy: A case study. *Behavioural and Cognitive Psychotherapy, 20*, 291–294.

Wells, A., & Matthews, G. (1994). *Attention and emotion: A clinical perspective.* Hove, UK: Erlbaum.

Wells, A., & Matthews, G. (1996). Modelling cognition in emotional disorders: The S-REF model. *Behaviour Research and Therapy, 34*, 881–888.

Wells, A., & Papageorgiou, C. (1995). Worry and the incubation of intrusive images following stress. *Behaviour Research and Therapy, 33*, 579–583.

Wells, A., & Papageorgiou, C. (1998a). Relationships between worry, obsessive–compulsive symptoms and meta-cognitive beliefs. *Behaviour Research and Therapy, 36*, 899–913.

Wells, A., & Papageorgiou, C. (1998b). Social phobia: Effects of external attention on anxiety, negative beliefs, and perspective taking. *Behavior Therapy, 29*, 357–370.

Wells, A., & Papageorgiou, C. (2001). Brief cognitive therapy for social phobia: A case series. *Behaviour Research and Therapy, 39*, 713–720.

Wells, A., & Sembi, S. (2001). *Metacognitive focused therapy for PTSD: Effectiveness of a new treatment approach.* Manuscript submitted for publication.

5

Emotional Schemas and Resistance

Robert L. Leahy

A common criticism of cognitive therapy is that it does not adequately address the importance of emotions in the therapeutic process. Cognitive-behavioral models do address the role of emotions in terms of cognitive and emotional priming effects (see Clark, Beck, & Alford, 1999; Riskind, 1989), activation of fear schemas (Foa & Kozak, 1986), modes (Beck, 1996), negative beliefs about emotions that impede the effects of exposure for posttraumatic stress disorder (PTSD) (Ehlers & Clark, 2000), mindfulness (Kabat-Zinn, 1995; Linehan, 1993b; Segal, Williams, & Teasdale, 2002) and anxiety sensitivity that makes some individuals far more aware and affected by their arousal and emotions than others (Taylor, 1998). In this chapter, I review a model of emotional schemas; indicate its relevance to depression and anxiety; examine how emotional schemas affect accessing emotions, self-disclosure, and emotional change; review how these schemas affect compliance with self-help (especially exposure); and indicate how these schemas affect the therapeutic relationship. Finally, I review some general strategies that are relevant in modifying emotional schemas and examine how these strategies are utilized in the treatment of a depressed, alcoholic patient.

A MODEL OF EMOTIONAL SCHEMAS

I have advanced a model of emotional schemas that attempts to describe the role of conceptions of emotions and strategies of emotional processing (Leahy, 2002). It is proposed that emotions such as fear, sadness, anxiety, and loneliness are universal experiences but that individual differences in the conceptualization of these emotions and strategies of response will determine how problematic these emotional experiences become. This "social cognitive" model (in which emotions are the object of cognition) is related to recent conceptualizations of intrusive thoughts and emotional arousal (see Papageorgiou & Wells, 1999; Purdon & Clark, 1993; Salkovskis & Campbell, 1994; Sookman & Pinard, 2002; Wells & Carter, 2001). For example, individuals with obsessive–compulsive disorder (OCD) interpret their intrusive thoughts as indicative of their loss of control, responsibility, and personal pathology. Attempts to suppress or avoid these thoughts lead to greater sense of shame, loss of control, and anxiety, further exacerbating the very thoughts that one attempts to eliminate. Similarly, a metacognitive model of worry proposes that individuals often believe that they must worry in order to solve or prevent problems and that this worry will lead to loss of control or personal harm, either physically or mentally (Wells, Chapter 4, this volume; Wells & Carter, 2001).

The model of emotional schemas that I have proposed argues the following points (Leahy, 2002):

- Unpleasant emotions—such as sadness, loneliness, fear, anxiety, and anger—are universal phenomena.
- Individuals differ as to their interpretations of the significance of these emotions.
- These interpretations reflect beliefs in the duration, controllability, extremity, complexity, pathology, and moral quality of the emotions and the individual experiencing them.
- Negative emotional schemas, as reflected by the foregoing interpretations, further exacerbate the intensity, negativity, and duration of the negative emotions.
- These negative interpretations inhibit expression, validation, and emotional processing.

Differences in Emotional Processing and Emotional Schemas

Current models of worry and rumination suggest that these problematic coping styles are maintained by emotional avoidance. Thus individuals who worry shift away from emotionally laden imagery toward more abstract linguistic content, and this abstract worry *reduces* physiological arousal temporarily (Borkovec, 1994; Mennin, Turk, Heimberg, & Carmin, in press). Indeed, a significant component of worry, as stated by many worriers, is that worry helps them focus on something less threatening (Borkovec, 1994). Modification of anxiety (or fear) may require activating the arousal of the feared stimulus so that the individual can access the negative cognitive content or fear schema (Foa & Kozak, 1986; Greenberg,

2002a), learn that the emotion or intrusive thoughts are not overwhelming (Clark, 2002; Purdon & Clark, 1993), and process the content in a manner that allows the individual to make sense of the experience. Pennebaker has defined "emotional processing" as decreased inhibition of emotion, increased self-understanding, and enhanced positive self-reflection (Pennebaker, Mayne, & Francis, 1997). A focus on emotional processing would include factors that operate once an emotion has been experienced. These factors include recognition and labeling of an emotion, attempts to inhibit or even magnify an emotion, hypervigilance and problem-solving strategies, expression or ventilation, reliance on a receptive and supportive audience, distraction, and examination of one's own thought distortions.

As we know, very few patients come to therapy complaining about illogical thoughts or the inadequate use of information. They come because they are distressed emotionally. Negative life events may activate cognitive and emotional strategies that interact reciprocally to determine outcome. For example, the individual who returns to her empty apartment, begins to notice a negative emotion, and believes that this emotion must be eliminated immediately lest it overwhelm her and last indefinitely may choose to cope by numbing herself with binge eating or alcohol. Her reliance on substance abuse or bingeing confirms her belief that her emotions cannot be tolerated.

A different individual may notice that she feels empty and lonely and may then ruminate, focusing on her negative mood and attempting to make *complete sense* of all of her feelings and reduce them to a simple formula. Failing this, she then believes that her emotional distress is a sign of something deeper and more problematic. Still another individual believes that she should never have emotional difficulties, feels ashamed and guilty, and isolates herself rather than finding opportunities for expression, validation, and clarification. Her isolation and lack of expression confirm her shame and guilt over her emotion, further complicating her depression.

I have attempted to depict a contrast between problematic and adaptive emotional processing by contrasting two individuals confronted with the same life event (Leahy, 2002). Consider the following two people: Worried Willy and Michael Mensch. Both learn that their desirable partners—both, coincidentally, named Mary—have just dumped them. Worried Willy, frustrated in his goal of attaining perfect romance, notices that he has become emotionally uncomfortable with this news. He recognizes that he is upset, but he has a hard time initially labeling the feelings. He notices that he is feeling angry, but he believes that he should not be angry with someone he presumably loves. He is afraid of expressing this anger, lest Mary find out and close off any chance of reconciliation. He believes that he cannot share his anger and sadness with others because they might view him as a burden. He finds it hard to understand why he is so sad, because he has only known Mary for 2 months, and he feels ashamed of being so "dependent" on her. He is further confused because he cannot reconcile his conflicting emotions, believing that you "either love someone or you hate them—but never both." He is afraid that his sadness and anger might go out of control, so he worries about his feelings and thinks that his unhappiness will last forever. He wonders if he is the entire cause of his unhappiness, believing that he does not have a right to be angry. He criticizes himself for being so "needy" and views his desire for Mary as a sign of his inferiority as a man. Worried Willy sits in his apartment, sipping a drink, focusing on how bad he is, reading the Book of Job, asking God, "Why me?" He no longer spends time with his friends, and he has missed work. Sometimes he wishes that he could just feel numb, and he finds that a few scotches will do the trick. Worried Willy looks at his worries as a sign of his weakness, claiming to himself that he should always be rational, as he has a law degree and did quite well on the licensing exam. He fears that his strong negative feelings will persist into the summer, ruining his experiences at the beach house that he dreamed of sharing with Missing Mary. Worried Willy is certain that no one shares these pathetic and confusing feelings and, therefore, he is reluctant to share them with others.

In contrast, Michael Mensch is fully aware of his range of feelings—anger, anxiety, sadness, and even a touch of hope. Initially upset with the news that Mary was gone, he recognized that his feelings were neither positive nor negative but simply "human"—a sign that he had the fullness of experience that gave his family the name "Mensch" generations ago. He is currently having dinner with his friend, Understanding Ed, with whom Michael feels confident that he can express his feelings and have a receptive audience. Michael finds that this expression helps him clarify his feelings, recognize that others might feel the same way, and helps him see that he has a right to feel a range of emotions. He recognizes that, with the breakup, it makes sense to have conflicting feelings, only because life and relationships are complicated. Thus he feels sad because he is losing a partner, angry because of her carelessness in telling him by e-mail, and relieved because she was "high maintenance" to begin with. Even though he may feel intense sadness at times, he knows that these feelings will not overwhelm him, that they can be controlled to some extent, and that they will not last forever. Consequently, although he enjoys a fine Guinness Stout with Ed, he does not feel a need to numb himself with a drinking binge. His view of the situation and his response is that the sadness he feels is due to both internal and external factors—that is, a consequence of the breakup and of his reliance on someone who was not that reliable. He feels sad, he recognizes, because intimacy and commitment are important to him and, although he will not have that with Missing Mary, he will look for it with someone else. Rather than sit at home ruminating about his situation, he has scheduled a number of possibly productive experiences, such as seeing friends, exercising, work, and a date with Jane. Michael likes to think of himself as rational, but he also balances this with the awareness that, like other people, he will feel bad after a breakup but that the feelings are simply a sign of being a "mensch" (Leahy, 2002).

Dimensions of Emotional Schemas

The emotional schema model proposes that there are 14 emotional schemas that are relevant to emotional processing. These schemas are not exhaustive, and some overlap may exist among them. However, if we review these schemas, we can see their potential relevance in both the maintenance of negative emotional experiences and in creating roadblocks in therapy. The 14 dimensions of the Leahy Emotional Schema Scale (LESS) are shown in Figure 5.1. A schematic depicting the hypothesized "emotional pathways" is provided in Figure 5.2.

As Figure 5.1 illustrates, individuals may conceptualize their emotions as incomprehensible, not similar to those of others (consensus), having a long duration, out of control, not related to their higher values, and shameful or guilt inducing. They may believe that they cannot accept or express these feelings and that they will not experience validation if they do express them. They may ruminate on how bad they feel, attempt to focus exclusively on rationality, and seek to simplify their feelings. Some may attempt to make themselves numb. Some may blame other people for these feelings. These problematic negative schemas for emotions make emotional processing or emotional regulation difficult, further prolonging emotional distress.

In Figure 5.2 we can see how the individual may pursue three separate paths, given an initially unpleasant emotion. The individual who first attends to his emotion (e.g., sadness) but who is able to normalize, express, and experience validation is less likely to maintain his sadness. In contrast, on the second pathway, emotional and cognitive avoidance, an individual might utilize bingeing, drinking, or dissociation to avoid negative feelings, further adding to the belief that negative emotions cannot be controlled or tolerated. This contributes to rumination and worry. The third path entails viewing emotions as incomprehensible, shameful, not similar to those that others have, and requiring simplification. These negative interpretations also contribute to rumination, worry, and the prolongation or escalation of negative feelings.

EMOTIONAL SCHEMAS, THEORIES OF EMOTIONS, AND DEPRESSION

Cognitive-behavioral therapy seeks to assist the patient in recognizing the difference between thoughts and feelings, to engage the patient in

FIGURE 5.1. Emotional Schema Questionnaire

We are interested in how you deal with your feelings or emotions—for example, how you deal with feelings of anger, sadness, anxiety, or sexual feelings. We all differ in how we deal with these feelings—so there are no right or wrong answers. Please read each sentence carefully and answer each sentence—using the scale below—as to how you dealt with your feelings during the past month. Put the number of your response next to the sentence.

Scale: 1 = very untrue of me
2 = somewhat untrue of me
3 = slightly untrue of me
4 = slightly true of me
5 = somewhat true of me
6 = very true of me

1. ___When I feel down, I try to think about a different way to view things.
2. ___When I have a feeling that bothers me, I try to think of why it is not important.
3. ___I often think that I respond with feelings that others would not have.
4. ___Some feelings are wrong to have.
5. ___There are things about myself that I just don't understand.
6. ___I believe that it is important to let myself cry in order to get my feelings "out."
7. ___If I let myself have some of these feelings, I fear I will lose control.
8. ___Others understand and accept my feelings.
9. ___You can't allow yourself to have certain kinds of feelings—like feelings about sex or violence.
10. ___My feelings don't make sense to me.
11. ___If other people changed, I would feel a lot better.
12. ___I think that there are feelings that I have that I am not really aware of.
13. ___I sometimes fear that if I allowed myself to have a strong feeling, it would not go away.
14. ___I feel ashamed of my feelings.
15. ___Things that bother other people don't bother me.
16. ___No one really cares about my feelings.
17. ___It is important for me to be reasonable and practical rather than sensitive and open to my feelings.
18. ___I can't stand it when I have contradictory feelings—like liking and disliking the same person.
19. ___I am much more sensitive than other people.
20. ___I try to get rid of an unpleasant feeling immediately.
21. ___When I feel down, I try to think of the more important things in life—what I *value*.
22. ___When I feel down or sad, I question my values.
23. ___I feel that I can express my feelings openly.
24. ___I often say to myself, "What's wrong with me?"
25. ___I think of myself as a shallow person.

(continued)

26. ___I want people to believe that I am different from the way I truly feel.
27. ___I worry that I won't be able to control my feelings.
28. ___You have to guard against having certain feelings.
29. ___Strong feelings only last a short period of time.
30. ___You can't rely on your feelings to tell you what is good for you.
31. ___I shouldn't have some of the feelings that I have.
32. ___I often feel "numb" emotionally—like I have no feelings.
33. ___I think that my feelings are strange or weird.
34. ___Other people cause me to have unpleasant feelings.
35. ___When I have conflicting feelings about someone, I get upset or confused.
36. ___When I have a feeling that bothers me I try to think of something else to think about or to do.
37. ___When I feel down, I sit by myself and think a lot about how bad I feel.
38. ___I like being absolutely definite about the way I feel about *someone else.*
39. ___Everyone has feelings like mine.
40. ___I accept my feelings.
41. ___I think that I have the same feelings that other people have.
42. ___There are higher values that I aspire to.
43. ___I think that my feelings now have *nothing* to do with how I was brought up.
44. ___I worry that if I have certain feelings I might go crazy.
45. ___My feelings seem to come out of nowhere.
46. ___I think it is important to be rational and logical in almost everything.
47. ___I like being absolutely definite about the way I feel about *myself.*
48. ___I focus a lot on my feelings or my physical sensations.
49. ___I don't want anyone to know about some of my feelings.
50. ___I don't want to admit to having certain feelings—but I know that I have them.

---

behavioral activation, to examine the costs and benefits of certain thoughts and behaviors, to evaluate the evidence and logic of negative beliefs, and to experiment with new ways of thinking and behaving (Beck, Rush, Shaw, & Emery, 1979; Leahy, 1997; Persons, Davidson, & Tompkins, 2001). An underlying assumption is that the patient will be able or motivated to distance him- or herself from unpleasant emotions in a manner sufficient to identify and modify dysfunctional thoughts. However, it is seldom the thoughts alone that are problematic—the patient is concerned about his or her emotions or feelings. The emotional schema model allows us to examine the patient's "theory of emotions," much as cognitive models of the mind (or metacognitive models) allow us to examine the patient's theories about intrusive thoughts, recurring traumatic imagery, the nature of worry, or the

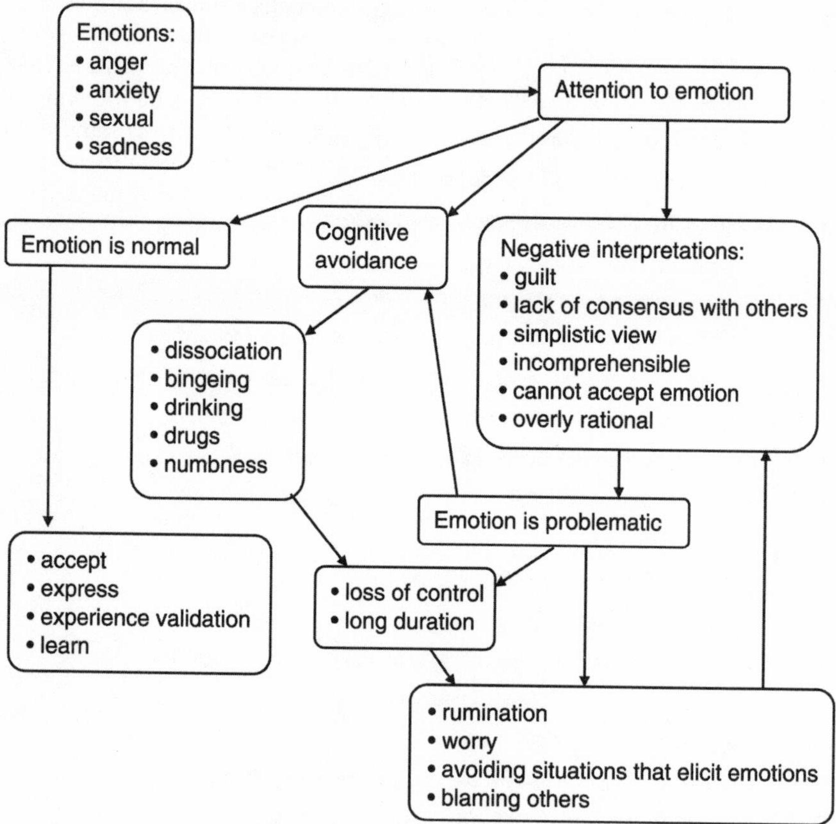

FIGURE 5.2. Metacognitive schematic of emotions.

significance of panic symptoms (Resick, 2001; Wells, 2002; Wells, Clark, & Ahmad, 1998).

Individual "theories" of emotion may contribute to the exacerbation of a negative emotion. The individual who believes that his emotional experience of depression is incomprehensible ("My depression makes no sense" or "I shouldn't be depressed") will believe that he is helpless in coping. Depressive thoughts may also elicit a sense of shame ("I will look like a loser to him") or guilt ("I am selfish—that's why I am depressed"), making it difficult to enter the therapeutic exchange. Theories of emotion based on "opening a can of worms"—such that awareness, acceptance, and expression are viewed as opening the floodgates of hell—will interfere with any attempts to elicit thoughts and feelings that are significant. For example, a depressed woman suffering from PTSD related to sexual victimization during her childhood believed that talking about her feelings would retraumatize her and that disclosure of these feelings would lead the therapist to devalue her. An alternative theory of emotions is that "other people cause me to have my feelings." For example, the husband who believes that all of his anger is caused by his wife's behavior will have little motivation for individual treatment and will be unlikely to comply with communication exercises in couples therapy. Finally, an anorectic woman who believes that her emotions are a sign of weakness and "messiness" and who views food restriction as exemplifying perfection will have little motivation to modify her starvation diet.

Emotional Socialization

A significant component of socialization is the acquisition of beliefs and skills regarding one's emotions. Emotional socialization includes the importance of mirroring or reflection of the emotional experience by the parent—for example, the "reflective gaze," labeling of feelings, and empathic response (Kohut, 1977). Another component is the predictability that the parent will respond to emotional distress, especially during and after brief periods of separation (Ainsworth, Blehar, Waters, & Wall, 1978; Bowlby, 1968; Guidano & Liotti, 1983). Eisenberg (Eisenberg & Fabes, 1994; Eisenberg, Fabes, & Murphy, 1996) and Gottman, Katz, and Hooven (1996); Katz, Gottman, and Hooven (1996) have identified several styles of emotional interaction between parent and child and within married couples. For example, Gottman et al. (1996) identify five meta-emotion philosophies: emotion coaching, high acceptance/low coaching, dismissing, disapproving, and dysregulation (Kennedy-Moore & Watson, 1999) . Emotion coaching assists the child in talking about emotions, labeling feelings, identifying rules for appropriate display of feelings, and elaborating problem-solving strategies. High acceptance/low coaching allows the child expression of emotion but does little to help identify, elaborate, or problem solve. In contrast, the dismissive strategy denies the significance of the child's emotions. Disapproving style entails criticism and overcontrol of the child's feelings, while the dysregulated parents are overwhelmed by their own emotions and reject the child's emotions. Gottman et al. (1996) find that emotional coaching assists the child in self-soothing of emotions.

Moreover, parents may assist or inhibit the child in developing appropriate display rules for emotions, knowledge of conflicting or ambivalent emotions, and regulation of emotion (Denham & Grout, 1993; Harter, 1999). Innate temperament (e.g., predisposal toward inhibition or activation of arousal) may also determine how emotional socialization occurs (Kagan, 1992). The child with a high level of arousal or activation may elicit more controlling and critical behavior in parents, contributing to the child's belief that his emotions are not acceptable to others. Finally, emotional socialization is not limited to childhood or adolescence. Certainly the current relationships in the patient's life also determine the patient's conceptualization and strategies about emotions. The patient with an alcoholic and paranoid husband may conclude that her emotions do not make sense to others, partly because her husband views her emotions as a personal attack on him.

In evaluating current roadblocks in therapy, it is often helpful to examine how the individual's earlier and current social environment has responded to his or her emotional expression. The clinician can inquire directly, "When you were a child, how did your parents respond to your feelings? Did they ask you about your feelings, criticize you, make you feel that your emotions were not important, or act like they were overwhelmed with how you felt? When you felt like you needed to be soothed or cared for, did you hesitate in approaching your parents? What thoughts did you have about approaching them? Did you find that your parents wanted you to comfort them or soothe them or understand them because they were going through a difficult time?" Similar questions can be asked about the current social environment—for example, how partners, friends, or family members respond to emotions.

Fear of Self-Disclosure

The therapeutic relationship is often a unique experience for patients with problematic emotional schemas—a relationship in which their emotions are the main focus in an accepting and supportive environment. However, it is also often intimidating, disappointing, and confusing. The intimidation is a consequence of the belief that one will be exposed, humiliated, misled, and judged: "If I tell you what I really feel, you will think I am a disgusting person." Disappointment may result from the patient's experience that her feelings are not understood, validated, or modified in the appropriate manner: "You don't really care about how I feel—all you want to do is change the way I think to go along with your beliefs." And self-disclosure may also be confusing, as the patient may believe that therapy is entirely based on self-expression but that cognitive-behavioral therapy involves testing and modifying beliefs and engaging in behavioral exposure: "I thought I could come here and just talk about my feelings."

A woman who presented with dysthymia, binge eating, and marital conflict expressed discomfort talking about her needs in therapy. When she began talking about her needs (for intimacy, affection, and support from her husband), she dissociated or changed the subject to something trivial. Her initial response to her needs was low awareness of her feelings, often numbed through bingeing or dissociation. When the therapist inquired as to her current state of mind prior to her dissociation, she indicated that, "It's selfish for me to be in therapy. I am just complaining." Further inquiry led to her disclosure that she felt ashamed and guilty for needing affection and understanding, that her mother and father used to tell her that she was selfish when she would talk about what she wanted, that no one else had these desperate needs like she did, that her needs were incomprehensible and no one would ever understand them. Consequently, she believed that there was no sense in expressing them. She further believed that once she allowed herself to feel any frustration with her relationship, she would lose control, decompensate, and never emerge from her depression and anxiety.

In this case, an emotional-schema case conceptualization was helpful to her. Part of this conceptualization was an examination of her early childhood environment and her current invalidating environment. Her mother had been a highly depressed and anxious individual, married to a distant husband who showed little affection. When the patient approached her mother with needs for affection and closeness, the mother distanced herself by claiming that she was selfish and did not appreciate how difficult the mother's life was. The mother then turned to the patient, who was 7 years old at the time, for "reverse parenting." When the mother was taken to the hospital for a 2-month stay during a major depressive episode, the patient attributed the loss to her own failure to take care of her mother and her belief that her needs were a burden. This pattern of self-sacrifice in relationships was currently reinforced in her life as an adult in her self-sacrificing behavior with her husband (whose alcohol abuse diminished his capacity to perform sexually) and her excessive work absorption.

The case conceptualization assisted her in recognizing that one of her major "therapy-interfering behaviors" (see Foertsch, Manning, & Dimeff, Chapter 12, this volume; Linehan, 1993a) was her denial of needs and her desire to terminate treatment. It was helpful to link her current dissociation and trivialization of her needs to her family-of-origin experiences with a mother who was overwhelmed and who, therefore, provided a "disorganized attachment system." She was able to recognize that experience, awareness, and expression of needs in her family of origin and also in her marriage was almost always disappointing, if not also punitive. Her style of coping with her own needs had been to refocus onto the needs of others and hope that they would not leave her.

Fear of Accessing and Describing Feelings

Although most patients pursue therapy because of their desire to modify emotions, negative emotional schemas may impede change. For example, the individual with the beliefs that strong negative emotions are shameful, not shared by others, or incomprehensible will have difficulty describing certain emotions to the therapist. A woman felt ashamed of describing her need that the therapist understand her angry feelings toward her daughter. Although her relationship with her daughter was difficult—due to problems attributable to both of them—she believed that the therapist would think less of her if she described these feelings, and she believed that her feelings did not make sense because her daughter would spend time with her. Her belief was that, once she began describing her feelings, it would become obvious that she was an undesirable person, that the therapist would reject her, and that this rejection would add to her belief that her feelings made no sense.

A successful business executive who feared crying began to describe the death of his daughter. As he struggled to hold back his emotion, the therapist asked him what he thought would happen if he let himself "go." He responded, "I'll just lose it. I won't stop." As he began to cry and talk about his feelings, his tension decreased, and he began to realize that his feelings made sense, that they were not shameful, and that they were self-limiting. Interestingly, this then led to a discussion of his purging through vomiting whenever he was angry or upset with his wife. His belief was that he had to get rid of his feelings in private rather than tell his wife that he felt hurt. It was further revealed that, as a child, he was often afraid of being physically assaulted by other adolescents—an earlier experience of being assaulted had led to panic attacks, humiliation by his father and brother for being frightened, and induced vomiting to modulate his anxiety.

THERAPEUTIC RELATIONSHIP

Emotional schemas are often difficult for therapists who are highly invested in being rational, technique oriented, "quick fix," or task oriented. Unfortunately, it may be that cognitive-behavioral therapy often appeals to therapists who find emotions and intensity unappealing. Emphasis on "rational disputation" or "challenging the patient's irrational shoulds" will often backfire with patients with problematic emotional schemas (Leahy, 2001).

Elicitation of emotion, empathy, and validation are key during the earliest phases of treatment (Greenberg, 2002b; Leahy, 2001; Safran, 1998). Indeed, it may be useful to tell the patient directly, "The most important thing in therapy will be your emotions—how you feel. It is important for you to know that you feel understood here, that your emotions have a safe place to be expressed, and that your emotions may contain information about you that is quite valuable." Greenberg's "emotional focused" approach has considerable value in the elicitation of emotions through experiential techniques, including imagery, memories, and mood induction. It can assist patients in recognizing that their emotions contain valuable information about their needs and cognitive schemata, rather than being an impediment to effective treatment.

Moreover, the emotional-schema approach presented here recognizes the essential importance of the therapeutic alliance (Safran, 1998; Stevens, Muran, & Safran, Chapter 14, this volume). Therapeutic ruptures often occur when emotional schemas are activated. For example, the patient's discussion of painful memories of traumatic experience may activate beliefs that the therapist is inducing even more emotional distress or that the therapist may not appreciate how difficult this recollection may be. Eliciting emotions may be important for modifying the thoughts and emotions involved but may also activate beliefs about the reliability, empathy, and protective qualities of the therapist.

The therapist's personal schemas may also interfere with emotional expression and emotional processing. I have identified a number of personal schemas held by therapists, including demanding-standards schemas, special/unique person schemas, rejection-sensitive schemas, abandonment, autonomy, and control schemas, and others (Leahy, 2001). The therapist who is highly committed to accomplishing "his tasks" in "his way" (demanding-standards and goal-inhibition/striving schemas) may find emotional expression in patients to be a frustrating, if not useless, process. This evaluation may be communicated inadvertently to the patient, with the impact experienced as, "He thinks I'm an emotional mess and a burden. I should keep my true feelings to myself." The therapist with personal schemas related to abandonment and rejection sensitivity may be reluctant to question the patient's negative beliefs associated with powerful emotions such as anger, lest the patient reject the therapist and leave. Consequently, the patient may experience this reluctance as indicative of the following: "My emotions are frightening to other people. I can intimidate people with my feelings. I can make them feel guilty."

Difficulties with Exposure

Cognitive-behavioral therapy involves a considerable degree of direct behavioral exposure as a method to test and evaluate negative thoughts. For example, the patient's belief that "women find me unattractive" may be tested by having the patient approach a number of women, begin conversations, and see what happens. Emotional schemas may affect how the patient experiences the suggestion to engage in this "risky" exposure. Some patients believe that the optimistic, action-oriented approach in cognitive-behavioral therapy suggests that the therapist will not understand how difficult this task is. Indeed, some patients who read popular self-help books believe that they are even more pathological, as others seem to find these tasks so easy. Shame, guilt, and beliefs that others do not share the same difficulties or feelings contribute to the patient's belief that if these self-doubts are expressed, then the therapist will not only fail to validate the feelings but also that the patient will be humiliated. Others fear that exposure to anxiety-provoking situations will result in loss of control, humiliation, and prolonged duration of negative feelings. A patient with obsessive–compulsive disorder feared that "contaminating" himself with dirt would make his anxiety escalate and never subside. In-session exposure, facilitated by the therapist's modeling of the contamination, helped the patient realize that the escalation of anxiety was temporary.

One patient believed that rumination was preparatory work for behavioral exposure—a process that prolonged her anticipatory anxiety prior to air travel. Fear of activating the imagery of air flight contributed to her belief that all anxiety and discomfort needed to be quelled, further contributing to her avoidance. Examining these beliefs about the dangers of exposure reduced her noncompliance with homework exposure by making it her goal to increase exposure enough to activate the fear so that she could learn that the fear decreases. Learning that fears that rise will also fall—and that this is the goal of exposure—allowed her to reframe anxiety during flight as an opportunity to learn that fears decrease with practice.

INTERVENTIONS AND STRATEGIES

In evaluating the emotional schemas, I have found that the LESS is a helpful interview tool for patients. After the patient has filled out the LESS, we can mutually examine beliefs about various emotional dimensions. I have listed below the emotional schemas that have proven to be associated with anxiety (and depression) and questions and interventions that can be utilized to modify the patient's emotional schema.

Comprehensibility

"Do the emotions make sense to you? What could be some good reasons why you are sad, anxious, angry, and so forth? What are you thinking (what images do you have) when you are sad? What situations trigger these feelings? If someone else experienced this, what kinds of different feelings could they have? If you think your feelings don't make sense right now, what does this make you think? Are you afraid that you are going crazy, losing control? Are there things that happened to you as a kid that might account for why you feel this way?"

Simplistic View of Emotions

"Do you think that having mixed feelings is normal or abnormal? What does it mean to have mixed feelings about someone? Aren't people complicated—so you could have different, even conflicting, feelings? What is the disadvantage of demanding that you have only one feeling?"

Guilt

"What are the reasons that you think your emotions are not legitimate? Why shouldn't you have the feelings that you have? Is it possible that others could have the same feelings in this situation? Can you see that having a feeling (such as anger) is not the same as acting on it (for example, being hostile)? Why are certain emotions good and others bad? If someone else had this feeling, would you think less of him? How do you know if an emotion is bad? What if you looked at feelings and emotions as experiences that tell you that something is bothering you—like a caution sign, a stop sign, and a flashing red light? How is anyone harmed by your emotions?"

Controllability

"Do you think that you have to control your feelings and get rid of the 'negative' feelings? What do you think would happen if you couldn't get rid of that feeling entirely? Is it possible that trying to get rid of a feeling completely makes that feeling too important to you? Are you afraid that having a strong feeling is a sign of something worse? Going crazy? Losing complete control? Isn't there a difference between controlling your actions and controlling your feelings?"

Consensus

"Exactly what feelings do you have that you think other people don't have? If someone else had these feelings, what would you think of them? Why do you think very emotional plays or movies or emotional novels or stories appeal to people? Do you think that people like to find out that other people have the same feelings? Is it normal to be upset, have fantasies, and so forth? If you are ashamed of your feelings and don't tell people, do you think that this keeps you from finding out that others have the same feelings?"

Rumination

"What are the advantages and disadvantages of focusing on how bad you feel? Do you think that if you keep thinking about it you will come up with a solution? Does your rumination (worry) make you worry that you can't control your worries? Try setting aside 30 minutes each day when you will intensely worry and set aside your worries until that time. Rephrase your worries into behaviors that you can carry out, problems that you can solve.

Distract yourself by taking action or calling a friend and talking about something other than your worries. Is there some 'truth' or 'reality' that you just refuse to accept?"

Acceptance of Feelings

"What will happen if you allow yourself to accept an emotion? Will you act on it (feeling–action fusion)? Do you fear that if you accept an emotion it won't go away? Or do you think that not accepting your emotions will motivate you to change? What are the negative consequences of inhibiting a feeling—excessive use of attention and energy? Rebound effect? Does the emotion conflict with a belief about good–bad feelings? If you deny that something bothers you, how could you fix the problem? Would you be willing to allow yourself to have an emotion and observe it rather than judge it or try to change it?"

CASE EXAMPLE

The patient ("Susan") was a divorced woman who sought treatment for anxiety, depression, low self-esteem, and recurring alcohol abuse. She had past treatment with fluoxetine, which she had discontinued a week before the intake, as she believed it was not helpful. Her Beck Depression Inventory (BDI) and Beck Anxiety Inventory (BAI) scores were 24 and 26, respectively, and she was abusing alcohol on a daily basis. Her worries consisted of the following: "I will get fired," "I'll always be alone," "My daughter is angry with me," "I'll run out of money and end up destitute," "My boss is angry with me," and "I'll get sick and have no one who will take care of me."

She had the following elevated scores on the LESS: lack of acceptance, guilt, low validation, simplistic thinking, loss of control, and rumination. Both parents had a history of depression; her father was bipolar, alcoholic and suicidal; both parents "didn't deal with emotions"; father would "hit us or stop talking" and dismiss her when she was upset; and mother was avoidant of any emotions: "The lesson I learned was that I wasn't supposed to have emotions." This experience of emotional socialization included dismissing, disapproving, and dysregulation, further contributing to her negative emotional schemas (Gottman, 1996a, 1996b). She described an intermittent history of bingeing, food restriction, and alcohol abuse. She indicated that she had always been afraid of showing anger when growing up, claiming that she feared being hit by her father. She worried about a variety of things and, when she began feeling anxious when alone, she would either drink or binge in order to get rid of her negative feelings.

Case Formulation

Susan was initially diagnosed with major depressive disorder, generalized anxiety disorder, and alcohol abuse. Her core cognitive schemas focused on her defectiveness as a person, and her interpersonal schemas suggested that people would evaluate her and reject her. Her emotional schemas were that her emotions were an indication of her defectiveness and that she had to get rid of them immediately by bingeing or drinking lest they consume her and land her in a mental hospital (like her father). Because she believed that her feelings were uniquely defective, she feared letting others know, further adding to her belief that she was inferior and that others would reject her. She believed that, if she cried, the therapist would think she was weak and that she would lose total control and decompensate. Her automatic thoughts included the following: "You think I'm a loser" (mind reading); "I'll end up destitute" (catastrophic fortune telling); "I'm a failure" (labeling); "I've ruined my whole life" (all-or-nothing thinking); and "Nothing I do has worked out" (discounting positives). Her beliefs about her worries (about money, work, and loneliness) were: "If I think about this, maybe I'll find a solution," "I'll be prepared," "I won't be disappointed (if I'm pessimistic)," and "The worry just happens to me. I have no control."

A case formulation based on emotional schemas is shown in Figure 5.3. Susan had initially low self-awareness of her emotions. She felt ashamed and guilty and believed that others did not share these feelings, that her emotions made no sense, and that she should have only one feeling—not conflicting feelings. She ruminated about her problems, believing that she had little control and that her feelings would last a long time. In addition, she found it difficult to express these feelings and expected little validation from others. Her pathological coping methods included isolation, alcohol abuse, bingeing, and nonassertiveness on her job or with family and friends.

Course of Treatment

The intake proved to be the initial intervention. Susan's responses on the LESS provided an opportunity to examine how she conceptualized and responded to her anxiety and depression. Her lack of acceptance, guilt, expectation of low validation, simplistic thinking, loss of control, and rumination on her emotions all became a focus of inquiry. I asked her, "What emotions can't you accept?" She responded, "My empty feelings. My anxiety and anger." Her beliefs were: "If I allowed myself to accept it, it will never go away"; "I've got to get rid of these feelings immediately"; and "I shouldn't be upset. I have a good life." This resulted in her belief that her feelings were incomprehensible—"Why do I feel so bad?"—further leading

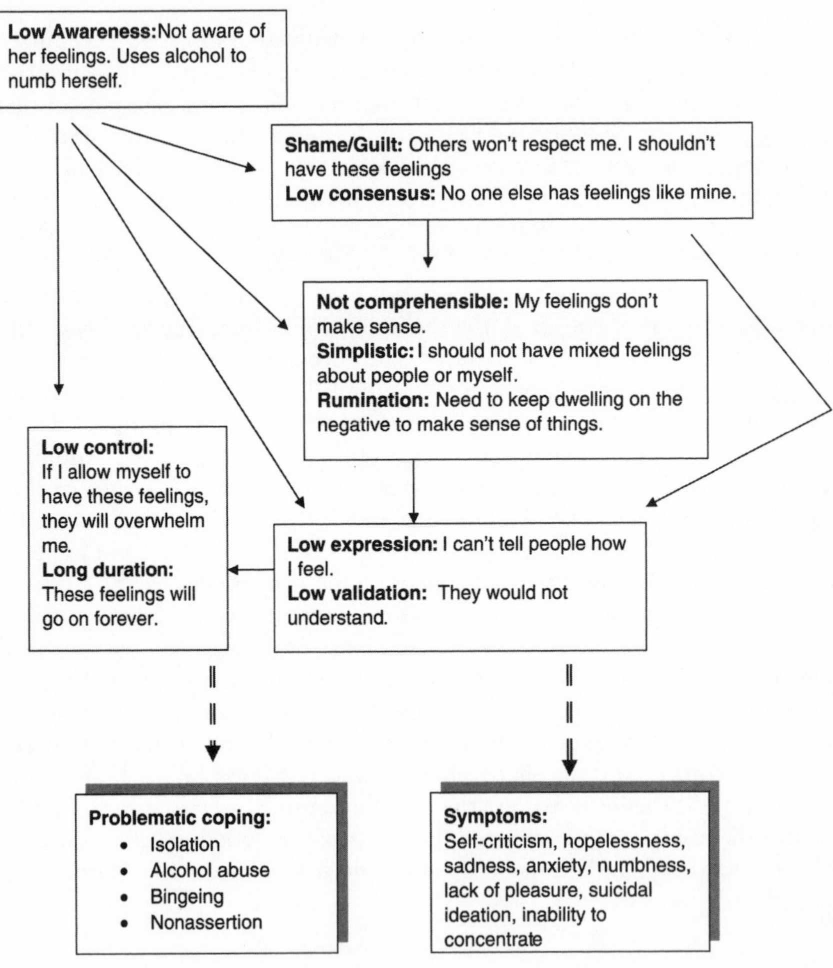

FIGURE 5.3. Emotional schemas case conceptualization.

her to believe that she had no control over her emotions except through drinking. Believing that her emotions were incomprehensible made her feel helpless about changing them. She believed that "if I don't drink, I'll just feel worse and worse." Her simplistic belief was that she should feel either happy or sad but never have mixed feelings about herself or anyone else: "Things should be clear." When alone, she would ponder how bad she felt, asking rhetorical questions: "Why is this happening to me?" We examined her belief that allowing herself to feel strong emotions would lead to decompensation:

THERAPIST: I noticed that you cried in the meeting today. What did you think I would feel about that?

SUSAN: I was afraid you'd think I was pathetic.

THERAPIST: What do you think now?

SUSAN: I feel you understand me. Maybe you're a nice person.

THERAPIST: But you also thought that if you let your feelings happen that you'd lose control and fall apart.

SUSAN: Yes. That didn't happen.

THERAPIST: And when you are home alone you think, "I have to get rid of this feeling or it will overwhelm me." What if you didn't try to deaden the feeling with alcohol? Have you ever not decided to drink?

SUSAN: Yes. I usually do something else. Read a book, watch TV. I used to exercise more.

THERAPIST: So there are different strategies to dealing with your feelings. Drinking is one of them. Let's examine the costs and benefits of these different ways of dealing with your emotions.

In order to make Susan's feelings comprehensible to her, we examined the genetic link in her family for psychiatric illness (parents both depressed, aunt was schizophrenic, grandmother was depressed). A biological vulnerability model, along with early family environment of criticism, withdrawal, and dismissal of emotions, was offered as an explanation of her current vulnerability. This proved helpful in allowing her to "make sense" of her feelings. A cognitive model helped her understand that, because she assumed she was defective, she would filter information to support that view and she would predict rejection, abandonment, and failure.

These interventions helped Susan reduce her guilt. Furthermore, her view that she should have only positive feelings toward her daughter was examined in terms of costs and benefits (the costs being that it was unrealistic, as her daughter was a complicated person). Double-standard technique was used ("If you had a friend who had some conflicts with her daughter and told you, 'There are things about her I like and things I don't like,' what would you think?"). This was helpful in reducing her simplistic view of emotions and people. Validation of her feeling sad because she missed her daughter helped reduce her guilt and increase her understanding of her emotions.

Because Susan used alcohol to neutralize her anxiety, the reduction of alcohol consumption was a key component in self-help outside of sessions. As long as she was using alcohol, she would not have access to her automatic thoughts and the use of rational responses. Her emotional schemas were central here: her simplistic beliefs about having only positive or only negative feelings, her beliefs that negative feelings would increase and overwhelm her, her guilt and lack of comprehension of her feelings, and her belief that rumination was the only alternative to drinking. Her first homework assignments included the following:

- Labeling her feelings: sad, anxious, anger, empty, curious, challenged, and so forth.
- Accepting feelings as part of being human ("I have to be strong" vs. "I should accept being human").
- Accepting ambivalence: "It's not realistic to expect to have only positive or negative feelings toward someone—including yourself. Having mixed feelings is a sign of being a complex person."
- Normalizing feelings: "It's normal to feel lonely sometimes. It's normal to miss my family."
- Finding control: "Set aside twenty minutes per day to worry." "When you feel down, distract yourself by taking a walk, making some plans, reading a book, exercising, or calling a friend."
- Reducing guilt: "You didn't decide on Tuesday afternoon at 3:15 to make yourself anxious and depressed. You didn't choose to have a problem. There are a lot of genetic factors, early childhood factors, that make you more vulnerable." "Being sad is not malicious."
- Reducing rumination: Utilize all the interventions under "finding control" and ask yourself, "What concrete things can I do that are pleasurable or meaningful now or in the next few days?"

In order to challenge Susan's worry, we utilized a number of metacognitive interventions:

- Distinguish between *productive* and *unproductive* worry: "Productive worry leads to concrete steps toward solving a problem. Unproductive worry is about what-ifs you can't really control."
- Distinguish worry from control: "Worry does not give you more control. If you imagine all the bad things happening, you may feel more out of control."
- Emotional reasoning: "Using your anxious feelings is not a good guide to what the real world is like. Just because you feel anxious doesn't mean bad things will happen."
- Illusory correlation: "You may believe that the reason terrible things haven't happened is that you worried about them. But it may be that terrible things generally don't happen anyway." "Aren't there some things that haven't happened that you didn't worry about?"

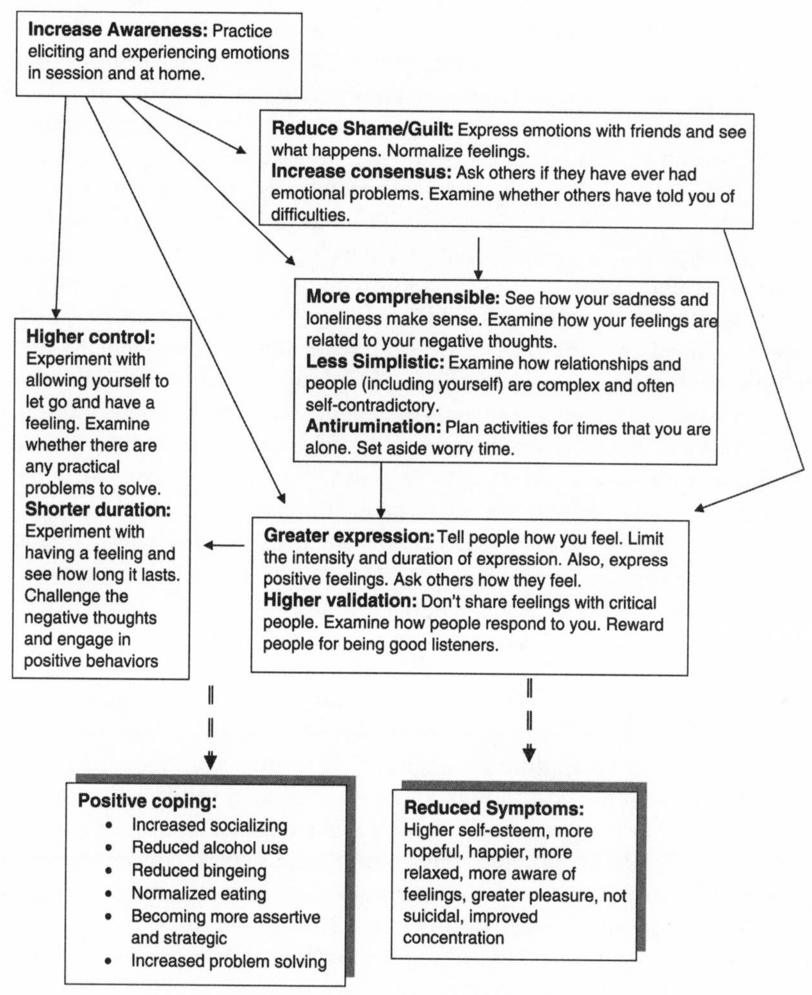

Increase Awareness: Practice eliciting and experiencing emotions in session and at home.
Reduce Shame/Guilt: Express emotions with friends and see what happens. Normalize feelings.
Increase consensus: Ask others if they have ever had emotional problems. Examine whether others have told you of difficulties.
More comprehensible: See how your sadness and loneliness make sense. Examine how your feelings are related to your negative thoughts.
Less Simplistic: Examine how relationships and people (including yourself) are complex and often self-contradictory.
Antirumination: Plan activities for times that you are alone. Set aside worry time.
Higher control: Experiment with allowing yourself to let go and have a feeling. Examine whether there are any practical problems to solve.
Shorter duration: Experiment with having a feeling and see how long it lasts. Challenge the negative thoughts and engage in positive behaviors
Greater expression: Tell people how you feel. Limit the intensity and duration of expression. Also, express positive feelings. Ask others how they feel.
Higher validation: Don't share feelings with critical people. Examine how people respond to you. Reward people for being good listeners.
Positive coping:
• Increased socializing
• Reduced alcohol use
• Reduced bingeing
• Normalized eating
• Becoming more assertive and strategic
• Increased problem solving
Reduced Symptoms:
Higher self-esteem, more hopeful, happier, more relaxed, more aware of feelings, greater pleasure, not suicidal, improved concentration

FIGURE 5.4. Emotional schemas case conceptualization: Interventions.

A schematic summary of these interventions is provided in Figure 5.4. The interventions began with the initial interview, utilizing the LESS as a method to elicit and identify Susan's negative emotional schemas (see Figure 5.3). This allowed her to increase her awareness of her emotions and her negative emotional schemas and coping. Her shame and guilt were reduced by normalizing her emotions, by encouraging her to share her feelings with others, and by utilizing the double-standard technique in role plays. As she inquired about others' problems, she increased her sense that she was not alone with these feelings. Her feelings became more comprehensible by virtue of recognizing and valuing the importance of relationships (from which she was isolating herself), by relating her feelings to her negative automatic thoughts, and by linking her predisposition to depression to her familial environment and genetic risk. Her simplistic view of herself and others was modified by normalizing mixed feelings and by recognizing that all of the "evidence" about self and other painted a more complicated picture. Reducing rumination and isolation was accomplished by activity scheduling, planning ahead, developing longer term plans, and normalizing uncertainty ("You can't know things for certain, but that does not mean that the outcome is bad"). She was able to experience higher sense of control and recognize that negative feelings could change by doing the following: practicing brief periods of "letting go" of feelings in session, observing and not judging feelings, challenging negative thoughts and planning positive activities to examine how she can modify her feelings, and developing a problem-solving strategy to deal with obtaining new work and a financial plan. More adaptive expression of feelings was encouraged by limiting the duration of expression and by focusing on problem solving and reporting positives as well as negatives. Finally, she was able to be more discerning about the people with whom she shared feelings and practiced rewarding people for being supportive.

Outcome and Prognosis

The combination of traditional cognitive therapy techniques (identifying assumptions or automatic thoughts and testing them utilizing cost–benefit analysis and examining evidence) with a metacognitive approach using the work of Wells (in press) and the emotional schemas conceptualization proved to be very helpful to this patient. Within 3 weeks, she had reduced alcohol use to twice per week (at lower levels), and within 4 weeks, she had discontinued use entirely. After nine sessions, her BDI score was reduced to 10 and her BAI to 9. She reported, after two sessions, sharing some of her difficulties with a friend, which led her to understand that other people had problems and that they could understand and validate her feelings. She became more appropriately assertive at work, rather than resentfully submitting to her boss and later withdrawing by staying home. This then led to some mutual problem solving with her supervisor that improved her status and security at work.

The prognosis for this patient is relatively good, but maintenance therapy or periodic booster sessions would be desirable. Her core schema of being defective and her belief that her emotions are shameful, incomprehensible, and uncontrollable have been effectively challenged. However, she has been reminded that she is vulnerable to emotional variation and that the desire to drink will likely reoccur. Rather than suggesting to her that we had achieved a "perfect cure," I decided to conceptualize our work as progress in self-acceptance and self-discovery.

REFERENCES

Ainsworth, M. S., Blehar, M. C., Waters, E., & Wall, S. (1978). *Patterns of attachment: A psychological study of the strange situation.* Hillsdale, NJ: Erlbaum.

Beck, A. T. (1996). Beyond belief: A theory of modes, personality and psychopathology. In P. Salkovskis (Ed.), *Frontiers of cognitive therapy* (pp. 1–25). New York: Guilford Press.

Beck, A. T., Rush, A. J., Shaw, B. F., & Emery, G. (1979). *Cognitive therapy of depression.* New York: Guilford Press.

Borkovec, T. D. (1994). The nature, functions, and origins of worry. In G. C. L. Davey & F. Tallis (Eds.), *Worrying: Perspectives on theory, assessment and treatment* (pp. 5–33). Chichester, UK: Wiley.

Bowlby, J. (1968). *Attachment and loss: I. Attachment.* London: Hogarth Press.

Clark, D. A. (2002). Unwanted mental intrusions in clinical disorders: An introduction. *Journal of Cognitive Psychotherapy, 16*(2), 123–126.

Clark, D. A., Beck, A. T., & Alford, B. A. (1999). *Scientific foundations of cognitive theory and therapy of depression.* New York: Wiley.

Denham, S. A., & Grout, L. (1993). Socialization of emotion: Pathway to preschoolers' emotional and social competence. *Journal of Nonverbal Behavior, 17*(3), 205–227.

Ehlers, A., & Clark, D. M. (2000). A cognitive model of posttraumatic stress disorder. *Behaviour Research and Therapy, 38,* 319–345.

Eisenberg, N., & Fabes, R. A. (1994). Mothers' reactions to children's negative emotions: Relations to children's temperament and anger behavior. *Merrill–Palmer Quarterly, 40*(1), 138–156.

Eisenberg, N., Fabes, R. A., & Murphy, B. C. (1996). Parents' reactions to children's negative emotions: Relations to children's social competence and comforting behavior. *Child Development, 67*(5), 2227–2247.

Foa, E. B., & Kozak, M. J. (1986). Emotional processing of fear: Exposure to corrective information. *Psychological Bulletin, 99,* 20–35.

Gottman, J. M., Katz, L. F., & Hooven, C. (1996). Parental meta-emotion philosophy and the emotional life of families: Theoretical models and preliminary data. *Journal of Family Psychology, 10*(3), 243–268.

Greenberg, L. S. (2002a). *Emotion-focused therapy: Coaching clients to work through their feelings.* Washington, DC: American Psychological Association.

Greenberg, L. S. (2002b). Integrating an emotion-focused approach to treatment into psychotherapy integration. *Journal of Psychotherapy Integration, 12*(2), 154–189.

Guidano, V. F., & Liotti, G. (1983). *Cognitive processes and the emotional disorders.* New York: Guilford Press.

Harter, S. (1999). *The construction of the self: A developmental perspective.* New York: Guilford Press.

Kabat-Zinn, J. (1995). *Wherever you go, there you are: Mindfulness meditation in everyday life.* New York: Hyperion.

Kagan, J. (1992). Temperamental contributions to emotion and social behavior. In M. S. Clark (Ed.), *Emotion and social behavior: Review of personality and social psychology* (Vol. 14, pp. 99–118). Thousand Oaks, CA: Sage.

Katz, L. F., Gottman, J. M., & Hooven, C. (1996). Meta-emotion philosophy and family functioning: Reply to Cowan (1996) and Eisenberg (1996). *Journal of Family Psychology, 10*(3), 284–291.

Kennedy-Moore, E., & Watson, J. C. (1999). *Expressing emotions: Myths, realities and therapeutic strategies.* New York: Guilford Press.

Kohut, H. (1977). *The restoration of the self.* New York: International Universities Press.

Leahy, R. L. (1997). *Practicing cognitive therapy: A guide to interventions.* Northvale, NJ: Aronson.

Leahy, R. L. (2001). *Overcoming resistance in cognitive therapy.* New York: Guilford Press.

Leahy, R. L. (2002). A model of emotional schemas. *Cognitive and Behavioral Practice, 9*(3), 177–190.

Linehan, M. M. (1993a). *Cognitive-behavioral treatment of borderline personality disorder.* New York: Guilford Press.

Linehan, M. M. (1993b). *Skills training manual for treating borderline personality disorder.* New York: Guilford Press.

Mennin, D. S., Turk, C. L., Heimberg, R. G., & Carmin, C. N. (in press). Focusing on the regulation of emotion: A new direction for conceptualizing and treating generalized anxiety disorder. In M. A. Reinecke & D. A. Clark (Eds.), *Cognitive therapy over the lifespan: Theory, research and practice.* New York: Guilford Press.

Papageorgiou, C., & Wells, A. (1999). Process and meta-cognitive dimensions of depressive and anxious thoughts and relationships with emotional intensity. *Clinical Psychology and Psychotherapy, 6,* 156–162.

Pennebaker, J. W., Mayne, T. J., & Francis, M. E. (1997). Linguistic predictors of adaptive bereavement. *Journal of Personality and Social Psychology, 72,* 863–871.

Persons, J. B., Davidson, J., & Tompkins, M. A. (2001). *Essential components of cognitive-behavior therapy for depression.* Washington, DC: American Psychological Association.

Purdon, C., & Clark, D. A. (1993). Obsessive intrusive thoughts in nonclinical subjects: I. Content and relation with depressive, anxious and obsessional symptoms. *Behaviour Research and Therapy, 31,* 713–720.

Resick, P. A. (2001). *Stress and trauma.* Philadelphia: Psychology Press.

Riskind, J. H. (1989). The mediating mechanisms in mood and memory: A cognitive-priming formulation. *Journal of Social Behavior and Personality, 4,* 173–184.

Safran, J. D. (1998). *Widening the scope of cognitive therapy: The therapeutic relationship, emotion and the process of change.* Northvale, NJ: Aronson.

Salkovskis, P. M., & Campbell, P. (1994). Thought suppression induces intrusion in naturally occurring negative intrusive thoughts. *Behaviour Research and Therapy, 32*(1), 1–8.

Segal, Z. V., Williams, M. J. G., & Teasdale, J. D. (2002). *Mindfulness-based cognitive therapy for depression: A new approach to preventing relapse.* New York: Guilford Press.

Sookman, D., & Pinard, G. (2002). Overestimation of threat and intolerance of uncertainty in obsessive compulsive disorder. In R. O. Frost & G. Steketee (Eds.), *Cognitive approaches to obsessions and compulsions: Theory, assessment, and treatment* (pp. 63–89). Amsterdam: Pergamon/Elsevier Science.

Taylor, S. (1998). *Anxiety sensitivity: Theory, research, and treatment of the fear of anxiety.* Mahwah, NJ: Erlbaum.

Wells, A. (in press). Meta-cognitive beliefs in the maintenance of worry and generalized anxiety disorder. In R. G. Heimberg, C. L. Turk, & D. S. Mennin (Eds.), *Generalized anxiety disorder: Advances in research and practice.* New York: Guilford Press.

Wells, A., & Carter, K. (2001). Further tests of a cognitive model of generalized anxiety disorder: Metacognitions and worry in GAD, panic disorder, social phobia, depression, and nonpatients. *Behavior Therapy, 32,* 85–102.

Wells, A., Clark, D. M., & Ahmad, S. (1998). How do I look with my mind's eye: Perspective taking in social phobic imagery. *Behaviour Research and Therapy, 36,* 631–634.

6

Avoidance of Emotion as an Obstacle to Progress

Stephen J. Holland

Cognitive-behavioral therapists have traditionally targeted negative emotion for change, and cognitive-behavioral techniques have proven remarkably effective in reducing negative emotion. However, for some patients, the inability or unwillingness to tolerate negative emotion and the self-protective maneuvers they employ contribute to and maintain the very symptoms they present. This tendency to avoid negative emotion may be carried into therapy, where it can create obstacles to progress. As a result, these patients may not benefit sufficiently from standard empirically supported treatments. Special attention may need to be paid to helping these patients cope more adaptively with their emotions in order to provide full relief for their presenting problems.

MODEL OF EMOTIONAL PROCESSING

Greenberg (2002; Greenberg & Paivio, 1997; Greenberg & Safran, 1987) provides a model of emotional processing that can be usefully integrated with cognitive theory. He proposes that emotion is a form of information processing. Emotions result from parallel processing of input from a number of sources, much of which takes place outside of awareness. The sum of this processing is a felt sense that provides information to the person about the impact of a situation on him or her as an organism. This process is adaptive because it allows for the rapid integration of a large quantity of information. Emotion also serves both to facilitate communication and to motivate action.

Emotion as a form of information can be contrasted with the process of logical thought that is the traditional target of cognitive techniques. According to Greenberg and Safran (1987), such thought is the product of a single track of linear processing involving symbolic representations (i.e., words). Of course, these two forms of information processing interact. Linear symbolic thought becomes one of the inputs in the complex processing that creates emotion, which is the reason cognitive techniques are effective

This integrated model suggests that for optimal adaptation, people need to be able to use both symbolic thought and emotion as sources of information. Faulty information processing in either the symbolic or the emotional system can lead to distortions in the appraisal of situations. However, problems may also arise when a person fails to adequately consider input from either system. As Linehan (1993) suggests, wisdom (or at least adaptive functioning) lies in the integration of thought and emotion. Nonetheless, some people emphasize one form of information at the expense of the other. We have all seen patients who try to think their way through every problem and patients who act as if their emotions were the only source of truth.

It is standard practice in cognitive therapy to teach patients to improve their attention to their cognitive processing (e.g., to notice their automatic thoughts). Noting the ways patients avoid and fail to attend to emotional information has been emphasized less. To be sure, some forms of emotional avoidance have received considerable attention in the cognitive-behavioral literature. Avoidance of anxiety is recognized as one of the maintaining factors in anxiety disorders, and exposure techniques have been developed to reverse this process. However, insufficient attention has been paid to avoidance of other emotions and the contribution such avoidance makes to the development and maintenance of psychological distress. At the same time, many of the cognitive and behavioral techniques that are useful in treating patients who avoid anxiety can be adapted to help patients deal with other avoided emotions.

PROBLEMS RESULTING FROM EMOTIONAL AVOIDANCE

Avoidance of emotion can create problems in at least three ways. First, the inability to tolerate negative emotion can make it difficult to access and change maladaptive thoughts and schemas. It is standard practice in cognitive-behavioral therapy to target "hot" cognitions—that is, cognitions that are associated with strong emotion. However, if patients can't stand the heat—that is, if they have difficulty tolerating the emotion and habitually avoid it—it becomes difficult to change their maladaptive beliefs.

The second problem with avoiding negative emotion is that in doing so patients deprive themselves of the adaptive functions of emotion: information, communication, and motivation. A patient who has trouble feeling angry may be unable to recognize when she is being harmed in a situation to take action to defend herself. A patient who cannot tolerate sadness may have difficulty identifying what he values and taking steps to preserve it. Patients who habitually avoid emotion may also have difficulty establishing close personal relationships, as such relationships typically depend on the communication and sharing of emotion.

Finally, the maneuvers that patients use to avoid emotion, both overt and covert, often have significant negative consequences. Active behaviors such as compulsive rituals, substance abuse, or excessive devotion to work will typically result in increased chaos and suffering. Passive avoidance of situations that put patients at risk for negative emotion—for example, intimate relationships or work challenges—can lead to restricted lives and reduced reinforcements.

Sometimes patients' maneuvers to avoid emotions involve distorted cognitions rather than overt behaviors. For example, a patient with social anxiety became very anxious when she entered her first romantic relationship. Before each date she found herself thinking that the man she was seeing was ugly. Once she was on the date and it was going well, she found the man very attractive. We came to understand that thinking her boyfriend was ugly served to protect her from her feelings of anxiety.

While standard cognitive theory emphasizes faulty information processing and maladaptive schemas as the primary source of cognitive distortions, a focus on emotional avoidance suggests that some distortions may serve to protect from negative emotion. Like all cognitive distortions, distortions that are motivated by emotional avoidance can have negative consequences for both mood and behavior. (In the example above, the patient had previously dismissed as unworthy and thereby avoided all potential romantic partners.)

IMPLICATIONS FOR THERAPY

Adopting the perspective that emotion is an important form of information processing has both practical and theoretical implications. On the level of theory, it suggests that our models of the development and maintenance of specific disorders may need to include more attention to problems in emotional processing. For example, many patients with panic disorder make catastrophic interpretations of their physical sensations in part because they fail to consider the more benign and accurate attribution that they are experiencing some emotion. Similarly, the intrusive thoughts and images experienced by patients with obsessive–compulsive disorder may, at least in some cases, represent a form of information from the emotional processing system that, rather than being valued as input, is regarded as threatening. Some depressed patients continue their relentless self-criticism, as painful as it is, in part because it may feel less upsetting than focusing on fears of loss in relationships or failure in work or academic endeavors.

On a practical level this perspective implies that clinicians need to (1) assess how patients cope with emotion and be alert for signs of emotional avoidance and (2) help patients identify, express, and cope with negative emotion when it is adaptive to do so. There are a number of techniques that can be useful in this process.

INTERVENTIONS

Orienting the Patient

The first step in helping patients deal more adaptively with emotion is to identify emotional avoidance and to bring such behavior to the patient's attention. This may be relatively easy when both the emotion and the avoidance maneuver occur in session. For example, a patient may begin to tear up and then attempt to hide the tears or change the subject. In such cases, the therapist may simply note the patient's behavior and ask what the patient was experiencing and why he or she tried to interrupt the emotional expression.

Often, however, the original emotion and/or the avoidance function of the patient's behavior may need to be inferred. For example, a patient may relate an event that has clear emotional implications without any sign of feeling. At a further remove, the patient may avoid certain topics altogether. Or the patient may behave in ways that are maladaptive (e.g., self-mutilation or substance abuse) and that appear to function to help avoid emotion. In such cases, the therapist will need to note the missing emotion, missing information, or maladaptive behavior and invite the patient to be curious about the lapse and whether there are any emotions that are being avoided.

Standard cognitive and behavioral techniques often provide good opportunities for observing emotional avoidance. For example, a patient may become visibly upset when asked to list evidence for a negative thought and then be unable to think of any further evidence. Often, when asked what has occurred, the patient will indicate that he or she was beginning to feel too upset and had to stop thinking about the subject. Similarly, patients may avoid a homework assignment because they fear it will be too emotionally overwhelming.

Functional Analysis

Once the patient's attention has been drawn to his or her avoidance of emotion, the next step is to begin a collaborative process of trying to identify the triggers, functions, and consequences of such avoidance. Among the factors to be considered should be (1) which emotion(s) the patient attempts to avoid; (2) under what circumstances; and (3) whether the avoidance is automatic or under conscious control. The patient's beliefs about emotion should also be explored. Typical maladaptive beliefs include:

- "To show emotions is weak."
- "If I allow myself to experience negative emotion it will be unbearable."
- "I won't be able to stop feeling bad."
- "I will be unable to control my actions."
- "I will go crazy."
- "The fact that I feel this way means I'm a bad person."
- "If I express negative emotion, others will reactive negatively (i.e., reject, attack, judge, ridicule)."
- "Experiencing negative emotion doesn't change anything and is pointless."

Leahy (2002) has found empirical support for the connection between maladaptive beliefs about emotion and psychopathology. Correlating scores on the Emotional Schema Scale with those on the Beck Depression Inventory (Beck & Steer, 1987) and Beck Anxiety Inventory (Beck & Steer, 1990), he found that increased depression was associated with guilt over emotions, the belief that one's emotions were not comprehensible, and the perception that emotions could involve loss of control and have long duration. Anxiety was associated with guilt, the belief that one's emotions were not comprehensible, simplistic views of emotions, a belief in lack of control, and less acceptance of emotions.

In addition, the patient's learning history regarding emotion should be explored. What messages was the patient given about emotion by caretakers and peers? What consequences have occurred in the patient's life when he or she has expressed emotion? Reactions to emotional expression by people in the patient's current life should also be assessed. Are the patient's fears of negative consequences based primarily in learning history, or do they also reflect some aspects of current reality?

For example, one patient who had the belief that his emotions made him weak was afraid to discuss with his wife how upset he felt about an insulting comment made to him by his father. When, as a behavioral experiment, he did talk to his wife, she was every bit as dismissive as he had feared. We then had to work on helping the patient feel entitled to emotional support even if his wife would not give it and on ways that he could assert his needs with her. (In this case, his wife eventually was able to respond more positively to his expressions of emotion, which helped improve both his mood and their marriage.)

Finally, it is important to help patients identify the positive and negative effects of their emotional avoidance. Such avoidance typically has short-term benefits, including a reduction in distress and interpersonal conflict, that are reinforcing. Often patients are aware of these immediate benefits, but they may be less aware of the negative long-term consequences of emotional avoidance. Clinicians must, therefore, help patients identify such consequences and possible links to the patients' presenting problems. It may take observation across a number of situations before such consequences become clear. For example, a patient who habitually avoids feelings of anger by not dealing with problems in his marriage may over time be helped to see that this behavior contributes to his sense of isolation and loneliness.

Once emotional avoidance has been identified and a collaborative agreement has been reached with the patient to target the problem, a number of techniques can be used to help the patient cope with emotion more adaptively. These techniques can be grouped into the following categories: cognitive challenges, coping skills training, response prevention, and exposure.

Cognitive Challenges

The goal of cognitive challenges is to modify patients' maladaptive assumptions and beliefs about emotion. For many patients, the first step in this process may be one of education. Patients who view emotions as threatening and/or shameful may need to be presented with a model of emotional processing that emphasizes the adaptive function of emotions. The model can be presented as an alternative hypothesis about emotions that can be tested along with the patient's beliefs.

When first confronted with evidence of emotional avoidance, patients often ask, "Why should I want to feel bad?" One possible answer is, "Of course, it makes sense that you don't want to feel bad. However, allowing yourself to feel (sad, angry, hurt, etc.) probably won't feel as bad as you expect, and trying to avoid feeling it actually makes you suffer more." This general principle can then be elaborated with specific examples from the patient's life (e.g., "Trying to prevent feeling hurt by avoiding intimate relationships has led to you feeling lonely and depressed, which reinforces your idea that you are unlovable").

A number of standard cognitive techniques can be used to directly challenge patients' maladaptive thoughts and assumptions about emotion. Patients can be asked to examine the evidence for their beliefs "What is the evidence that if you allow yourself to feel sad you won't be able to stop crying? Has this ever happened? Do you know anyone who spent his or her whole life in tears?"). Double standards can be examined ("Would you tell a friend she never has the right to be angry?"). Patients can be asked to define terms ("What do you mean when you say that showing emotion is weak? How do you define weakness and strength? Can someone be emotionally vulnerable at times and still be strong in other ways? Could the ability to tolerate rather than avoid emotion be a sign of strength?"). Patients can be asked to examine the advantages and disadvantages of their beliefs. As part of this process patients can be assigned to track the consequences of emotional experience and expression versus avoidance between sessions.

Similarly, behavioral experiments can be set up ("You predicted that your wife will think less of you if you tell her you sometimes feel anxious. In the next week tell her about something you feel a little anxious about and see how she reacts.") Overgeneralization and catastrophizing should also be addressed. Some people in the patient's current life may react negatively or otherwise punish him or her for emotional expression. The patient can be encouraged to view the consequence of such judgments realistically and to test whether the reaction of one individual is really representative ("How is your life affected if this person thinks you are weak for crying? If person *A* thinks you are weak, does this mean that everyone does?") In some cases, patients may need to be encouraged to seek out new sources of emotional support and/or to end aversive relationships.

Developmental analysis can also be helpful in modifying maladaptive beliefs. Patients can be asked to recall what they were taught about how to deal with emotions while growing up or when they first remember forming their current beliefs. Experiences with family members and/or peers can then be explored and the logic of the received beliefs challenged.

In many cases, the method of dealing with emotion that is currently problematic will turn out to have once been adaptive. Helping patients understand this can reduce shame and allow them to begin to consider coping skills that might be more useful in their current lives. For example, a gay man in his 30s described being picked on and harassed by peers during middle and high school. He believed, probably correctly, that had he shown how hurt he was by these attacks, his emotional reactions would have been used against him as further evidence that he was a "sissy." Not showing or even allowing himself to be fully aware of his reactions was adaptive at the time, but it interfered with his ability as an adult to maintain intimate relationships.

Empathy can be a useful tool in challenging patients' maladaptive beliefs about emotions. Patients often fear that their emotions are incomprehensible, intolerable, or "crazy," and that expressing them will lead to retaliation, rejection, or other negative interpersonal consequences. When the therapist is able to communicate to the patient an accurate understanding of how the patient is feeling (even if the emotion is strongly aversive and/or the therapist believes it is based on a faulty appraisal), the patient may begin to modify these beliefs.

Coping Skills Training

In addition to challenging beliefs about emotion, it can be helpful to teach patients more adaptive coping skills. Without such alternative skills it may be hard for patients to give up or modify their avoidance behaviors. Depending on the patients' needs and deficits, training in relaxation, distraction, mindfulness, problem solving, communication skills, anger management, and assertiveness may all be helpful.

For some patients, the problem may not be that their preferred method for dealing with unpleasant emotion is problematic in and of itself but rather that they use one form of emotional coping inflexibly in all situations. For example, occasionally buying oneself something nice when one is feeling down can be adaptive. Going on a shopping spree every time one has a negative emotion, on the other hand, is not. Patients should be encouraged to develop a menu of coping skills.

Response Prevention

Another important technique for helping patients cope with negative emotion is response prevention. In essence, patients need to stop using their typical maladaptive ways of avoiding emotion. For some patients, this will mean helping to eliminate obvious destructive behaviors, such as substance abuse, binge eating, or self-mutilation. For others (or at other times in therapy), response prevention will involve blocking subtle moves away from emotion in the moment-to-moment process of a therapy session. Thus behaviors such as hiding tears or suddenly changing the subject may be noted, and the patient may be encouraged to move back toward the emotions. This process will often have to be repeated many times over the course of therapy.

Special attention will need to be paid to cognitive distortions that function to help avoid emotion. Initially such thoughts may be challenged using standard techniques. However, once a thought has clearly been identified as self-protective, it will often be more useful to simply note it and encourage the patient to focus instead on the emotion and thoughts that are being avoided.

For example, a man who complained of depression spent hours berating himself as a bad person because he failed to take action on certain projects. Cognitive challenges did little to alter this pattern. At the same time, the patient never actually took steps to begin these projects. When this apparent contradiction was pointed out, the patient said that, while it felt awful to berate himself, it was better than the anxiety he felt when he contemplated taking action because he was sure he would fail at anything he attempted. Once we had identified the self-flagellating thoughts as a form of avoidance, we began to interrupt them in session and move directly to addressing the patient's underlying fears of incompetence.

Exposure

Finally, patients who habitually avoid emotion will need to be exposed to their own emotions and to the thoughts and situations that trigger them. This process has several goals: (1) to help patients realize that they can tolerate negative emotion and that the consequences of doing so are less aversive than the consequences of avoidance; (2) to alter maladaptive beliefs that can be accessed only when the emotion is activated; and (3) to help patients use emotion for its adaptive functions of information, communication, and motivation.

In some situations, exposure to avoided emotions can be accomplished in planned exercises. For example, a session may be set aside for discussing an emotional topic that is typically avoided. The process may be similar to the "retelling" used in treatment for posttraumatic stress disorder, in which the patient's narrative is recorded and the patient is assigned to listen to it repeatedly (Foa & Rothbaum, 1998; Leahy & Holland, 2000). Alternatively, patients may be assigned to tolerate a distressing emotion or situation *in vivo* between sessions for a set period of time without using typical coping mechanisms. Gestalt techniques, such as the empty-chair exercise (Greenberg & Safran, 1987), can also facilitate emotional exposure.

Often, however, the relevant emotion cannot be elicited on demand. When this is the case, the process of exposure will depend on taking advantage of opportunities that present themselves during the flow of sessions. Simply calling attention to subtle signs of emotion can increase the patient's awareness of his or her emotion and facilitate exposure. Empathic reflection of the therapist's own emotional response can also be useful, as can gestalt techniques, such as having patients focus on bodily sensations when they are emotional or repeating an emotionally charged phrase (Greenberg & Safran, 1987).

Finally, it should be noted that the therapeutic relationship can be used to promote emotional exposure. Aspects of the relationship will often trigger emotionally laden schemas. Discussing patients' reactions to interactions with the therapist can be a potent technique for accessing avoided emotion and challenging fears about its expression. This is particularly true when a patient's maneuvers to avoid such emotion begin to directly interfere with the process of therapy.

WHEN TO TARGET EMOTIONAL AVOIDANCE

One important question still to be considered is how to determine whether to target an emotional reaction for change or for exposure. The first criterion is whether the reaction appears to be based on a realistic appraisal of the triggering situation. If, instead, the reaction is based on faulty information processing, the emotion should be targeted for change using standard cognitive and behavioral techniques. Alternatively, emotion based on realistic assessment should be treated using exposure and adaptive coping skills. Sometimes, both realistic and unrealistic reactions will be triggered by the same event and will require different interventions. For example, a woman with a chronic debilitating medical condition that frequently required hospitalization missed her son's wedding due to one of her periodic flare-ups. Her disappointment and sadness at missing the event were empathized with and targeted for exposure and coping. However, her guilt and self-hatred for something over which she had no control were targeted for change.

The second basis for deciding whether to target emotion for change or for exposure is the manner in which the patient currently copes with the emotion and the consequences of such coping. An emotion that is based on faulty appraisal may still be targeted initially for exposure if the patient's attempts to avoid the emotion prevent cognitive change or lead to self-destructive behaviors.

Another important question is how to integrate a focus on emotional avoidance with standard empirically supported treatments. There are at least two ways in which this integration can be done. First, emotional avoidance can be targeted when it is impeding progress that would be expected using standard techniques. Second, emotional avoidance may be addressed when the standard treatment has been successful in reducing symptoms of an Axis I disorder but additional problems exist that appear related to how the patient handles emotion. The following case examples illustrate each of these approaches.

CASE EXAMPLES

Case Example 1

Tom was a 24-year-old man who complained of depression following the breakup of a long-standing relationship. He indicated that he had always assumed he would marry his ex-girlfriend, Sara, but that the breakup had been messy and had included his having an affair with another woman. He worried that he was unattractive and incapable of having a relationship and that he would always be alone. He scored in the moderately depressed range on the Beck Depression Inventory (Beck & Steer, 1987), and his symptoms interfered with his performance in graduate school. He denied any prior history of depression.

Tom initially responded well to standard cognitive therapy for depression (Beck, Rush, Shaw, & Emery, 1979; Leahy & Holland, 2000; Persons, Davidson, & Tompkins, 2001). Within 3 months his scores on the Beck Depression Inventory were averaging in the mild range, and he was doing better in school. However, over the following 2 months Tom remained mildly depressed. In addition, he had several brief bouts of increased depression, each triggered by some disappointment in dating. Tom was also having difficulty getting started on his graduate thesis.

In trying to understand why treatment had bogged down, two things emerged that pointed to emotional avoidance. First, I noticed that Tom was not using thought records when he was most upset. Tom said he was afraid that if he wrote down his thoughts, he would become too emotional and would not be able to get himself out of it. This fear was targeted by teaching him additional coping skills (relaxation and distraction), followed by cognitive challenges and the assignment to test his belief by writing his thoughts the next time he was upset.

Second, I realized that, although Tom identified the breakup as the trigger for his depression, he had actually told me very little about his relationship or how it had ended. When I asked about this, Tom said that he still found it upsetting to think about the breakup. I suggested to Tom that we conceptualize the breakup as a traumatic event that he had yet to come to terms with. We agreed to set up a 90-minute session to have Tom tell the story of the breakup as an exposure exercise.

As it turned out, once Tom started he had a lot to say, and it took four 90-minute sessions to complete the story. Tom reported that he and Sara had met early in college and had done a lot of typical college drinking and partying together. Tom found Sara beautiful and exciting and had fallen in love with her. Over time Tom became uncomfortable with some of what he and Sara were doing, which had begun to include experimenting with drugs and group sex. As they approached the end of college, Tom was focused on getting into graduate school, while Sara had no specific plans. Tom began to feel that Sara was more interested in partying than in him or their relationship. After college, their differences continued to grow, and Tom eventually began to have doubts that Sara was being faithful.

It was in this context that Tom became interested in a woman in his graduate program who appeared to embody more of what he was looking for—stability and a focus on career. They become briefly involved, leading Tom to break up with Sara. However, the other woman was not interested in a relationship. The affair ended, and Tom felt devastated.

What was most striking in the telling of this story was that Tom appeared to have been largely unaware of his emotions or the reasons for his actions. He seemed particularly unaware of how hurt and angry he felt about some of Sara's behavior. As I reflected the situation back to him with empathy and validation, Tom began to be able to better identify what he had been feeling and why. This allowed him to see the events leading up the end of his relationship with Sara as comprehensible. He no longer viewed their breakup as an unpredictable catastrophe or as the result of his inability to maintain a relationship, both of which thoughts had left him feeling hopeless and depressed. Instead, he began to believe that, even though he regretted some of the things he did, he had had good reason to question and eventually end the relationship. This allowed him to feel more confident about his ability to learn from what had happened and to find a more suitable partner.

After these four extended sessions, we returned to weekly 45-minute meetings. Tom's depression improved rapidly, and his scores on the Beck Depression Inventory held steady in the normal range. He began dating more actively and without the emotional ups and downs he had experienced earlier. In addition, he began to make progress on his thesis. Two months later, Tom elected to stop therapy, indicating that his goals had been met.

In treating Tom, I focused on emotional avoidance after he failed to show adequate response to standard cognitive-behavioral therapy for depression. Emotional avoidance contributed to Tom's problems at two stages. First, during his relationship with Sara, Tom was unable to use his emotions as information. As a result, he had difficulty making sense of his own actions and the sequence of events that led to the end of the relationship. Then, during therapy, avoiding emotion made it difficult to access and modify the beliefs that maintained his depression. Emotional exposure, combined with cognitive challenges, coping skills, and response prevention, allowed Tom to tolerate his negative emotion long enough to examine and challenge these beliefs. Consequently, he was able to construct a realistic understanding of what had happened that allowed him to mourn the end of his relationship with Sara and to move forward with hope.

Case Example 2

This second case illustrates the use of techniques that target emotional avoidance during extended treatment following the successful use of empirically supported treatment for symptom relief. Sally was a college junior referred by her university counseling center because of panic attacks. Her first attack had occurred a year earlier. Since that time she had suffered several panic attacks per month and worried almost constantly about having another attack. Her primary fear was that her throat would close and she would be unable to breathe. She avoided a number of situations and when she was most anxious she would spend nights and weekends at her parents' house, about an hour away from school.

Sally was treated using standard cognitive-behavioral techniques for panic disorder (Barlow & Cerney, 1988; Clark, 1986; Leahy & Holland, 2000), including distraction, cognitive restructuring, and exposure. Within 3 months she had stopped having panic attacks and had completed all the items on her exposure hierarchy, except for being more than a few hours from her parents' home. At that point, we discussed whether to begin tapering sessions. Sally indicated that she wanted to continue meeting weekly to address two concerns: (1) her relationship with her mother, and (2) her relationships with men.

Sally's mother was her primary safety figure. Consequently, Sally spent a great deal of time with her. She spoke to her mother daily by phone and would often call her in the middle of the night when she felt panicked. Although she reported feeling emotionally close to her mother, Sally also viewed her as overcontrolling and unwilling to treat Sally as an adult with her own wishes and judgments. Thus frequent verbal arguments occurred between the two.

Sally had never had a romantic relationship of any length, in spite of the fact that she received a lot of positive attention from male peers. Because many of her friends had formed stable relationships over the previous few years, Sally found her own lack of a relationship upsetting. She typically had at least one man "interested" in her. She would flirt and string him along without ever really getting involved. Many of the men in Sally's social circle would not date her because of her reputation for "playing" people. On the rare occasion that Sally did not have anyone interested in her, she became quite anxious and insecure.

Sally reported that her parents' marriage was rocky. Her father was a senior partner in a large law firm who was rarely home. Her mother was angry at what she saw as her husband's neglect. Sally also felt ignored by her father and shared in her mother's anger at him. When her father did make some overture to Sally, she would typically rebuff him, and he would quickly withdraw. Sally's mother appeared to recruit her daughter as an ally in her discontent. Sally's younger brother, still in high school, sided with the father.

As we continued to work on Sally's panic symptoms and began to explore the issues of Sally's relationships with her family and with men, a pattern of emotional avoidance began to emerge. For example, we did an exposure exercise in which Sally related the story of her first panic attack. This had happened in her sophomore year of college, less than a week after a man she had liked had "dumped" her. She was in the shower getting ready to go out with friends, when she began to feel her throat close and became afraid that she would not be able to breathe. She managed to meet her friends as planned. However, the bar they went to was hot and smoky. Sally again began to fear she would be unable to breathe and had a full-blown panic attack. A friend took her back to the dorm, and Sally went home for the weekend. As she told this story, it became clear that as Sally had been standing in the shower, she had been feeling sad and had been on the verge of tears. In essence, she had been "all choked up." However, she had not recognized the feeling as sadness and had, therefore, misinterpreted it as a dangerous physical symptom.

Another indication of emotional avoidance came as Sally discussed her relationship with her father. In general, she described him with disdain. Occasionally, however, she would be visibly upset about some event in which she felt he had failed her. When I would call attention to the emotion, Sally would quickly close down. Sally appeared to cope with the hurt she felt in relation to her father by attempting to denigrate him and to deny his importance to her.

About 6 months into treatment, Sally had a brief relapse of panic. The first intervention was to encourage Sally to use the techniques she had found helpful in the past. Thus the relapse was used as an opportunity to strengthen Sally's coping skills. This intervention quickly brought the panic attacks under control. We then explored what had triggered the panic. Sally had become interested in a fellow student named Bob, whom she found very attractive. She believed that he was attracted to her as well but was not sure. Sally wanted to pursue a relationship with Bob, but she had become anxious for several reasons. First, she knew she would have to give up the pseudo-relationship she had maintained with the latest man she had been stringing along. She feared that if Bob rejected her, she would be alone and would become anxious and depressed. In addition, she was afraid that if she liked Bob more than he liked her, she would appear weak and pathetic. I pointed out to Sally that her fear of her own emotions—being depressed if she felt rejected or appearing weak for liking someone more than he liked her—had apparently triggered her relapse.

Sally did begin a relationship with Bob. Because he was a senior, they had only a couple of months together before he graduated. They continued to see each other frequently over the summer. In the fall, Bob moved to a city several hours away, and Sally visited him periodically. Treatment during this time focused on helping Sally cope with her anxiety as she became more involved with Bob and felt more emotionally vulnerable and then as she began to feel Bob becoming physically and emotionally more distant.

Eventually Bob told Sally he had started seeing someone else. Suddenly, the whole tone of the therapy shifted. Up until this point, the therapeutic relationship had been predominantly positive and collaborative. Now, it seemed I could do nothing right. When I attempted to help Sally challenge her beliefs that this rejection meant that there was something wrong with her and that she would always be alone, she refused to participate. When I tried to be empathic about how hurt she felt, she said I was making her feel worse. When I asked her what she wanted to work on, she said she didn't know. When I sat and said nothing, she grew angry.

After several sessions like this, I finally talked to Sally about my sense that nothing I did felt useful to her. Sally, in turn, expressed anger that I had allowed her to render me helpless. She began talking about how angry she was at her father for allowing her to push him away and how she always sought to be in control of men she dated so she would not get hurt.

This interaction proved to be a turning point in the therapy. We were then able to look at Sally's attempts to push away and control the men in her life as a self-protective maneuver meant to allow her to avoid feeling hurt. Sally began to see that this behavior resulted in confirming her fear that she would be alone and that no man would care for her. Subsequently, several changes began to take place in Sally's life. For the first time, she expressed some positive feelings for her father, and she reported some tentative attempts to connect with him, such as meeting him for lunch. Interestingly, around this time, Sally's parents decided to begin couple therapy. Sally also began to discuss her sadness about ending college and saying good-bye to her friends and to make plans for her future. She decided to attend a graduate program in another state. This move would take her far enough away that it would be impractical to get home for a night if she had a panic attack. In essence, Sally began to allow herself more distance from her mother while still retaining some of the emotional closeness that she valued. When we ended therapy around the time of Sally's graduation, she had been panic free for over a year.

In this case, emotional avoidance did not present an obstacle to the initial treatment of Sally's panic symptoms. However, once her symptoms had improved, Sally elected to use therapy to address some interpersonal issues. It was at this point that it became apparent that emotional avoidance played a role both in the development of her panic attacks and in preventing Sally from achieving age-appropriate goals, such as increased autonomy from her parents and the development of a romantic relationship. Her emotional avoidance eventually played out in the therapeutic relationship in a way that allowed us to examine both its function and consequences. As a result, Sally not only was able to eliminate her panic attacks but also began to make changes in her relationships with her family and with men.

SUMMARY

Patients who habitually avoid negative emotion may pose challenges for therapists attempting to use standard empirically supported treatments. A number of techniques—including cognitive challenges, skills training, response prevention, and exposure—can be used to help patients cope more adaptively with emotion. Directly targeting emotional avoidance in this way can help patients achieve better outcomes in terms of both symptom relief and increased effectiveness in meeting life goals.

REFERENCES

Barlow, D. H., & Cerney, J. A. (1988). *Psychological treatment of panic*. New York: Guilford Press.

Beck, A. T., Rush, A. J., Shaw, B. F., & Emery, G. (1979). *Cognitive therapy of depression*. New York: Guilford Press.

Beck, A. T., & Steer, R. A. (1987). *Manual for the revised Beck Depression Inventory*. San Antonio, TX: Psychological Corporation.

Beck, A. T., & Steer, R. A. (1990). *Beck Anxiety Inventory manual*. San Antonio, TX: Psychological Corporation.

Clark, D. M. (1986). A cognitive approach to panic. *Behaviour Research and Therapy, 24*, 461–470.

Foa, E. B., & Rothbaum, B. O. (1998) *Treating the trauma of rape: Cognitive-behavioral therapy for PTSD*. New York: Guilford Press.

Greenberg, L. S. (2002). *Emotion focused therapy: Coaching clients to work through their feelings*. Washington, DC: American Psychological Association.

Greenberg, L. S., & Paivio, S. (1997). *Working with emotion in psychotherapy*. New York: Guilford Press.

Greenberg, L. S., & Safran, J. D. (1987). *Emotions in psychotherapy*. New York: Guilford Press.

Leahy, R. L. (2002) A model of emotional schemas. *Cognitive and Behavioral Practice, 9*, 177–191.

Leahy, R. L., & Holland, S. J. (2000). *Treatment plans and interventions for depression and anxiety disorders*. New York: Guilford Press.

Linehan, M. M. (1993). *Skills training manual for treating borderline personality disorder*. New York: Guilford Press.

Persons, J. B., Davidson, J., & Tompkins, M. A. (2001). *Essential components of cognitive-behavior therapy for depression*. Washington, DC: American Psychological Association.

Part III

Specific Populations

7

Psychosis

Gillian Haddock
Ronald Siddle

It is now reasonably well established that cognitive-behavioral therapy for schizophrenia is a valid treatment option for patients experiencing chronic treatment-resistant psychosis (Rector & Beck, 2001). In addition, there is growing evidence that patients experiencing acute, recent onset, and dual diagnoses can also benefit from cognitive-behavioral approaches (Haddock et al., 1999; Lewis et al., 2002; Barrowclough et al., 2001). However, the application of cognitive-behavioral therapy to psychosis has been influenced by a range of factors that have resulted in a form of cognitive-behavioral therapy that differs somewhat from that adopted in the neurosis field. This may be a result of the complexity in the symptoms and problems that the psychotic patient can present with; within the wide spectrum of schizophrenia, one patient may not resemble the next in any presenting symptomatology, characteristics, or problems. This situation has caused some difficulties in establishing a cognitive-behavioral model from which to drive treatment. As a result, some researchers and clinicians have focused on developing models and treatments for the individual symptoms of psychosis (e.g., paranoid delusions; Bentall & Kinderman, 1998) rather than for the overall schizophrenia syndrome and/or on developing treatments that can be adapted to suit a range of difficulties that may present in psychosis, for example, coping strategy enhancement (Tarrier et al., 1998) or social skills training (Halford & Hayes, 1992). Recently, the main trials evaluating cognitive-behavioral therapy for psychosis have assessed the effectiveness of comprehensive treatment packages that incorporate specific treatments for individual symptoms, such as hallucinations and delusions, and that also offer general cognitive-behavioral strategies for coping and treating other aspects of the disorder, for example, depression, low self-esteem, poor social skills, and negative symptoms (see Tarrier et al., 1998). Some of these approaches have been borrowed directly from the cognitive-behavioral treatments developed for neurotic symptoms, and some have developed from psychopathological models of psychosis and of specific psychotic symptoms. The following heuristic model illustrates how these factors have been incorporated into a pragmatic guide for assessment and treatment in therapy, taking into account the neurodevelopmental, social, and cognitive factors that are thought to be important in the development and maintenance of psychosis.

As can be seen from Figure 7.1, the Manchester model assumes that there are certain predisposing factors that can influence the development of psychosis and that interact with familial and social factors leading to the onset of psychosis. The psychosis will then continue to develop until the patient (or others) brings the problem to the attention of a service agency. It is

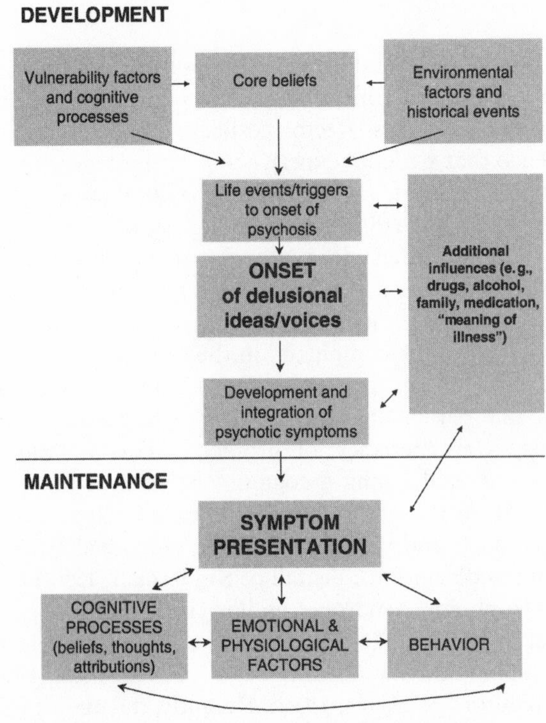

FIGURE 7.1. The Manchester model of cognitive-behavioral therapy.

at this point that a range of interventions will begin. Predominantly, the intervention will not be cognitive-behavioral therapy but will involve a combination of psychopharmocological and psychosocial interventions, for example, supported work or programs, occupational therapy, or group programs. Cognitive-behavioral therapy is offered sporadically and inconsistently within service agencies because psychosis is primarily considered to be a biological disorder that will respond to biological treatments and because cognitive-behavioral therapy has only recently become a viable treatment option that is backed up by positive research findings (Rector & Beck, 2001). Issues relating to the setup of services are discussed in more detail in the next section.

THE PROGRESSION OF TREATMENT

Engagement

The Manchester model of cognitive-behavioral therapy illustrated previously provides a summary of the areas of potential assessment and intervention. However, the application of cognitive-behavioral therapy is extremely dependent on the therapist's ability to engage the patient in any sort of dialogue about his or her problems and subsequently to engage the patient in a cognitive-behavioral treatment program. The degree to which this is possible when working with psychotic patients is extremely variable, but it is by far the most important roadblock to overcome. A number of reports of trials evaluating cognitive-behavioral therapy for psychosis have commented on the problems of engaging this population (Barrowclough et al., 2001; Lewis et al., 2002). For example, substance use and florid psychotic symptoms may interfere with the patient's ability to engage in a therapeutic dialogue. This does not mean that important work cannot be carried out. It is usually possible to provide some aspect of therapy to even the most difficult patient. Additionally, once patients are engaged in treatment, dropouts can be relatively low. Engagement issues are discussed throughout this chapter, specifically in relation to particular patient groups.

Assessment Strategies

The degree to which assessment strategies are utilized depends on a number of factors. The purpose of assessment is to gain a comprehensive cognitive-behavioral account of the patient's main problem or problems. With psychosis, the problem list can be extremely long; therefore, the therapist has to balance the need to keep the patient engaged with a wish to ensure that the assessment is as comprehensive as possible. Ideally, the therapist should aim to gain a complete overview of the patient's difficulties covering mental state, social and familial functioning, and history of illness and symptoms, as illustrated in the top half of Figure 7.1. This investigation should be followed by collaborative prioritizing of the key problems and needs for further assessment. This would usually mean focusing in on one or two areas, such as distressing voices or paranoia, for further assessment.

The continued assessment should explore the nature and phenomenology of the psychotic symptoms and their cognitive, behavioral, emotional, and physiological correlates (e.g., the nature of the thoughts and beliefs about symptoms, the physiological arousal symptoms associated with them, and the patient's behavioral responses to them). This is the ideal approach. However, the degree to which this is possible is extremely dependent on the patient, and the therapist may not always be able to achieve this, particularly with the patient groups previously described. Some patients may even find it difficult to describe their experiences in a way that is understandable to the therapist, and responses may be inconsistent from one meeting to another. In this case, sometimes focusing in on one main symptom or problem rather than attempting to get a comprehensive assessment is sensible. This procedure may engage the patient and may allow the therapist to provide some relief from the symptom as an engagement strategy. The patient may then be helped to engage in further assessment and therapy. Sometimes, general questions such as, "What brought you into the hospital this time?" or "What happened last time you were ill?" can help to give an overview of the sort of problems that contribute to a worsening of the patient's problems. Even if the therapist is not able to engage the patient in a cognitive-behavioral therapy treatment program, an intervention could focus on identifying early signs and stressors that contribute to a relapse and on implementing a staying-well program with the patient and/or care givers and staff. The main purposes of assessment are to open up discussions with the patient about his or her symptoms, to allow the therapist opportunities to normalize symptoms, to educate the patient where necessary, and to generate enough information to get a collaborative formulation of the patient's difficulties. Normalization strategies might involve illustrating how psychotic symptoms may arise as a result of chronic sleep deprivation or following a bereavement. The purpose of these strategies might be to present understandable reasons for the patient becoming psychotic given the stressful circumstances that he or she was exposed to preceding the psychotic breakdown. This strategy can help some patients to feel that they can gain an understanding of their psychoses and begin to see that there may be aspects of their psychoses that could be influenced by cognitive-behavioral dimensions of their symptoms that could be modifiable.

Formulation

A shared formulation or understanding of the patient's key problems or symptoms is fairly crucial to the further progression of cognitive-behavioral therapy. However, the complexity of that formulation can be extremely variable. It is not necessary to have a formulation that explains the origin, development, and maintenance of the patient's psychosis in order to provide effective and useful therapy. Such a formulation may be helpful to some patients, but often a simple collaborative formulation in terms of the factors that contribute to the maintenance of the patient's key symptom or problem is sufficient (see the lower half of Figure 7.1, illustrating how symptoms may be maintained by cognitive, behavioral, and emotional factors). For example, negative thoughts attacking a person's self-worth may be triggered in situations in which a patient gets into conflicts in close relationships. These negative thoughts may then trigger voices that are similar in content themes to the thoughts. These voices in turn will contribute to changes in mood and arousal states that may result in avoidance strategies for future situations that trigger the thoughts, such as close emotional relationships. As a result, the individual will reduce his or her opportunities to engage in social interactions that might provide evidence to disconfirm the feelings of being worthless and the opportunities to engage in activities that might increase his or her self-worth.

The formulation also needs to take into account that patients will already have been trying to make sense of their symptoms and will have been doing this since the symptoms began. Some of these explanations may be wrong, some may be delusional, and some may be accurate. The formulation needs to take account of patients' explanations, as they are often sensitive about mental health workers whom they perceive to be trying to disprove their delusional ideas. Some of the difficulties include: insufficient information given by the patient despite the therapist's sensitive and empathic exploration; delusional material interfering with patient's responses; a patient's difficulty in understanding basic abstract ideas; or a patient's unwillingness to consider other than his or her own explanation of symptoms. However, collaboratively generating a simple formulation can usually be achieved in even the most difficult therapeutic encounter, as long as the patient is engaged enough to stay in the room with you. The following transcript illustrates this:

THERAPIST: When you hear your voices say you are a useless person and don't deserve to live, what do you think of that? Do you think it's true?

CHARLOTTE: I know it's true, they've been saying it for years.

THERAPIST: And how does that make you feel?

CHARLOTTE: Same as usual, I'm always depressed, I am useless. I've never had a boyfriend. I've got no money, I've got no job. There's no point in doing anything. Whatever I do, I'm still useless. The aliens are right.

THERAPIST: If you had a job, money, and a boyfriend, would what the voices say be true then?

CHARLOTTE: No, but they might say other things then.

Even from this sort of short transcript, it is possible to put together a miniformulation that might help to engage the patient in some cognitive-behavioral therapy work. For example, the therapist could illustrate to the patient how the voices have an impact on her thoughts ("I am useless, I've got no job," etc.), how she feels (depressed) and how they affect her behavior (she doesn't do anything because there is no point). This type of miniformulation does not challenge Charlotte's delusional belief that the voices are aliens from outer space. However, it does allow the therapist to lead her toward the idea that if she could influence her own thoughts, feelings, and behavior, then it may matter less what the voices actually said. That is, if she were able to improve her life, then the voices may still say she is useless, but she may not agree with them. Once engaged in this approach, more sensitive questioning may allow further exploration of the delusional beliefs.

Interventions

Once the intervention stage is reached, it is likely that the patient is engaged in a therapeutic approach to some extent. The extent to which the therapist has been able to assess and formulate the patient's key problems will determine the sorts of interventions that are possible, although the range of interventions available to practitioners of cognitive-behavioral therapy with patients with psychoses is as extensive as in the field of neurosis. Table 7.1 summarizes some of the common strategies used in cognitive-behavioral therapy for psychosis.

The extent to which the strategies can be employed depends on the level of engagement reached with the patient, the patient's cognitive abilities, and the degree to which psychotic phenomena interfere with treatment. For example, a potential problem in using guided discovery is that a number of patients simply do not have the cognitive capability to make the links needed to gain from guided discovery. However, this is usually the minority of patients. Many are able to make thought, feeling, and behavior links and are able to focus on key cognitions in the same way that other patient groups are. Therapists should be aware that key cognitions also include perceptions, beliefs, and attributions that are derived from psychotic beliefs. Nevertheless, these phenomena have very similar characteristics to those generated by patients with neuroses and can be managed similarly.

The use of behavioral experiments is an important aspect of most cognitive-behavioral interventions in psychosis. The aim is to collaboratively generate situations in which the patient can test his or her delusional beliefs with a view that the findings reduce the strength of the belief. However, these should be carried out only with reference to the formulation and should be the result of collaborative planning with the patient—that is, the

TABLE 7.1. Common Cognitive-Behavioral Strategies Used for Psychotic Symptoms

Ongoing monitoring	Guided discovery
Early intervention/relapse prevention	Focus on key cognitions
Coping strategy enhancement	Homework setting
Schema work	Behavioral experiments
Medication compliance enhancement	Social skills training
Distraction/counterstimulation	Belief modification
Focusing/concurrent monitoring	Rational responding
Activity scheduling	Social skills training
Psychoeducation	

experiment should be the result of the patient's desire to test his or her beliefs, not of the therapist's persuading him or her to do so. Patients often like to know whether their "delusional" beliefs are definitely true or not. This is a common dilemma for patients. They may know that their beliefs are fantastic or ridiculous and know that other people think this, too, and would like the opportunity to explore this idea with a therapist who is not trying to persuade them that they are delusional. This means that some experiments should be set up in a way that attempts to "prove" that the patient is right in his or her delusions rather than trying to weaken the patient's beliefs. When the evidence collected during a behavioral experiment does not fit in with the patient's delusions, then it is the therapist's job to help the patient to process this information. In addition, delusional beliefs may be serving an important function for the person—for example, grandiose or paranoid beliefs may make the person feel special or important in some way (even if the consequence is that he or she is persecuted). Careful thought needs to go into whether it is appropriate to intervene using behavioral experiments that might reduce the patient's conviction in his or her belief, as doing so may also reduce self-esteem and result in a worsening of the patient's mental health.

However, even when set up well, these types of experiments may be influenced by factors outside our control. For example, a recent patient believed that an intelligence organization was plotting to harm him. The people from the organization were following him and planning to attack him. The therapist and patient reviewed the previous few months to investigate whether there were potential times at which the organization could have attacked him but did not. This process revealed that there had been very few opportunities, as the patient had rarely been out over the previous few months because of his fear. A behavioral experiment was set up to find out whether the patient really would be attacked by the organization if he went out, with the assumption that this would be unlikely to happen. However, the patient was mugged during the following week, and he interpreted this as the work of the organization. It is possible to reduce the potentially catastrophic impact of this event by anticipating these types of occurrences when planning experiments, even if the possibility of something occurring is very slight. This possibility can then be discussed with the patient beforehand and the findings incorporated into the formulation.

Accordingly, it is important that the experiment be set up in such a way that the findings can be interpreted as the therapist intends; that is, that the findings provide evidence that weakens rather than strengths the belief or that the patient cannot dismiss the evidence. Sensitive discussion about what evidence the patient thinks will influence the strength of his or her belief (in either direction) is important when setting up the experiment.

Behavioral experiments are almost always set up as part of some sort of homework task (or between-session work). However, patients without psychotic illness do not always do homework, and patients with psychosis are perhaps just as likely not to do it. Problems such as poor concentration and memory and negative symptoms may reduce the likelihood that tasks will be completed. Anxiety about the task may also affect participation, particularly if the task is a behavioral experiment intended to introduce doubt into delusional ideas. However, homework is a key component of cognitive-behavioral therapy and is essential to maximize the generalizability of the intervention. Homework should be clearly discussed within the session. Fuller participation will be obtained if the homework arises from something discussed in the session and if the patient can see the rationale for the task. The instructions for the patient should be unambiguously outlined, and, whenever possible, complex tasks should be rehearsed in session. Written or audiotaped instructions are helpful. Patients should be given the opportunity to explain what they expect they will discover from the task and how that will help. If the patient's responses indicate a degree of confusion or errors, these ought to be rectified before the patient leaves the session so that he or she can derive benefit from the task. Homework tasks must always be checked on the next available opportunity, as it is entirely possible that patients will discover a whole range of unexpected things from their homework task. The following example illustrates this. A young man who had a diagnosis of schizophrenia lived in a shared house with a couple of other men who also had schizophrenia. During therapy it emerged that the young man believed that other people could hear the voices he heard. An experiment was set up that involved questioning his housemates about whether they could also hear the patient's voices. Unfortunately, the task was not fully clarified. The voices started one evening when the patient was watching TV, and he asked the man sitting near him, "Carl, do you hear the voices?" Carl, who also was a hallucinator, responded that he did, hence providing support for the young man's belief about his voices. Fortunately, this situation was followed up quickly in the next session, and more specific tasks were planned with the patient to explore his voices. The patient asked Carl about his voices the next time he heard them and this time, when Carl responded that he could hear the voices, the young man went on to ask Carl what they said. Because Carl's voices did not have the same content as the patient's, a slight hint of doubt regarding the voices was introduced.

SPECIFIC CLINICAL FACTORS AND ENGAGEMENT IN COGNITIVE-BEHAVIORAL TREATMENT

Negative Symptoms

Specific clinical factors such as the negative symptoms of social withdrawal and apathy can reduce the degree to which the patient is able to attend and engage in therapy. Even while in treatment, the patient may be unable to do between-session work, and the patient may get fewer opportunities to test delusional ideas using behavioral experiments if he or she has limited social contact or exposure to the outside world. In practice this means ensuring that the therapy takes place in an environment that is easily accessible, and it can mean assisting or bringing the patient into therapy. Short sessions with few agenda items and short- and long-term goal setting can be crucial in engaging patients with negative symptoms. Much repetition, summaries, and clear information sharing can be essential. Activity scheduling, such as that used in treatment programs for depression, can be extremely useful in gradually increasing patient's activity levels and in encouraging patients to interact socially to test delusional ideas. In addition, as negative symptoms of schizophrenia can be extremely difficult for relatives or caregivers to cope with, involving a patient's extended family network in therapy in some way can be helpful. Relatives may assist with activity scheduling strategies and may welcome advice and information on the nature and management of negative symptoms. For example, caregivers sometimes misperceive problems with motivation and apathy as a result of laziness rather than as part of their relative's illness. As a result they might react by encouraging or putting pressure on the patient to do more. Sometimes they may nag and criticize the person. Providing relatives with information about negative symptoms and how they might affect their relative can help them to change their attributions to ones that are less likely to result in criticism or exerting pressure. They learn that the person's illness is the cause of the low motivation (external and uncontrollable explanations for the symptoms) and that the person is not inherently lazy (internal and controllable explanations for the symptom). This may reduce the level of stress within the family and lead to lower expressed criticism from relatives about the causes of the negative symptoms.

Explanations of Symptoms or Insight

The degree to which the patient agrees with the mainstream explanation for his or her psychotic experiences can be an additional factor that can influence the extent to which patients will engage with a therapist (or any other service provider). A difficult problem arises if patients do not believe that they have any sort of mental illness and that services provides are inflicting a schizophrenia diagnosis and its treatment on them. Patients detained under the Mental Health Act often present in this way. There are also many patients who are happy to go along with diagnostic labels and accept treatment but who have conflicting beliefs regarding specific symptoms. A patient like this, Eleanor, had a range of psychotic symptoms. She had grandiose beliefs that she had been chosen by the world leaders to have a special mission in life. She also heard unpleasant critical voices from people in the world who knew that she had been specially chosen but who were trying to undermine her. She had been admitted to the hospital many times when these voices appeared to overwhelm her. She had also attempted suicide as a result of the intense distress they were causing her. Eleanor also believed she had schizophrenia, but she did not think that the psychotic symptoms were related to it. She thought that her schizophrenia was a biological disorder that made her feel depressed and made it difficult for her to have a job and to build good relationships. As a result she was happy to engage in therapy and take medication. However, there were a number of potential blocks to engaging her. First, as she believed she was adequately treated for her problem of schizophrenia and that her other problems were real things that mental health professionals could do nothing about, she saw no point in talking to someone about her difficulties. Second, her distress about the critical voices was linked directly to her beliefs that she was a special person, and this was very important for her self-esteem. So, even though her voices had caused much disruption and distress in her life, they were important in maintaining one of the few positive things she had in her life. Similarly, some types of religious attributions for symptoms can also make engagement difficult and perform an important function for the person. For example, a person who believes his or her voices are a gift or punishment from a higher spiritual entity may be little motivated to challenge or investigate alternative origins and may feel that a therapist is not the person with whom to discuss these issues.

There are a number of strategies that can help to engage people with these types of difficulties. It is extremely important that the therapist is accepting of the patient's beliefs and their possible reality. If the patient does not believe that he or she has schizophrenia, the therapist can agree that he or she may be right. The therapist can then focus on helping the patient understand why some people think that he or she does have schizophrenia and, perhaps more important, why the patient is sure that he or she does not have this illness. Sometimes it can be helpful to act as an advocate for patients within the agency and to help the patient to discuss his or her ideas in an atmosphere in which his or her unusual beliefs will not be dismissed as being mere symptoms of mental illness. The therapist may need to take the role of the "third person," that is, someone who neither agrees nor disagrees with the agency's views on mental illness or the patient's views on the origins of his or her symptoms (Haddock, Lowens, Brosnan, Barrowclough, & Novaco, 2003). If patients are detained in a hospital, a helpful engagement strategy is to suggest that one purpose of therapy may be to explore the reasons why they are being detained and, often more important for the patient, what can be done to get them out of the facility. For some people this can be a powerful motivator.

For those patients like Eleanor who are happy to participate in usual treatment but who can see no rationale for engaging in a talking treatment, a different approach can be helpful. Motivating strategies can include helping the whole mental health team to use a consistent model of psychosis when talking to the patient about his or her illness. This may mean discussing schizophrenia in the context of a stress vulnerability model in which factors other than biological ones can be important. This does not mean telling him or her that the symptoms are caused by schizophrenia, but it may involve illustrating to him or her that environmental stressors may have an impact on his or her experiences even if the experiences are "real." It is usually possible for even extremely deluded patients to understand that if they feel depressed or anxious, their experience of their "psychotic" experiences may seem worse. They may then be more motivated to look at how they can relieve their depression and anxiety and improve their lives. Thus the therapist has an opportunity to discuss the symptoms in more detail in terms of how they make the person feel, what impact they have, and how they affect the person's beliefs about him- or herself, the world, and others. Once patients are engaged in this way, generally they will soon notice that "talking therapy" can have an impact on making them feel better, and this realization can lead the way to discussing symptoms and beliefs in more detail.

Thought Disorder

Very few patients are so severely thought or speech disordered that it is impossible to engage them in therapy. As a rule of thumb, we usually do not pursue engaging people unless we feel they are able to give informed consent to take part in initial discussions about becoming involved in therapy. However, for many patients, extreme thought disorder may be restricted to the most acute part of their illness or relapse and often may reduce significantly during the first few days of drug treatment. Thought disorders such as flights of ideas, severe perseveration, and loosening of associations are likely to prevent a proportion of patients from participating fully in therapy. However, thought disorder worsens under conditions of emotional distress or when discussing material that has high emotional salience (Haddock, Bentall, Lowens, & Wolfenden, 1996). As a result, it may be possible to lessen thought disorder by helping the patient to reduce his or her arousal and to limit the amount of discussion of emotionally salient material during initial sessions. As the therapist becomes used to the patient's way of communicating, the thought-disordered speech often becomes more understandable. In addition, treatment of the thought disorder itself can become the main focus of therapy, sometimes as a precursor to work on delusions or hallucinations. This could take the form of using audio feedback of the patient's speech and monitoring of thought disorder. These techniques can help patients to identify and clarify communication difficulties (Kingdon & Turkington, 1994) and lead to improvements in speech and thought disorders.

Sensory Impairments, Cultural Factors, and Engagement

Little has been written about carrying out cognitive-behavioral therapy with people who have severe sensory impairments. It is likely that deafness may be a significant roadblock to participating in a talking therapy. However, manualized treatments are used widely, and there is no reason why a manual could not be incorporated into a treatment program. Similarly, blindness will inhibit the degree to which usual therapy materials can be used; however, this problem could be overcome by using tape recordings of self-help materials and handouts and by producing information in Braille. A learning disability may also be a hindrance to engaging in therapy, and an inability to read may make using written materials more difficult. However, these difficulties can be overcome to a certain extent. Doing cognitive-behavioral therapy with people with a learning disability is discussed in more detail in the next section. Finally, it is usually important to carry out therapy with a person whose first language is consistent with your own. Although it is not impossible to do therapy with someone who has excellent second language skills, it is possible that the subtleties of their language may be missed and that specific cultural meaning and values may not be understood. This consideration is especially pertinent in psychosis, in which there may be only subtle differences between what is delusional and what is a belief that is in keeping with social norms. Matching patients and therapists who have common cultural and language backgrounds is helpful. However, certainly in the United Kingdom, this is not always possible, and some patients might not receive any therapy if this condition were adhered to strictly. Making sure to become as familiar as possible with the patient's individual background and culture is essential for a therapist. The patients themselves can often be very helpful in this regard.

SPECIFIC PATIENT GROUPS AND ENGAGEMENT

There are a number of psychotic patient groups for which engagement is particularly difficult—for instance, patients who have substance use problems (Barrowclough et al., 2001; Haddock, Barrowclough, et al., 2003), those detained against their will in hospitals (Haddock, Lowens, et al., 2003), and those who have learning disabilities (Haddock, Lobban, Hatton, & Carson, 2003). Specific strategies that have been shown to be effective in engaging these groups are discussed in the following sections relating to specific groups.

Patients with Substance Abuse

Many people with schizophrenia are using and abusing alcohol and drugs, as well as experiencing psychotic ideas. There are some whose problems are made worse by the drugs or alcohol, and some who are merely prevented from full participation in therapy by the effects of these substances on attendance, concentration, or disinhibition within the sessions. In psychosis, there may be number of reasons for patients' ongoing use of illicit substances. Reduction in anxiety and distress about symptoms may be one reason. However, other factors are particularly pertinent to this group. Many psychotic patients have limited access to social interactions. Drug use may increase the patient's ability to become involved in interactions and may also provide access to a social group for patients who previously had none. In addition, many patients report boredom and negative symptoms as being significant problems for them; drug and alcohol use can serve as methods to reduce these problems. More than one patient has reported the beneficial effect of amphetamines on their ability to "get up and go" and to be able to do things that "normal" people find easy. Without the drugs the sedative effect of medication can be difficult to cope with for some. It is important for therapists to recognize the positive benefits that many patients gain from substance use, even if the negative consequences of their use appear very severe.

A recent trial carried out by our group at the University of Manchester showed significant benefits for an integrated cognitive-behavioral therapy and motivational interviewing treatment program delivered to schizophrenic patients with substance use problems and their caregivers (Barrowclough et al., 2001; Haddock, Barrowclough, et al., 2003). The treatment integrated a cognitive-behavioral therapy program aimed at remediating persistent and distressing hallucinations and delusions (see Haddock and Tarrier, 1998) with a motivational interviewing approach (Miller & Rollnick, 1991) adapted from the substance use field that was directed at increasing and developing motivation for changing substance use. A caregiver/family intervention based on Barrowclough and Tarrier's (1992) approach was modified to incorporate aspects of the motivational style. For example, the education phase of the intervention included information about the motivational interviewing model for relatives. Later treatment sessions involved helping relatives to adopt a "motivational" style in their interactions with their relative that was dependent on the particular motivational stage their relative was in. Patients were initially difficult to involve in cognitive-behavioral therapy and usually had a history of poor engagement with other services. However, motivational interviewing was extremely helpful in getting people to engage in therapy and, once engaged, patients tended to remain involved in a course of therapy (for example, only one person dropped out of the treatment program described here). As a result, this strategy has been used with other difficult-to-engage patient groups with some success.

Patients Detained in Hospitals or Those with a History of Violence or Aggression in Service Agencies

Those patients who are legally detained in hospitals or who have a history of violence or aggression within service agencies are also a group that present particular challenges to a cognitive-behavioral therapy therapist. Generally, like the substance user group, they have had a poor history of engagement with services, and treatment is likely to have been forced on them. Motivational strategies and befriending approaches can be extremely useful in setting up therapeutic relationships with this group of patients. In addition, presenting oneself as being separate from the clinical management team can be helpful (if the multidisciplinary team agrees). Agreement may need to be reached concerning level of confidentiality about the therapy sessions; for example, agreeing that material discussed is not passed on to the clinical team unless the therapist believes there is a risk to the patient or to other people. Often inpatients are concerned that if they discuss their symptoms with a member of the staff they will be detained longer or be transferred to more secure settings. They are often also worried that discussion of problems may delay their discharge from the facility or reduce the amount of leave or time allowed out of the ward. Therapists need to be prepared to offer a number of nonspecific engagement sessions. These sessions will help the patient become used to seeing someone regularly with whom they can discuss their problems and to see that the benefits of therapy outweigh the potential disadvantages in terms of risk of further incarceration. Many patients in these types of settings have never had any type of meaningful therapeutic involvement despite having a long history of contact with mental health services. This situation may take some time to overcome. However, once they are involved in talking regularly to a therapist, the therapist can take steps toward helping them to agree to a plan of cognitive-behavioral therapy treatment. At this stage a tentative problem list can be created between therapist and patients. As pointed out earlier, such a list may often include goals such as "getting out of the hospital" or "changing medication," as well as more symptom-specific ones, such as "reducing the distress of my voices." In addition, as patients also are likely to have a history of violence or aggression within service agencies that has contributed to their detention, it is likely that discussion and intervention in this problem area is going to form part of the intervention. In order to address these issues, we have combined the cognitive-behavioral therapy approach for treating persistent psychotic symptoms, a cognitive-behavioral therapy approach for treating anger (see Novaco, 1994), and a motivational interviewing style (Miller & Rollnick, 1991) into an integrated package for treating patients in secure or forensic settings. The treatment approach allows for a long engagement phase in which motivational strategies are employed to increase the patient's motivation to work in therapy on his or her aggression or anger problems, as well as his or her psychosis. In addition, the cognitive-behavioral formulation of anger and psychosis is integrated with the assumption that both will interact and contribute to the expression of aggression. Structured work with staff is also incorporated to tackle incorrect and/or negative attributions about the patient's aggression and to increase the generalizability of the approach. This approach has been described more fully in a small study of individual cases (see Haddock, Lowens, et al., 2003).

Patients with Learning Disabilities

Despite the developments within some dual-diagnosis groups, those patients who have schizophrenia and a coexisting learning disability have not generally been offered treatment with cognitive-behavioral therapy and usually have been excluded from research trials. Several factors may account for this exclusion. For example, historically, services for people with learning disabilities have been delivered separately from mainstream mental health services. There is also a widespread underreporting of mental health problems in people with learning disabilities and a consequent lack of referral to mental health professionals. The reason may be the difficulties of applying standard diagnostic instruments to people with learning disabilities, but it also may be related to beliefs among clinicians that patients with learning disabilities do not have the capacity to benefit from cognitive treatments (Caine & Hatton, 1998). Nevertheless, there is some evidence that cognitive-behavioral therapy can be applied successfully with people with learning disabilities (see Stenfert-Kroese, Dagnan, & Loumidis, 1997), although, to our knowledge, there is only one published case study describing the application on cognitive-behavioral therapy techniques to a patient with psychosis (Legget, Hurn, & Goodman, 1997). Recent work being carried out between the University of Manchester and the University of Lancaster is evaluating the effectiveness of a modified cognitive-behavioral therapy for psychosis program for people with schizophrenia and a mild to moderate learning disability (Haddock, Lobban, et al., 2003). The approach includes a preparatory phase that is designed to assess the patient's ability to make thought, feeling, and behavior links using vignettes of real situations (based on Dagnan, Chadwick, & Proudlove, 2000). For example, a typical event–emotion vignette would be, "It's Johnny's birthday and he receives a present. How would he feel?" A typical emotion–thought vignette would be, "It's Johnny's birthday, and he thinks everyone has forgotten it. How would he feel?" This information is then used by the therapist to tailor a preparatory phase that is appropriate to the patient's level of understanding and that includes a training element to help the patient make the thought, feeling, and behavior links that are important when carrying out cognitive-behavioral therapy. This stage is supplemented by the use of materials that are appropriate to the level of understanding of the patient, such as tape-recorded material rather than written materials for patients who cannot read. Finally, the approach takes particular account of environmental and caregiver factors. Many people with learning disabilities will be living with relatives or caregivers due to the nature of their difficulties. The challenging behavior that is associated with mental health problems and learning disability may cause particular stresses between patients and caregivers that can be tackled using the family intervention approaches that have been used in the non–learning disability field.

CONCLUSIONS

The difficulties in carrying out cognitive-behavioral therapy for psychosis are related to multiple issues covering the specific symptoms the patient has, the additional problems the patient has on top of the psychosis (dual diagnosis), and the environment in which the patient lives and presents to service agencies. As a result, the strategies needed to overcome these problems should be focused on all these areas. It should be particularly emphasized that the difficulties do not always lie within the patient. Many mental health service agencies are not set up to deal well with the needs of some patients, and further developments are needed to address this problem. For example, despite the literature recommending that people with a dual diagnosis of psychosis and substance use should be given both substance use and mental health services, few mental health services in the United Kingdom are set up to do this. The result is often that patients are treated by only one service that does not have the specialist knowledge to deal with their unique problems. There is a similar lack of integrated services for other dual-diagnosis groups. However, recent research studies and service developments are starting to address this problem. One area in which there is a dearth of research or treatment is personality disorder and psychosis. In addition, although we know cognitive-behavioral therapy can be an effective treatment for psychosis and can be applied with very difficult patient groups, very little cognitive-behavioral therapy is offered in routine care for psychotic patients. Many mental health staffs do not have basic training in cognitive-behavioral therapy, and even if they do, the degree to which they have the skills to deal with challenging clients can be limited. For all of the interventions with the patient groups described herein, expert supervision was essential even for the most experienced therapists. Further work is necessary in order to ensure that service planners are aware that when new treatment strategies are developed specialist staff members must be trained to a high standard and that services may need to be configured differently to allow the treatment to be delivered in optimal circumstances.

REFERENCES

Barrowclough, C., Haddock, G., Tarrier, N., Lewis, S., Moring, J., O'Brien, R., et al. (2001). Randomized controlled trial of motivational interviewing, cognitive behavioral therapy, and family intervention for patients with comorbid schizophrenia and substance use disorders. *American Journal of Psychiatry, 158,* 1706–1713.

Barrowclough, C., & Tarrier, N. (1992). *Families of schizophrenic patients: A cognitive behavioural intervention.* London: Chapman & Hall.

Bentall, R. P., & Kinderman, P. (1998). Psychological processes and delusional beliefs: Implications for treatment of paranoid states. In T. Wykes, N. Tarrier, & S. Lewis (Eds.), *Outcome and innovation in psychological treatment of schizophrenia* (pp. 119–144). Chichester, UK: Wiley.

Caine, A., & Hatton, C. (1998). Working with people with mental health problems. In E. Emerson, C. Hatton, J. Bromley, & A. Caine (Eds.), *Clinical psychology and people with intellectual disabilities* (pp. 210–230). Chichester, UK: Wiley.

Dagnan, D., Chadwick, P., & Proudlove, J. (2000). Toward an assessment of suitability of people with mental retardation for cognitive therapy. *Cognitive Therapy and Research, 24*(6), 627–636.

Haddock, G., Barrowclough, C., Tarrier, N., Moring, J., O'Brien, R., Schofield, N., et al. (in press). Randomized controlled trial of cognitive-behavior therapy and motivational intervention for schizophrenia and substance use: 18-month, career and economic outcomes. *British Journal of Psychiatry.*

Haddock, G., Bentall, R. P., Lowens, I., & Wolfenden, M. (1996). The effect of emotional salience on the thought disorder of schizophrenic patients. *British Journal of Psychiatry, 167,* 618–620.

Haddock, G., Lobban, F., Hatton, C., & Carson, R. (2003). Cognitive-behaviour therapy for psychosis and mild learning disability: A case series. *Clinical Psychology and Psychotherapy.*

Haddock, G., Lowens, I., Brosnan, N., Barrowclough, C., & Novaco, R. W. (2003). Cognitive-behaviour therapy for inpatients for psychosis and anger problems within a low secure environment. *Behavioural and Cognitive Psychotherapy.*

Haddock, G., & Tarrier, N. (1998). Assessment and formulation in the cognitive behavioural treatment of schizophrenia. In N. Tarrier, A. Wells, & G. Haddock (Eds.), *Treating complex cases: The cognitive behavioural therapy approach.* London, Wiley.

Haddock, G., Tarrier, N., Morrison, A., Hopkins, R., Drake, R., & Lewis, S. (1999). A pilot study evaluating the effectiveness of individual cognitive-behavioural interventions in early psychosis. *Social Psychiatry and Psychiatric Epidemiology, 34,* 255–258.

Halford, W. K., & Hayes, R. L. (1992). Social skills training with schizophrenic patients. In D. Kavanagh (Ed.), *Schizophrenia: An overview and practical handbook* (pp. 374–392). London: Chapman & Hall.

Kingdon, D. G., & Turkington, D. (1994). *Cognitive-behavioral therapy of schizophrenia.* Hove, UK: Erlbaum.

Legget, J. M., Hurn, C., & Goodman, W. (1997). Teaching psychological strategies for managing auditory hallucinations: A case report. *British Journal of Learning Disabilities, 25,* 158–162.

Lewis, S., Tarrier, N., Haddock, G., Bentall, R. P., Kinderman, P., Kingdon, D., et al. (2002). Randomised controlled trial of cognitive-behaviour therapy in early schizophrenia: Acute phase outcomes. *British Journal of Psychiatry, 181,* 91–97.

Miller, W. R., & Rollnick, S. (1991). *Motivational interviewing: Preparing people to change addictive behavior.* New York: Guilford Press.

Novaco, R. W. (1994). Anger as a risk factor for violence among the mentally disordered. In J. Monahan & H. J. Steadman (Eds.), *Violence and mental disorders: Developments in risk assessment* (pp. 21–59). Chicago, IL: University of Chicago Press.

Rector, N., & Beck, A. T. (2001). Cognitive behavior therapy for schizophrenia: An empirical review. *Journal of Nervous and Mental Disease, 189*(5), 278–287.

Stenfert-Kroese, B., Dagnan, D., & Loumidis, K. (Eds.). (1997). *Cognitive behavioural therapy for people with learning disabilities.* London: Routledge.

Tarrier, N., Yusupoff, L., Kinney, C., McCarthy, E., Gledhill, A., Haddock, G., & Morris, J. (1998). Randomised controlled trial of intensive cognitive behaviour therapy for chronic schizophrenia. *British Medical Journal, 317,* 303–307.

8

Bipolar Disorder

Cory F. Newman

Therapists who treat patients suffering from bipolar disorder can expect to have to deal with problematic episodes as a matter of course, as it is the exception to the rule that bipolar disorder is treated free of complications. For starters, bipolar disorder is difficult to diagnose accurately early in the course of the illness, when pharmacologic and psychosocial interventions may have their most positive, enduring impact. For example, the prevalence with which young children and adolescents develop bipolar disorder is still not well known (Berenson, 1998; Carlson, 2000; Weller, Weller, & Fristad, 1995). Some youngsters who evince symptoms that in adulthood would be considered signs of hypomania or mania are thought to have conduct disorders or attention-deficit/hyperactivity disorder (Barton, 2001; Bowden & Rhodes, 1996; Geller & Luby, 1997; Schneider, Atkinson, & El-Mallakh, 1996; West, McElroy, Strakowski, Keck, & McConville, 1995). Thus a golden opportunity for early intervention in bipolar disorder may be missed. Young adults who experience their first hypomanic or manic episode may not seek therapy and may later enter treatment only when they have plummeted into a clinical depression. Thus there is the risk that the given diagnosis will be major depression rather than bipolar disorder, which may lead to incomplete and even inappropriate treatment (e.g., antidepressant monotherapy, which may trigger a "switching" episode into mania; see Bauer et al., 1999). Given that only one manic episode—perhaps amid numerous depressive episodes—is necessary for a diagnosis of bipolar disorder (American Psychiatric Association, 1994), it is easy to see how the correct diagnosis can be missed. In this manner, the very first roadblock that therapists face is diagnostic accuracy and its attendant implications for early intervention.

Another fundamental difficulty in initiating the proper treatment for bipolar disorder is the propensity for patients to deny that they have the disorder (Jamison, 1995). If they are feeling depressed, they may insist that their problem is a clinical depression, which is arguably less stigmatic than full-fledged bipolar illness. They may therefore minimize the importance of past incidents of hypomanic or manic behavior, perhaps omitting them altogether in self-report at intake. Similarly, patients with bipolar disorder who are experiencing hypomania or mania may never think to seek therapy, owing to the fact that they are feeling so good at the time. It may be necessary for their friends, relatives, or other loved ones to cajole them into seeking the care of a mental health professional.

Assuming that the would-be patient actually makes it into a session with a mental health professional, the intake evaluation may reveal that symptom episodes have been occurring for many years. Perhaps the patient has been in and out of counseling many times in the past or has tried (and discontinued) a panoply of psychotropic medications and/or has been hospitalized on one or more occasions. Even more distressing, the patient may have a history of suicide attempts.

The purpose of this introduction is to convey that bipolar disorder is a serious adversary for patients, for important others in their lives, and for their treatment providers as well. Professionals who enter into a therapeutic relationship with patients with bipolar disorder need to find a way to maintain hope in the face of difficulties and to model optimism and perseverance in spite of setbacks. They must also be willing to deal with clinical crises, with patients' attempts at premature flight from therapy, with real and idiosyncratic difficulties with medications, and with other therapy-interfering behaviors.

COMMON ROADBLOCKS IN CONDUCTING COGNITIVE THERAPY COMBINED WITH MEDICATIONS

In particular, the high likelihood that the patient is on medications—or will need to be on medications for the long run—presents a number of challenges. Whether the patients receive their cognitive therapy and pharmacotherapy from one or multiple clinicians, a greater degree of difficulty in the delivery of the appropriate care is introduced into the treatment of bipolar disorder, as the following illustrates.

Coordination of Care with Another Professional

Bipolar disorder, similar to other conditions such as schizophrenia (in which biochemical abnormalities are well-established etiological and maintaining factors), almost always requires pharmacotherapy as part of the overall treatment plan (Goodwin & Jamison, 1990). Thus, unless the therapist is a psychiatrist, he or she will need to work in parallel with at least one other mental health professional in treating bipolar disorder. There is nothing inherently problematic with this situation in theory. In fact, it may be argued that having two professionals simultaneously treating a patient can be quite advantageous, inasmuch as they can provide greater vigilance and supervision in dealing with the clinical complications so common in bipolar disorder. In practice, however, the situation can be fraught with difficulties, from "benign" instances in which the psychiatrist and the nonpsychiatric therapist do not communicate with each other (and thus do not actively coordinate care) to more problematic instances in which the two professionals may unwittingly or deliberately undermine the patient's confidence in or compliance with the other's treatment recommendations. Thus it may be said that an unfortunate and needless roadblock in the care of patients with bipolar disorder is the insufficient collaboration between the clinician in charge of the pharmacotherapy and the one in charge of the cognitive therapy.

In order to provide patients with bipolar disorder with the advantages of multidisciplinary care minus the potential drawbacks (see Wright & Thase, 1992), the pharmacotherapist and the cognitive therapist need to create a plan of cooperation. Although very little has been written about this important topic, a new and promising model has recently been developed, based on the dual-provider care of chronically, severely depressed individuals (Moras & DeMartinis, 1999). The authors' manual states explicitly that "It is crucial to coordinate providers' interventions so that a consistent 'message' and intervention strategy [are] being given to the patient at all times" (p. 5). In the Moras and DeMartinis consultation model, points of disagreement or contention between the pharmacotherapist and cognitive therapist are dealt with in planned communications (e.g., phone calls, e-mails in which the patients' names are coded for confidentiality, or meetings in person if possible) so that a satisfactory resolution of clinical issues can be reached prior to their next sessions with the patient. Further, the model mandates communication between the providers in response to a number of clinical incidents, such as (but not limited to) the patient's failure to show up for a session, increased suicidality, therapy-interfering behaviors, negative feelings expressed about the other clinician, and so on.

Problematic Beliefs about Medication

Many patients with bipolar disorder have a difficult time coming to terms with the biochemical abnormalities inherent in their disorder, and they may either resent and/or reject the need for medication. As patients with bipolar disorder who go off their medications are at high risk for symptomatic relapse (Silverstone & Romans-Clarkson, 1989; Strober, Morrell, Lampert, & Burroughs, 1990), their negative beliefs about pharmacotherapy are high-priority roadblocks that need to be hurdled in order for therapy to proceed with the best chance of success.

Before we as therapists can persuade our patients to collaborate positively in their pharmacotherapy, we need to be open to hearing their complaints about the medications. Not all negative reactions to medications are cognitive distortions. We cannot merely patronize our patients by giving them rote platitudes about the need to take their pills without also striving to understand their fears, misgivings, and opinions about the matter. Therapists have to remember that pharmacotherapy, like psychotherapy, is an inexact science, and sometimes the patients have adverse reactions to their medications that signify that a change is necessary. We also have to bear in mind that few people would ever volunteer to take medications such as lithium or divalproex unless their health or their very lives depended on it. Part of our job is to empathize with this reality and to help our patients to come to terms with the fact that the stakes are indeed very high.

At the same time that we are trying to understand our patients' legitimate complaints about the side effects of their medications, we are also on the lookout for overt statements (or implicit beliefs) indicating that patients misunderstand the purpose, function, effects, and/or meaning of their pharmacotherapy. When therapists spot such misapprehensions, it is important to address the issue head on, with tact and care. The following is a short sampling of some problematic beliefs that patients with bipolar disorder sometimes entertain about their medications (see Newman, Leahy, Beck, Reilly-Harrington, & Gyulai, 2001; Wright & Schrodt, 1989):

- "Medication will turn me into a different person and cause me to lose my 'true' self."
- "Medication will take away all my creativity and energy."
- "I might get addicted to my medication and wind up being worse off."
- "Taking medications means that my doctors are 'controlling' me."

It is important for therapists to identify and address such beliefs as they would any other maladaptive belief in cognitive therapy. For example, therapists can help their patients to reframe beliefs such as the aforementioned, to look for the evidence that supports or refutes such beliefs, and to do the all-important behavioral experiment of trying the medications for an appropriate length of time before passing judgment so that the patients see for themselves whether or not their fears are coming true. Sometimes it is useful simply to offer psychoeducational materials[1] of the sort that would dis-

[1] The Lithium Information Center at the Madison (Wisconsin) Institute of Medicine is an excellent resource for pamphlets on lithium and other pharmacologic agents. The overarching Web site through which one may contact this center is: *www.miminc.org*.

abuse patients of the mistaken notion that medications such as lithium could be "addictive." At other times it is helpful to direct them to the writings of Kay Jamison (1993, 1995), who argues eloquently that one's intelligence and creative process suffer far more from the complications and dementing process of an inadequately controlled bipolar illness than from the salubrious effects of the proper pharmacotherapy.

When patients express the belief that their medications take away their "true self," they are often overlooking some very important data that need to be brought to their attention in a tactful way. For example, some of the behavior of which the patients may be most ashamed may have occurred during previous bouts of uncontrolled mania. Would the patients aver that this medication-free, undercontrolled behavior reflected the best of their ideals? On the other hand, patients may have experienced periods of symptom quiescence owing (at least in part) to following their prescriptions. In the absence of depression or mania, the persons may have been free to live their lives as they would do so normally, without the obvious yoke of a serious illness encumbering their actions, judgment, and capabilities. Our hope is to demonstrate that an active, untempered manic-depressive illness itself is perhaps the greatest threat to the patients' identity, not its pharmacotherapy.

Therapists should also be on the lookout for problematic beliefs that patients maintain about the interaction between the prescription of medications and the therapeutic relationship. For example, a patient may believe that by taking his medications faithfully he is being unduly "controlled" by his therapists. Thus, issues of choice and autonomy need to be addressed—for example, to what degree this patient believes he is giving up his freedom by "following doctor's orders" and to what degree he is giving up his freedom if his moods go unchecked. Similarly, a patient may believe that if she tries a medication that does not bring about a full remission of the illness, this means that the therapist does not care and/or is not competent; thus there is little or no point in continuing in a collaborative therapeutic relationship. It is a very sensitive issue—but one that warrants addressing—that some degree of trial and error is involved even in the best of therapeutic relationships, indeed, in any relationship. Thus, medication difficulties do not have to damage the patient's and therapist's mutual quest to help the patient achieve a substantial remission.

Symptom "Breakthrough" in Spite of Faithful Adherence to Treatment

Patients with bipolar disorder sometimes have the disconcerting experience of engaging in treatment with energy, commitment, and hope, only to have symptoms break through once again nonetheless. This can be extraordinarily demoralizing for patients, especially if it happens more than once. Similarly, patients whose medications and ongoing cognitive therapy are succeeding in keeping them out of full-blown manic or depressive episodes may still experience subsyndromal symptoms and lament the fact that for all their participation in treatment they are still not symptom free (see Gitlin, Swendsen, Heller, & Hammen, 1995: Keller et al., 1992; Robb, Cooke, Devins, Young, & Joffe, 1997).

As a result, some patients adopt a problematic shift in their approach to their treatment—to wit, that if they are going to have to deal with residual and/or breakthrough symptoms of bipolar disorder, then they are not going to volunteer their participation in treatment. This reaction, born of understandable frustration, represents "all-or-none" thinking at its pernicious worst. When patients with bipolar disorder experience setbacks in symptomatology, it does not logically follow that treatment is useless. There are alternative hypotheses to consider, such as the idea that residual and breakthrough symptoms require an adjustment in medication(s) and/or in the treatment plan, not an abandonment of either. Similarly, it is reasonable to posit that with steadfast perseverance with the full treatment regimen, even during periods of symptom exacerbation, the combined forces of cognitive therapy and pharmacotherapy can help keep the patient's condition from worsening even further and may be a boon to a quicker recovery from the episode. Sadly, if the patients act on their all-or-none beliefs by slacking off or neglecting their treatment, they may produce the self-fulfilling prophecy of worsening their condition, an outcome that they may attribute erroneously to such factors as "life being hopeless" or their illness being "beyond anything anyone can do."

Therapists need to educate their patients that their responses to treatment will not be perfect and that the symptoms that stubbornly persist or worsen in spite of taking their medications and learning the tools of cognitive therapy perhaps require reassessments and modifications in their treatment, not a hopeless dismissal thereof. In the process of discussing this concept with their patients, therapists must be highly sensitive to the frustration and even grief that patients with bipolar disorder experience when they are trying their best and are still not feeling optimally well. Therapists would do well to keep in mind that our goal is not merely to help patients to reduce or eliminate active symptom episodes but to help them improve the quality of their lives overall.

Negative Reactions to Side Effects

Yet another roadblock to successful treatment is the situation in which patients are experiencing tangible benefits from the overall treatment regimen but the specific side effects from their medication(s) are difficult to bear. At times, this is not merely a subjective impression—there is an objective, medical necessity to discontinue a medication that otherwise is doing a great job. For example, a patient may be very pleased with his initial response to lamotrigine (Lamictal), only to have to discontinue it in response to a severe rash—a rare but serious side effect of lamotrigine (Buzan & Dubovsky, 1998; Calabrese et al., 1999).

More frequent than the preceding example are those instances in which no medical necessity exists to discontinue a medication but the patient wishes to do so nonetheless. If therapists simply exhort such patients to stay on their medications, they run the risk of getting into power struggles with their patients or losing them from treatment. The approach that is more compatible with the tenor of cognitive therapy is to engage the patients in a careful weighing of the pros and cons of being on medications and being off them (see Wright & Schrodt, 1989). This strategy involves two-way psychoeducation. First, the patients are invited to explore their own pasts, and to tell the therapist about previous experiences in being on and off medications, for better or worse, respectively. Second, the therapist informs the patient about what to expect from the pharmacotherapy—for example, that side effects may predominate at the start but that therapeutic effects will be more prominent over the subsequent few weeks. Such information may prevent patients from assuming erroneously that their new medicine is more trouble than it is worth before ever seeing what benefits actually could accrue.

In any event, medication side effects can be a troublesome roadblock in the treatment of bipolar disorder (Bauer & McBride, 1996), and cognitive therapists must be alert to address this issue, even if the therapist cannot give direct advice without the official endorsement of the prescribing physician. By being willing to look at the data, rather than just instructing patients to take their medications without question, therapists strengthen the therapeutic relationship, assist the patients in getting the proper adjustments in their pharmacotherapy, and provide an appropriate model for an open-minded, empirical approach to treatment. Patients are then perhaps more receptive to an examination of their beliefs about their medications and their side effects to see if they may be judging the medications harshly and/or prematurely.

Belief That Problems Are "All Biochemical"

Although many patients—for some of the reasons described earlier, as well as others—are reluctant to treat their symptoms pharmacologically, others take a contrasting view. These are the patients who understand well that bipolar disorder has a strong biochemical component but who take this knowledge to the extreme and believe erroneously that psychosocial factors are irrelevant. Such patients may be willing to engage in pharmacotherapy but are less inclined to take part in cognitive therapy, believing that "talking about the illness doesn't do anything."

Before we quickly pass judgment on this "anti–cognitive therapy" belief, we would do well to understand how the patients have come to this conclusion. Many will tell us that when they feel the crushing depths of depression or the wild ecstasy of full-blown mania, they are impervious to the entreaties of others, including therapists. In their experience, extremes of mood operate on their own timetable, without rhyme or reason, resulting in the patients' not being able to alter their functioning by dint of will, reason, or knowledge. They will tell their therapists flat out that when they are depressed, no words can either console or cajole them out of their vegetative, morbid, hopeless, and helpless states. Similarly, these patients maintain steadfastly that when they are manic, they are beyond anyone's control and restraint, including their own. Thus, they reason, talk therapy is superfluous.

In response to this belief (which may or may not be overtly articulated by the patients), therapists need to introduce four lines of discussion into the therapeutic agenda: (1) the connection between mind and body, (2) the role of life events in influencing depressive and manic reactions, (3) the importance of recognizing early warning signs (or "prodromes") of impending symptom episodes, and (4) the usefulness of psychological coping skills in managing an illness.

The Mind–Body Connection

Therapists can teach their patients with bipolar disorder the concept of "diathesis–stress." Many medical maladies involve a combination of genetic–biochemical predisposition, and the activation of this potential illness through subjective stressors. The key word here is "subjective," and this is where talk therapy such as cognitive therapy comes in. If patients can learn methods to reconstrue their cognitive triad (views of oneself, the world, and one's future; see Beck, 1976) in a more constructive, hopeful way, there is reason to believe that the biochemical effects can be muted. If patients are interested, they can be made aware of some of the data in the field of obsessive–compulsive disorder (OCD) treatment, in which psychosocial and pharmacologic treatments resulted in similar changes in glucose metabolism in the brain, as seen via PET scans (Baxter et al., 1992). Additionally, patients can be introduced to the behavioral medicine literature, in which (for example) psychosocial methods often are used successfully to combat chronic pain (Dowd, 2001; Eimer & Freeman, 1998; Turk & Feldman, 2000). Thus cognitive therapy and medications can both work on the "biochemical problem."

Life Events and Bipolar Symptoms

One of the chief functions of cognitive therapy is to help patients deal with life events that tax their coping skills. Likewise, cognitive therapy helps patients to learn ways to steer clear of avoidable difficult life events. As there is a substantial literature on the hazardous impact of stressful life events on the onset of both depressive and manic episodes (e.g., Alloy, Reilly-Harrington, Fresco, Whitehouse, & Zechmeister, 1999; Hammen & Gitlin, 1997; Johnson & Miller, 1997; Johnson & Roberts, 1995; Reilly-Harrington, Alloy, Fresco, & Whitehouse, 1999), it is particularly important for patients with bipolar disorder to simplify their lives as much as they can while they are in vulnerable states. For example, one of the principles outlined by Newman and colleagues (2001) is that people who are experiencing labile emotions should try to refrain from making big life decisions until their moods are on solid ground again. By averting potentially stressful life demands and consequences (such as from an impulsively quit job, an abandoned relationship, or a major financial investment), patients can help reduce the chances that harmful biochemical changes will occur or worsen.

Recognition of Prodromes

There is evidence that patients with bipolar disorder who are taught to identify the early warning signs of their mood abnormalities—especially in the manic direction—benefit in a number of ways that would not be predicted by the periodicity of the mood swings alone. In particular, studies such as those conducted by Smith and Tarrier (1992), Palmer and Williams (1997), Lam and Wong (1997), and Perry, Tarrier, Morriss, McCarthy, and Limb (1999) collectively have found that patients who have learned this self-assessment skill are more apt to maintain fidelity to their pharmacotherapy, to show more willingness to moderate their activity level, and to demonstrate greater adeptness in social functioning. Further, they are less likely to go into the hospital than those patients who are less well prepared to spot their prodromal symptoms. Thus, a psychosocial model of therapy such as cognitive therapy has much to offer even the patient who has seemingly inevitable mood swings.

Benefits of Learning Psychological Skills

A familiar refrain from cognitive therapists who find themselves defending the efficacy of their approach against those who maintain that only somatic treatments can help serious psychiatric disorders is "Pills don't teach skills." It is not enough to regulate someone's neurotransmitters; one must also teach the patient to navigate life's demands more effectively. Many patients with bipolar disorder, in the absence of effective psychosocial treatment, make their mood problems worse by taking an all-or-none view of their condition (e.g., "Now that I have made a bad decision, everything is ruined, so I might as well throw caution to the wind and do whatever I please") and by failing to engage in the principles of "damage control" (e.g., "There is no way I can solve this problem, so I'm not even going to try anymore"). Cognitive therapy helps patients with bipolar disorder to keep problems contained as much as possible by teaching the patients to utilize psychological skills such as rational responding, problem solving, assertiveness, and tactful communication. Even if one takes the position that mood swings are biologically autonomous phenomena, it is still reasonable to hypothesize that the *amplitude* and *duration* of these swings can be attenuated to the extent that the patients use powerful self-help skills (such as those just mentioned) in the process.

ROADBLOCKS HAVING TO DO WITH PESSIMISM, FATALISM, AND HELPLESSNESS

Patients who battle bipolar disorder face a tough, long-term fight. Although the reward for persevering through this struggle can be nothing short of a rescued life, the process can be grueling and demoralizing at times. Patients with bipolar disorder sometimes grow weary and cynical about ever being able to get a leg up on their illness, and they lapse into despair.

Stigma, Denial, and Shame

It is very difficult to admit that one has bipolar disorder and to deal with its ramifications, and it is very easy to deny it. Part of the problem, as mentioned earlier, is the difficulty in making an early diagnosis of the illness. By the time people have come to the realization that they actually have a bipolar illness, they may have believed for years that they simply had bouts of depression, or attention-deficit problems, or a "temperamental nature." There is still a stigma attached to bipolar illness—the brave attempts by talented, accomplished persons who have disclosed their manic–depression to the public notwithstanding—and this adds to the patient's dread in coming to terms with what it means to have bipolar disorder (see Corrigan, 1998; Lundin, 1998).

It is extremely unfortunate that persons with bipolar disorder often have to face the prospect of subtle and not-so-subtle discrimination in terms of employment, advanced schooling, housing, and the attitudes of some family, friends, and acquaintances (Corrigan, 1998). Arguably, however, the worst form of stigma is *self-stigma* (Newman et al., 2001), which involves people maintaining judgmental views about themselves (e.g., "I'm a chronic loser"), feeling ashamed of their illness, and withdrawing from relationships and opportunities for success in life. Although it may be true that therapists and their patients cannot change (i.e., humanize and demystify) society's views of mental illness in one fell swoop, they can begin this process one person at a time, starting with the patients themselves.

Although there are many ways that patients with bipolar disorder demonstrate their self-stigmatic beliefs, some of the most common—and problematic—are (1) constant, frequent, implicit, and explicit self-labeling in denigrating ways; (2) shunning involvement in support groups; (3) refusal to engage in treatment, as it "reminds" them of their illness; and (4) assuming they will fail and thus giving up before they try to achieve important goals.

Self-Labeling

One of the ways that stigma harms people is by robbing them of their individuality. The person becomes lumped in with a group, and that group is assumed to have uniformly undesirable qualities. In the case of bipolar disorder, the person becomes "a manic–depressive," rather than someone who has strengths, weaknesses, hopes, and dreams, just like anybody else—and who happens to be struggling with a serious psychiatric illness that needs long-term treatment. When therapists hear their patients engaging in self-stereotyping, they should take the cue to ask the patients to take stock of themselves more completely, such as by taking inventory of their interests, relationships, accomplishments, philosophies of life, and goals. Thus the patient who heretofore has dubbed herself a "manic–depressive sad sack" may now view herself as a "sardonic, poetic, animal-loving naturalist who likes New Age music, peace and quiet, and intellectual conversation—and who needs treatment for bipolar disorder."

Shunning Involvement with Support Groups

Some patients with bipolar disorder are fortunate (or skilled) enough to have sufficient social support within their families or among their longtime companions and friends. However, even these people, and especially those who do *not* have such positive, interpersonal attachments, should be apprised of the availability of support groups, as social support has been shown to be a boon to the well-being of patients with bipolar disorder over the course of their illness (Johnson, Winett, Meyer, Greenhouse, & Miller, 1999). These include such organizations as the National Alliance for the Mentally Ill (NAMI) and the National Depressive and Manic–Depressive Association (NDMDA),[2] each of which have hundreds of chapters through-

---

[2] *www.nami.org*; *www.ndmda.org*.

out North America and beyond. When individual patients balk at the suggestion that they attend meetings of groups such as these, it may be a sign that the patients themselves are buying into stigma. Upon questioning, a patient may admit that he does not want to "associate with a bunch of social misfits." Clearly, the patient who says this is not evaluating people with bipolar disorder as individuals and is not accepting membership in the now-devalued group. This problem needs to be addressed in session so that the patients can see the potential benefits in meeting with people who understand the illness firsthand and who may have a lot to offer in terms of support and suggestion, without assuming that everyone in the group has a global adaptive functioning (GAF) rating in the lower ranges.

Treatment Refusal

When patients miss sessions, are absent from treatment for significant stretches, and/or are less than diligent in taking their prescribed medications, it represents a most significant and fundamental roadblock to treatment. When such a patient actually attends a cognitive therapy session, the therapist needs to seize the moment and address the issue of self-stigma. In other words, it is vital to put forth the hypothesis that at least one of the reasons that the patients are refusing to engage in treatment is that they do not wish to be reminded of their illness and do not want to face the realization of its implications. Often, patients will admit that they feel stigmatized by taking medication or by sitting in a therapist's waiting room. However, they fail to see the irony in their decision to avoid treatment. If they engage in treatment, the stigma may be theirs alone to manage, because their public behavior will be normative as a result of their pharmacotherapy and cognitive therapy. However, by neglecting their therapies, they run the very great risk of making their symptoms worse, and doing so in ways that will be quite conspicuous to others. Thus they will fulfill the prophecy of their fear of stigma. The conclusion is clear—involvement in the proper treatment reduces the risk of shameful, regretful public occurrences. By "reminding themselves" that they are battling bipolar disorder, patients lessen the likelihood that they will unwittingly remind others.

Giving Up Too Soon

Patients with bipolar disorder face the balancing act of needing to take their illness and their treatment seriously without letting the disorder become a reason to abandon the pursuit of personal goals. Although bipolar disorder can disrupt people's lives, it does not have to diminish their capacity for love, learning, faith, striving, and contributing to humankind. Unfortunately, when patients have experienced significant losses and interruptions in their life's trajectory, they can grow to feel helpless and thus may choose to withdraw from active participation in the world. This is a major roadblock for therapy, for it is the patients' steadfast pursuit of meaningful activities and goals that can help them to weather their periodic setbacks and to continue their quest for joy and a sense of mastery. Again, the therapist's task is to help the patients view *themselves* as being in charge of their lives—not the bipolar illness, nor the treatment, and certainly not a cruel Fate. One of the basic components of this approach is to encourage and assist patients in formulating and striving toward personal goals, taking the bipolar disorder and its treatment into account but not as exclusion criteria for having a life.

It should be noted that cognitive therapy itself takes an approach to treatment that is inherently empowering for patients and thus combats stigma (Lam, Jones, Hayward, & Bright, 1999). Patients are active participants in their treatment; they engage in self-help assignments between sessions, collaborate in the treatment plan, and become more and more autonomous in setting the session agenda as therapy progresses. Such a model for therapy promotes self-efficacy, hopefulness, and self-acceptance.

Hopelessness and Suicidality

Bipolar disorder can be lethal. Conservative figures place the lifetime suicide rate for people with manic–depression at 15% (Simpson & Jamison, 1999), and this high figure includes those who receive treatment. There are many hypotheses as to why this is the case (see Newman et al., 2001). First, the depressive episodes can be particularly crushing, made even worse by the realization of the damage that has been wrought by a previous manic episode (Jamison, 1995). Regardless of whether or not there is a qualitative difference between the subjective despair of the bipolar depressive patient and the unipolar depressive patient, there are issues pertaining to the course of the illness and its psychosocial impact that may account for the suicidogenic nature of bipolar disorder.

For example, in a study of completed suicides, the histories of those with unipolar depression were compared with those who had bipolar disorder (Isometsä, Heikkinen, Henriksson, Aro, & Lonnqvist, 1995). The bipolar sufferers were found to have had relatively more divorces, longer treatment histories, and more hospitalizations than those with unipolar depression. In other words, though both groups of individuals had subjective reasons for wanting to kill themselves, the patients with bipolar disorder may have actually had more objective, negative life events leading up to the suicide. Thus, therapists must be prepared to help patients with bipolar disorder come to terms with very real losses in their lives and in doing so still maintain hopefulness for an improved future. Further, patients with bipolar disorder face a war against mood abnormalities on two fronts and thus may feel frightened of the prospects of mania whenever they emerge from a depressive episode. This means that they find little sense of security, no matter what the state of their moods. The cyclical course of the illness makes it even more difficult for patients with bipolar disorder to trust that they will "settle into" a normal life for any substantial period of time before another episode interferes with their important life roles, such as student, employee, spouse, or parent. The collective result may be a sense of resignation and hopelessness.

The data are very clear that hopelessness is downright dangerous. Simply put, the construct of hopelessness (e.g., as measured by inventories such as the Beck Hopelessness Scale; Beck, Weissman, Lester, & Trexler, 1974) is a very important factor in predicting who will be at risk for suicide (Beck, Brown, Berchick, Stewart, & Steer, 1990; Beck, Brown, Steer, Dahlsgaard, & Grisham, 1999; Beck, Steer, Beck, & Newman, 1993). It has also been found that hopelessness is an important predictor of suicide risk even during those times when patients are not in the active episodes of a mood disorder (Young et al., 1996). In other words, a patient's baseline propensity for hopelessness (in everyday life) is potentially as important to assess as the sensitivity to increased hopelessness patients may show in active phases of their mood disorder. Thus, whether a patient with bipolar disorder is actively suicidal or not, clinicians can stay one step ahead of potential crisis by routinely monitoring their patients' views about the future, including their goals and plans.

A thorough overview of antisuicidality techniques for bipolar disorder is beyond the scope of this paper (for a more complete review, see Ellis & Newman, 1996; Newman, in press). Suffice it to say that it is helpful to do as many of the following as possible:

1. Assess the patient's hopelessness on a regular basis, both during and between active symptom episodes.
2. Assess and rigorously discuss the evidence for and against the patient's beliefs about suicide, such as, "My loved ones would be better off without me," "The only way to solve my problems is to get rid of them by dying," "I can only stop my emotional pain through ceasing to be," and "I hate myself, and I deserve to die," among others.
3. Increase the patients' engagement in activities that put them in contact with appropriate social supports.
4. Encourage the patients' involvement in activities that represent the "simple pleasures" of life and that create a mild to moderate sense of "mastery" (including the accomplishment of restraining oneself from impulsive actions that could cause harm).
5. Assist the patients in developing, improving, and utilizing problem-solving and communications skills.
6. Examine the pros and cons of living and dying for the patients themselves and for the loved ones left behind, now and in the distant future.

All of these strategies create attachments to life and gnaw away at the metaphorical rope that would pull patients ever closer to suicide. The goal is not merely to survive—it is to live a better life and to take the leap of faith that by working hard in therapy (and by taking the proper medications) patients can actively improve their lot to a significant degree.

ROADBLOCKS PERTAINING TO CONTROL AND AUTONOMY

Sometimes individuals with bipolar disorder view their treatment as interfering with their freedom to conduct their lives as they see fit. They may resent the fact that they have to go for frequent therapy appointments, that they have to take medications and get blood tests, or that they have to monitor their medication side effects, not to mention their moods, thoughts, and behaviors.

Reluctance to Relinquish the "Highs"

Some patients with bipolar disorder do not wish to pursue the therapeutic goal of inhibiting their hypomanic and manic states, arguing that the "highs" provide them with unmatched joy, energy, power, creativity, and insight. In some respects this aspect is similar to the allure of certain illicit drugs (e.g., stimulants such as amphetamines or cocaine), whereby the intense, immediate gratification is so compelling that people are willing to damage their lives in order to pursue the extreme euphoric states again and again. Jamison (1995) notes that a manic high is extremely seductive and that therapists would do well to acknowledge the sacrifice that patients with bipolar disorder are being asked to make when they undertake treatment to moderate their moods.

One of the ways to address this problem is to look at the flip side of the mania—namely, the inevitable depressive crash. Therapists can explain to their patients that the goal of treatment is not to rob them of joy but rather to spare them the misery of the aftermath of mania. As Jamison (1995) has explained with such poignant clarity, individuals in a manic state scarcely realize the damage they are doing to their lives, and they may seem not to care, but the ensuing depressive episode makes it abundantly clear what horrors they have wrought—credit cards tapped out, relationships damaged via angry outbursts and sexual improprieties, jobs impulsively quit, the backlash of public humiliation, impossible schemes in progress, and so on. As with illicit drug abuse, the price is simply too high. The pursuit of "normal" degrees of happiness can avert the misery described here, but the excessive highs of mania must be a target of intervention.

Another way to deal with patients' desire to keep their occasional manic states is to look at their beliefs about their moods and about treatment. For example, some people believe they cannot be creative if they are not manic. Others will contend that the only way to catch up with all the obligations and demands to which they could not attend while they were depressed is to maximize their manias. They then stay up all night, cram all their tasks and projects into a short space of time, and try desperately to get as much out of life as they can until the next depressive crash. Others take a more libertarian approach, believing that they have a basic right to their moods and that well-meaning others should leave them alone to live their lives as they see fit.

Such beliefs can be evaluated just as any other potentially problematic belief in cognitive therapy. The therapist does not use heavy-handed methods to browbeat the patients into accepting treatment but rather uses more subtle, collaborative means, such as by taking a historical view of the patient's life for clues about the pros and cons of mania and the pros and cons of active engagement in treatment. Similarly, they can look at the quality of the patients' most important relationships and how mood swings affect these personal ties. Therapists can assist their patients in looking for evidence that they can experience a sense of happiness, energy, creative thinking, and connection to important others without the consequences, if they are willing to compromise. Once again, the works of Jamison (1993, 1995) are valuable resources. In *Touched With Fire* (1993), patients can read compelling arguments about how certain great writers and artists actually lost more than they gained as a result of uncontrolled mania in their lifetimes. In *An Unquiet Mind* (1995), Jamison stresses—from both an expert professional and an "expert patient" point of view—that there is much to enjoy in life without deliberately taking the hellish risks associated with full-blown mania.

It may also be possible to appeal to the patients' care and concern for their loved ones—to wit, that it would be in the best interest of their parents, spouses, children, and so forth if they invested themselves optimally in their treatment. If the patients grew up in a household with a manic–depressive parent, this argument may be that much more compelling. For example, the patient whose father had uncontrolled bipolar disorder may have had a miserable childhood of turmoil and crisis. However, the patient may be able to spare his own children the same horrors by transcending his father, through adhering to his pharmacotherapy and cognitive therapy.

Family Issues

Bipolar disorder is often a family affair, either because more than one more person in the family has the diagnosis (Brent, Bridge, Johnson, & Connolly, 1996; Coryell, Endicott, Andreason, & Keller, 1985; DePaolo, Simpson, Folstein, & Folstein, 1989), or because the family member who is symptomatic gets into negative interactions with the others. Both the patients and their family members suffer from the effects of the bipolar disorder, especially when they live together. For example, family members may have to contend with their manic–depressive relative's excessive spending, irritability, reckless behavior, legal troubles, sexual infidelity, and risk for self-harm, among other major problems. In turn, the individuals with bipolar disorder often have to contend with family members hounding them to go to sleep at night, to take their medications, to get off the phone or computer, to be quiet, to act "more responsibly," to "go see the doctor," and other similar (seemingly overcontrolling) directives. In such cases, both the patients with bipolar disorder and their families are under increased stress, and their negative interactions can escalate and aggravate each other further (Miklowitz & Goldstein, 1997).

When persons with bipolar disorder become involved in conflictual relationships with their families, feelings of blame, shame, frustration, anxiety, and helplessness may abound. The parties may each make negative attributions about the other, such as when the patient believes his parents enjoy making his life miserable with their restrictions, whereas the parents believe that their son's mania is deliberately spiteful behavior that he could stop "if he wanted to" (Miklowitz, Wendel, & Simoneau, 1998; Wendel & Miklowitz, 1997). Such a scenario can create significant roadblocks in therapy, as patients may drop out of treatment to reassert "control" against family members or may relapse due to an exacerbation of stress at home. They may also spend their time in session railing against family members rather than focusing on themselves.

First, therapists need to try to comprehend the family interactions through the eyes of their patients and to communicate this understanding. Having done so, therapists then have more leverage to ask their patients to try to view the contentious situations from their family's position. The goal is to spread around the responsibility for the problems at home, while also rejecting the notion that anybody is acting out of malice. Rather, it is often true that families are acting out of anxiety, that the patients are acting out of a sense of being controlled, and that all are experiencing frustration and desperation. Second, therapists can assist patients in learning some basic communication and interpersonal problem-solving skills (see Dattilio & Padesky, 1990), often by utilizing role playing in session. Third, the therapist should be brave enough to consider inviting the relatives (e.g., spouse, parents) to sessions, along with the patient, for couple or family therapy, with the consent of the patient. Here, therapists have the advantage of making a direct assessment of family interactions and can test interventions *in vivo*, with the relevant parties present.

Many patients with bipolar disorder experience conflicts with family members over their medications. The problems run the entire gamut, from families who actively discourage their relatives with bipolar disorder from being on medications (perhaps as a result of their own denial or in response to the implied stigma for the family) to those who are so frightened of the patients' extreme symptoms that they overbearingly micromanage the patients' use of medications to the point that the patients become resentful.

In the event that a patient is in fact going through some conflict with family members over taking medication, it is reasonable to assume that the patient may perceive the therapist's approach to the pharmacotherapy in a similar light. For example, a patient who asserts herself at home with her domineering husband may be met with his snappy retort, "You're getting manic again—you had better take your medications!" This patient may then feel unduly controlled and patronized in similar fashion by her therapist, who—unlike the husband in this example—is actually well intentioned in asking questions and making suggestions about the patient's pharmacotherapy. If the therapist understands that the patient's husband uses his wife's bipolar diagnosis and involvement in pharmacotherapy as a weapon to demean and punish her when she questions his "authority," he or she will be in a position to express accurate empathy in the course of discussing the sensitive issues surrounding the medication.

Patients' Belief That Treatment May Be Stopped

When patients seek treatment for their bipolar disorder, it is unlikely that they are eager to sign on for a lifetime of treatment. They may be hopeful that a circumscribed period of therapy and/or medication will cure them, whereupon they can leave treatment and go about their business without the burden of the illness or the treatment. This is understandable but not the way bipolar disorder works.

Treatment is long term, by necessity. When patients "feel better," it is a positive development but not a signal that therapy and/or medications should stop (Goodwin & Jamison, 1990; Jamison & Akiskal, 1983). Unfortunately, many patients with bipolar disorder find out the hard way that they are *not* "fine" and that their improved condition is just that—an improved *condition* that continues to require care. If they leave treatment, it is likely that before long they will become symptomatic again, and they may suffer needless setbacks that can be demoralizing and sometimes dangerous.

As part of the psychoeducation process at the start of therapy, therapists should apprise their patients with bipolar disorder of the need for a longitudinal approach to care. Periods during which the patients are feeling stable and hopeful can be times to hypothesize that the medications are doing their job properly (and therefore should be continued), as well as times to work on maintenance-of-gains issues in therapy. The hope is that when patients begin to show signs of improvement, they will not abandon their medication or their cognitive therapy. Rather, they will stay the course with their medications, and they will utilize cognitive therapy sessions at least in the manner of booster sessions. Thus, needless relapses may be averted.

REFERENCES

Alloy, L. B., Reilly-Harrington, N. A., Fresco, D. M., Whitehouse, W. G., & Zechmeister, J. S. (1999). Cognitive styles and life events in subsyndromal unipolar and bipolar disorders: Stability and prospective prediction of depressive and hypomanic mood swings. *Journal of Cognitive Psychotherapy: An International Quarterly, 13,* 21–40.

American Psychiatric Association. (1994). *Diagnostic and statistical manual of mental disorders* (4th ed.). Washington, DC: Author.

Barton, L. (2001). Attention deficit hyperactivity disorder (ADHD) and bipolar disorder in children and their coexisting comorbidity: A challenge for family counselors. *Family Journal: Counseling and Therapy for Couples and Families, 9*(4), 424–430.

Bauer, M. S., Callahan, A. M., Jampala, C., Petty, F., Sajatovic, M., Schaefer, V., et al. (1999). Clinical practice guidelines for bipolar disorder from the Department of Veterans Affairs. *Journal of Clinical Psychiatry, 60,* 9–21.

Bauer, M. S., & McBride, L. (1996). *Structured group psychotherapy for bipolar disorder: The life goals program.* New York: Springer.

Baxter, L. R., Schwartz, J. M., Bergman, K. S., Szuba, M. P., Guze, B. H., & Mazziotta, J. C. (1992). Caudate glucose metabolic rate changes with both drug and behavior therapy for obsessive–compulsive disorder. *Archives of General Psychiatry, 49*(9), 681–689.

Beck, A. T. (1976). *Cognitive therapy and the emotional disorders.* New York: International Universities Press.

Beck, A. T., Brown, G., Berchick, R. J., Stewart, B. L., & Steer, R. A. (1990). Relationship between hopelessness and ultimate suicide: A replication with psychiatric outpatients. *American Journal of Psychiatry, 147,* 190–195.

Beck, A. T., Brown, G. K., Steer, R. A., Dahlsgaard, K. K., & Grisham, J. R. (1999). Suicide ideation at its worst point: A predictor of eventual suicide in psychiatric outpatients. *Suicide and Life-Threatening Behavior, 29*(1), 1–9.

Beck, A. T., Steer, R. A., Beck, J. S., & Newman, C. F. (1993). Hopelessness, depression, suicidal ideation, and clinical diagnosis of depression. *Suicide and Life-Threatening Behavior, 23,* 139–145.

Beck, A. T., Weissman, A., Lester, D., & Trexler, L. (1974). The measurement of pessimism: The Hopelessness Scale. *Journal of Consulting and Clinical Psychology, 42,* 861–865.

Berenson, C. K. (1998). Frequently missed diagnoses in adolescent psychiatry. *Psychiatric Clinics of North America, 21*(4), 917–926.

Bowden, C. L., & Rhodes, L. J. (1996). Mania in children and adolescents: Recognition and treatment. *Psychiatric Annals, 26*(7, Suppl.), S430–S434.

Brent, D. A., Bridge, J., Johnson, B. A., & Connolly, J. (1996). Suicidal behavior runs in families: A controlled family study of adolescent suicide victims. *Archives of General Psychiatry, 53,* 1145–1152.

Buzan, R. D., & Dubovsky, S. L. (1998). Recurrence of lamotrigine-associated rash with rechallenge. *Journal of Clinical Psychiatry, 59*(2), 87.

Calabrese, J. R., Bowden, C. L., McElroy, S. L., Cookson, J., Anderson, J., Keck, P. E., et al. (1999). Spectrum of activity of lamotrigine in treatment-refractory bipolar disorder. *American Journal of Psychiatry, 156*(7), 1019–1023.

Carlson, G. A. (2000). Very-early-onset bipolar disorder: Does it exist? In J. L. Rapoport (Ed.), *Childhood onset of "adult" psychopathology: Clinical and re-*

search advances. American Psychopathological Association Series (pp. 303–329). Washington, DC: American Psychiatric Press.

Corrigan, P. W. (1998). The impact of stigma on severe mental illness. *Cognitive and Behavioral Practice, 5,* 201–222.

Coryell, W., Endicott, J., Andreason, N., & Keller, M. (1985). Bipolar I, bipolar II, and nonbipolar major depression among the relatives of affectively ill probands. *American Journal of Psychiatry, 142,* 817–821.

Dattilio, F. M., & Padesky, C. (1990). *Cognitive therapy with couples.* Sarasota, FL: Professional Resource Exchange.

DePaolo, J. R., Simpson, S. G., Folstein, S., & Folstein, M. (1989). The new genetics of bipolar affective disorder: Clinical implications. *Clinical Chemistry, 35*(7), B28–B32.

Dowd, E. T. (2001). Cognitive hypnotherapy in the management of pain. *Journal of Cognitive Psychotherapy: An International Quarterly, 15*(2), 87–97.

Eimer, B. N., & Freeman, A. M. (1998). *Pain management psychotherapy: A practical guide.* New York: Wiley.

Ellis, T. E., & Newman, C. F. (1996). *Choosing to live: How to defeat suicide through cognitive therapy.* Oakland, CA: New Harbinger.

Geller, B., & Luby, J. (1997). Child and adolescent bipolar disorder: Review of the past ten years. *Journal of the Academy of Child and Adolescent Psychiatry, 36,* 1168–1176.

Gitlin, M. J., Swendsen, J., Heller, T. L., & Hammen, C. (1995). Relapse and impairment in bipolar disorder. *American Journal of Psychiatry, 152,* 1635–1640.

Goodwin, F. K., & Jamison, K. R. (1990). *Manic-depressive illness.* New York: Oxford University Press.

Hammen, C., & Gitlin, M. J. (1997). Stress reactivity in bipolar patients and its relation to prior history of the disorder. *American Journal of Psychiatry, 154,* 856–857.

Isometsä, E., Heikkinen, M., Henriksson, M., Aro, H., & Lonnqvist, J. (1995). Recent life events and completed suicide in bipolar affective disorder: A comparison with major depressive suicides. *Journal of Affective Disorders, 33*(2), 99–106.

Jamison, K. R. (1993). *Touched with fire: Manic-depressive illness and the artistic temperament.* New York: Free Press.

Jamison, K. R. (1995). *An unquiet mind: A memoir of moods and madness.* New York: Knopf.

Jamison, K. R., & Akiskal, H. (1983). Medication compliance in patients with bipolar disorder. *Psychiatric Clinics of North America, 6,* 175–192.

Johnson, S. L., & Miller, I. (1997). Negative life events and time to recovery from episodes of bipolar disorder. *Journal of Abnormal Psychology, 106,* 449–457.

Johnson, S. L., & Roberts, J. (1995). Life events and bipolar disorder: Implications from biological theories. *Psychological Bulletin, 117,* 434–439.

Johnson, S. L., Winett, C., Meyer, B., Greenhouse, W., & Miller, I. (1999). Social support and the course of bipolar disorder. *Journal of Abnormal Psychology, 108,* 558–566.

Keller, M. B., Lavori, P. W., Kane, J. M., Gelenberg, A. J., Rosenbaum, J. F., Walzer, E. A., & Baher, L. A. (1992). Subsyndromal symptoms in bipolar disorder: A comparison of standard and low serum levels of lithium. *Archives of General Psychiatry, 49,* 371–376.

Lam, D. H., Jones, S. H., Hayward, P., & Bright, J. A. (1999). *Cognitive therapy for bipolar disorder: A therapist's guide to concepts, methods, and practice.* Chichester, UK: Wiley.

Lam, D. H., & Wong, G. (1997). Prodromes, coping strategies, insight and social functioning in bipolar affective disorders. *Psychological Medicine, 27,* 1091–1100.

Lundin, R. K. (1998). Living with mental illness: A personal experience. *Cognitive and Behavioral Practice, 5,* 223–230.

Miklowitz, D. J., & Goldstein, M. J. (1997). *Bipolar disorder: A family-focused treatment approach.* New York: Guilford Press.

Miklowitz, D. J., Wendel, J. S., & Simoneau, T. L. (1998). Targeting dysfunctional family interactions and high expressed emotion in the psychosocial treatment of bipolar disorder. *In-Session: Psychotherapy in Practice, 4*(3), 25–38.

Moras, K., & DeMartinis, N. (1999). *Provider's manual: Consultation for combined treatment (CCM-P) with treatment resistant, depressed psychiatric outpatients.* Unpublished manuscript, University of Pennsylvania, Philadelphia.

Newman, C. F. (in press). Reducing the risk of suicide in patients with bipolar disorder: Interventions and safeguards. *Cognitive and Behavioral Practice.*

Newman, C. F., Leahy, R. L., Beck, A. T., Reilly-Harrington, N. A., & Gyulai, L. (2001). *Bipolar disorder: A cognitive therapy approach.* Washington, DC: American Psychological Association.

Palmer, A. G., & Williams, H. (1997). *Early warning signs.* Unpublished manuscript.

Perry, A., Tarrier, N., Morriss, R., McCarthy, E., & Limb, K. (1999). Randomised controlled trial of efficacy of teaching patients with bipolar disorder to identify early symptoms of relapse and obtain treatment. *British Medical Journal, 318,* 139–153.

Reilly-Harrington, N. A., Alloy, L. B., Fresco, D. M., & Whitehouse, W. G. (1999). Cognitive styles and life events interact to predict bipolar and unipolar symptomatology. *Journal of Abnormal Psychology, 108,* 567–578.

Robb, J. C., Cooke, R. G., Devins, G. M., Young, L. T., & Joffe, R. T. (1997). Quality of life and lifestyle disruption in euthymic bipolar disorder. *Journal of Psychiatric Research, 31(5),* 509–517.

Schneider, S., Atkinson, D. R., & El-Mallakh, R. S. (1996). CD and ADHD in bipolar disorder. *Journal of the American Academy of Child and Adolescent Psychiatry, 35(11),* 1422–1423.

Silverstone, T., & Romans-Clarkson, S. (1989). Bipolar affective disorder: Causes and prevention of relapse. *British Journal of Psychiatry, 154,* 321–335.

Simpson, S. G., & Jamison, K. R. (1999). The risk of suicide in patients with bipolar disorders. *Journal of Clinical Psychiatry, 60*(Suppl. 2), 53–56.

Smith, J., & Tarrier, N. (1992). Prodromal symptoms in manic depressive psychosis. *Social Psychiatry and Psychiatric Epidemiology, 27,* 245–248.

Strober, M., Morrell, W., Lampert, C., & Burroughs, J. (1990). Relapse following discontinuation of lithium maintenance therapy in adolescents with bipolar I illness: A naturalistic study. *American Journal of Psychiatry, 147,* 457–461.

Turk, D. C., & Feldman, C. S. (2000). A cognitive-behavioral approach to symptom management in palliative care: Augmenting somatic interventions. In H. M. Chochinov & W. Breitbart (Eds.), *Handbook of psychiatry in palliative medicine* (pp. 223–239). New York: Oxford University Press.

Weller, E. B., Weller, R. A., & Fristad, M. A. (1995). Bipolar disorder in children: Misdiagnosis, underdiagnosis, and future directions. *Journal of the American Academy of Child and Adolescent Psychiatry, 34*(6), 709–714.

Wendel, J. S., & Miklowitz, D. J. (1997, November). *Attributions and expressed emotion in the relatives of patients with bipolar disorder.* Poster presented at the annual conference of the Association for the Advancement of Behavior Therapy, Miami Beach, FL.

West, S. A., McElroy, S. L., Strakowski, S. M., Keck, P. E., Jr., & McConville, B. J. (1995). Attention-deficit hyperactivity disorder in adolescent mania. *American Journal of Psychiatry, 152,* 271–273.

Wright, J., & Schrodt, R. (1989). Combined cognitive therapy and pharmacotherapy. In A. Freeman, K. Simon, L. Beutler, & H. Arkowitz (Eds.), *Handbook of cognitive therapy (pp. 276–282).* New York: Plenum Press.

Wright, J., & Thase, M. (1992). Cognitive and biological therapies: A synthesis. *Psychiatric Annals, 22,* 451–458.

Young, M. A., Fogg, L. F., Scheftner, W., Fawcett, J., Akiskal, H., & Maser, J. (1996). Stable trait components of hopelessness: Baseline and sensitivity to depression. *Journal of Abnormal Psychology, 105,* 155–165.

9

Posttraumatic Stress Disorder: A New Algorithm Treatment Model

Mervin R. Smucker
Brad K. Grunert
Jo M. Weis

The recent burgeoning of studies in the trauma literature offers clinicians a better grasp today of how to treat individuals suffering from posttraumatic stress disorder (PTSD) than even a decade ago. Trauma research and treatment have been expanded from their early focus on war-related PTSD to include victims of physical assault, sexual assault, death threats (e.g., holdups at gun point, kidnappings), terrorist attacks, industrial accidents, occupational injuries, vehicular accidents, and natural disasters. Although the preponderance of trauma outcome studies has found cognitive and exposure-based therapies that focus on emotional processing of the trauma material to be the most effective treatments for PTSD (Sherman, 1998), evidence also exists that some patients have not responded to such treatments (Bryant, 2002; Grunert, Weis, & Rusch, 2000).

To date, little effort has been put forth attempting to understand or explain cognitive-behavioral therapy failures with PTSD. Instead of exploring questions of when and under what circumstances specific cognitive-behavioral interventions are most likely (or least likely) to be effective with particular trauma characteristics, proponents of such treatments have tended to assert that if the empirically demonstrated treatment is not working, then it is not being adequately implemented. The possibility that specific empirically supported cognitive or exposure-based treatments may not be appropriate for all types of traumas or PTSD sufferers has not been adequately explored or addressed in the scientific literature. Currently, no cognitive-behavioral treatment models are available that examine or attempt to predict which specific interventions would be best suited for which particular trauma types and characteristics. As such, practicing clinicians have been given little in the way of constructive guidelines on how to overcome PTSD treatment roadblocks or how to proceed when the cognitive-behavioral treatment being applied with a particular patient is ineffective.

PROLONGED IMAGINAL EXPOSURE TREATMENT FOR PTSD

Although the positive effects of exposure treatment with PTSD have been widely cited (Foa & Meadows, 1997; Grunert, Matloub, Sanger, & Yousif, 1990; Grunert & Dzwierzynski, 1997), nonresponders to exposure have also been noted (Grunert, Smucker, Weis, & Rusch, 2003). Because exposure therapy is poorly tolerated by a number of PTSD sufferers, it has remained limited in clinical practice (Becker & Zayfert, 2001; Grey, Young, Holmes, 2002). A recent clinician survey (Becker, Zayfert, & Anderson, in press) revealed that a majority of licensed doctoral-level psychologists trained in cognitive-behavioral therapy are either reluctant to use or refrain from using exposure treatment for PTSD because of concerns of symptom exacerbation and/or retraumatization. The reportedly high dropout rate of PTSD patients who undergo exposure treatment is likewise troubling. According to a recent outcome study (Zayfert, Becker, Gillock, & Schnurr, 2001), over 40% of participants with PTSD who were treated with exposure therapy dropped out of treatment.

WHEN FEAR IS NOT THE PRIMARY PTSD EMOTION

A fundamental assumption behind the use of exposure treatment with trauma patients is that *fear* is the predominant PTSD emotion and *avoidance* is the primary coping strategy (Foa & Kozak, 1986). To be sure, exposure treatment has a long history of well-documented and demonstrated success in the treatment of phobic disorders, in which the interplay of fear and avoidance is critical to developing and sustaining phobic anxiety. However, the assumption that fear is always the predominant emotion that underlies, perpetuates, and maintains a patient's PTSD response may need to be reexamined. A perusal of the trauma literature would suggest that PTSD is more complex than a phobic disorder and that nonfear emotions are often primary components of PTSD. Prominent PTSD-related emotions other than fear that have been reported in the literature include anger, guilt, shame, disgust, and mental defeat (Brewin, Andrews, & Rose, 2000; Dunmore, Clark, & Ehlers, 1999; Ehlers, Mayou, & Bryant, 1998; Foa, Riggs, & Massie, 1995; Grey, Young, & Holmes, 2002; Lee, Scragg & Turner, 2001; Leskela, Dieperink, & Thuras, 2002; Novaco & Chemtob, 2002).

In a recent study, Grunert et al. (2003) found that 14 exposure treatment sessions led to an exacerbation of PTSD-related clinical symptoms in an industrial accident victim, in whom *anger* was identified as the predominant emotion underlying and perpetuating the PTSD. The patient subsequently made a full and complete recovery from PTSD after just one session of imagery rescripting and reprocessing therapy (IRRT)—an imagery-based, cognitive restructuring treatment that activated, modified, and processed the victim's PTSD-related anger cognitions. In the same study, two exposure sessions were found to exacerbate the symptoms in the treatment of a second industrial accident victim, in whom *guilt* was identified as the predominant PTSD-related emotion. This patient, likewise, made a dramatic recovery from PTSD after one IRRT cognitive restructuring session that activated, challenged, modified (in imagery), and processed his PTSD-related cognitions of guilt.

These findings are especially noteworthy in light of the many outcome studies published by Grunert and colleagues over the past 15 years reporting on the efficacy of exposure treatment with victims of industrial and vehicular accidents who suffer from PTSD (e.g., Grunert et al., 1990; Grunert, Devine, Smith, et al., 1992; Grunert, Devine, Matloub, et al., 1992; Grunert & Dzwierzynski, 1997). In a retrospective analysis of exposure studies published by Grunert and colleagues since 1988 (Grunert & Grunert, 2003) a striking pattern was noted between victims of PTSD who successfully responded to exposure treatment and those for whom it failed:

1. When *fear* was the predominant PTSD emotion and *avoidance* the primary coping strategy, exposure therapy was successful in about 90% of the cases.
2. When the predominant PTSD emotion was not fear (e.g., anger, guilt, shame, disgust), exposure therapy was successful less than 20% of the time.

These findings suggest that different cognitive-behavioral interventions may need to be applied to the treatment of fear than to the treatment of other negative emotions. This notion is reinforced by brain studies showing that the underlying neural substrates of fear are different from those of other negative emotions. Recent neurobiological research has found that *limbic structures* (e.g., the amygdala) are involved in the processing of fear, whereas *higher cortical structures* (e.g., the frontal neocortex) are involved in the processing of more complex negative emotions, such as guilt, shame, disgust (Beauregard, Lévesque, & Bourgouin, 2001; Damasio, 1998).

RATIONALE FOR AN ALGORITHMIC PTSD TREATMENT MODEL

In spite of recent advances in the treatment of PTSD, numerous treatment questions continue to plague clinicians as they attempt to "find their way" through the maze of possible interventions:

1. Should the clinician always begin the treatment of PTSD with exposure?
2. What does the clinician do when exposure appears ineffective or contraindicated?
3. When are cognitive restructuring (CR) interventions useful in the treatment of PTSD, what type of CR interventions are most effective, and under what conditions?
4. When are imagery interventions useful as part of CR?
5. When are CR interventions used to complement exposure, and when is exposure used to complement CR?
6. What does the clinician do when neither exposure nor CR is effective?

To date, such questions have not been adequately addressed in the PTSD treatment literature. Nor have PTSD outcome studies differentiated between the nature and type of traumas experienced by their participants—for example, between victims of a Type I or Type II trauma (Terr, 1991) or between human-perpetrated and non-human-perpetrated traumas. Similarly, the trauma victim's age has not been adequately examined in terms of its likely effect on treatment outcome. Equally striking is the absence of research examining the link between a patient's most salient or predominant PTSD-related emotions (e.g., fear, anger, guilt, self-blame) and treatment outcome.

DESCRIPTION OF AN ALGORITHMIC PTSD TREATMENT MODEL

Our own clinical experience and preliminary research findings suggest that roadblocks encountered with treatment-recalcitrant patients with PTSD do not reflect the inherent inefficacy of the cognitive-behavioral treatment itself but are the function of a "mismatch" between the cognitive-behavioral interventions being applied and the specific trauma characteristics of the patient. In order to more effectively address PTSD treatment roadblocks, we have developed an algorithmic treatment model designed to aid the clinician in determining which type of cognitive-behavioral interventions are likely to be the best fit for which specific PTSD characteristics. This model examines the specific, unique trauma characteristics of each traumatized individual (see Table 9.1).

TABLE 9.1. Assessing Trauma Characteristics in Accordance with the PTSD Algorithm Treatment Model

1. Nature of trauma (e.g., physical/sexual assault, occupational injury, vehicular crash)?
2. Type of trauma: Type I versus Type II trauma (single versus multiple or repeated events)?
3. Number and duration of traumatic events?
4. Age of trauma victim?
5. Human perpetrated (intentional, unintentional) versus non-human perpetrated?
6. Victim–perpetrator relationship?
7. Perceived severity of trauma (e.g., life threatening)?
8. Emotional state at time of trauma (e.g., degree of emotional numbing, dissociation)?
9. Trauma coping responses (peritrauma, posttrauma)?
10. PTSD symptoms (past, current)?
11. Predominant PTSD emotions and related cognitions?
12. Other trauma-related emotions and cognitions?
13. Previous trauma(s) experienced?

According to the PTSD algorithm treatment model, *exposure therapy* is the recommended treatment with those who have experienced a Type I trauma, whose predominant PTSD emotion is *fear*, and whose primary coping strategy is *avoidance*. If the Type I posttraumatic symptoms involve intrusive, fear-based visual memories (e.g., recurring flashbacks), then prolonged imaginal exposure (PE) is recommended to both activate the trauma memory and offer *corrective information* via flooding and habituation (Foa & Kozak, 1986). In PE, imagery is used to activate the fear memory and associated affect by visualizing and verbalizing the entire traumatic event from beginning to end. An audiotape is made of each exposure session and given to the patient for daily listening as a means of enhancing exposure and habituation between sessions. Exposure treatment may also consist of *in vivo* exposure or a combination of imaginal and *in vivo* exposure (Grunert et al., 1990).

If progress is not noted after several sessions, the clinician assesses (1) exposure compliance, (2) the degree to which avoidance behaviors are interfering with treatment, and (3) whether a PTSD-related emotion other than fear is more predominant and needs to be processed first. By contrast, if the PTSD symptoms begin to abate within several sessions, the clinician assesses whether any maladaptive, secondary trauma-related emotions and cognitions exist that need to be targeted and processed. If such secondary cognitions can be accessed visually, imagery interventions are employed that directly challenge and modify the trauma-related beliefs—for example, imagery rescripting and reprocessing therapy (Smucker, 1997; Smucker & Dancu, 1999; Smucker, Dancu, Foa, & Niederee, 1995), cognitive restructuring within reliving (Grey, Young, & Holmes, 2002), or imagery modification (Beck, Emery, & Greenberg, 1985). If such secondary trauma-related cognitions are linguistically stored and cannot be accessed visually, verbal cognitive restructuring interventions that target maladaptive attributions and beliefs are recommended.[1]

By contrast, when the predominant PTSD emotions are other than fear, *cognitive restructuring interventions* are used to process trauma-related emotions and provide corrective information. This involves identifying, challenging, modifying, and linguistically processing the traumatic cognitions (e.g., transforming traumatic imagery into adaptive imagery, replacing maladaptive trauma-related beliefs with adaptive beliefs). Exposure is now used not for habituation but for enhancing cognitive restructuring by activating the trauma memory so that critical, trauma-related cognitions can be identified, challenged, and modified. Once the intrusive traumatic images have ceased and/or have lost their emotional impact and the patient is able to create adaptive imagery at will (e.g., mastery imagery, self-calming imagery), the clinician assesses whether maladaptive trauma-related beliefs remain that require further cognitive and emotional processing. Frequently, Type II trauma victims will continue to be plagued with maladaptive beliefs (e.g., faulty attributions, self-deprecating schemas) about their traumatization long after the disturbing, intrusive images of the traumatic event have abated. For this, cognitive restructuring interventions that actively identify, challenge, and modify their trauma-related beliefs are recommended.

CLINICAL CASE EXAMPLES

Case Example 1 (Work-Related Sexual Harassment)

PJ, a 51-year-old female employed as a manager for a national firm, was on medical leave for 5 months at the time of her referral. She had been sexually harassed by her regional manager while he was in town to review her office's performances and practices 6 months earlier. During the review, the regional manager insisted on conducting closed-door meetings with PJ and became quite upset if any of her staff interrupted for any reason. During their meetings, the regional manager repeatedly brushed his leg against

[1] This aspect of the PTSD algorithm treatment model is consistent with Brewin's (2001) dual-representation model of PTSD in which separate memory systems underlie imagery-based memories (SAM) versus language-based memories (VAM).

hers, bumped shoulders with her, and touched her hands and wrists. He further insisted that she dine with him each evening so that they could finish more of their business. PJ felt "violated" and "assaulted" by her boss's behavior and, by the end of the 5-day review, was feeling quite traumatized by the entire experience.

At intake, PJ was taking Prozac (60 mg) and trazodone (75 mg) daily. Evaluation data confirmed the diagnosis of PTSD. In addition to experiencing daily intrusive flashbacks involving her boss, PJ complained of sleep disturbance, loss of concentration, hypervigilance (including fears of seeing her boss again), startle reaction, and inability to work. She also avoided contact with office coworkers.

The clinician's initial conceptualization of PJ's trauma characteristics, in accordance with the PTSD algorithmic treatment model (see Table 9.1), was as follows: (1) sexual harassment; (2) Type I trauma; (3) single, 5-day event; (4) age 51; (5) human-perpetrated; (6) employee–boss relationship; (7) mild–moderate severity (not life threatening); (8) high emotional upset, no dissociation or emotional numbing at time of trauma; (9) trauma coping responses: (a) peritrauma—behavioral paralysis, endurance; (b) posttrauma—avoidance, withdrawal; (10) PTSD symptoms: recurring flashbacks, nightmares, chronic hypervigilance, startle reaction, loss of concentration, depression; (11) predominant PTSD emotion and related cognitions: *fear* ("He wants to have sex with me"); (12) other trauma-related emotions and cognitions: *self-blame* ("I should be able to stop him"), *powerlessness* ("I'm trapped and unable to defend myself"), *embarrassment* ("I'm being publicly humiliated"), *anger* ("He shouldn't be able to get away with this"); (13) No previous traumas reported.

Because PJ's predominant PTSD emotion appeared to be fear and her primary coping strategy avoidance, PE was chosen as the treatment. PE focused on the most upsetting harassment experiences that PJ experienced during her boss's 5-day review. She described working with her boss for hours in a small office area, during which he repeatedly bumped her leg and touched her arm and hand. PJ felt there was nothing she could do without jeopardizing her job. At the end of the day he informed her that they had more work to do and that they would be having dinner at an "intimate" restaurant with small tables and a cigar bar. PJ described how her boss continued to touch and bump her during dinner and how trapped, ashamed, and humiliated she felt. After dinner, her boss took her into the cigar bar and sat down at a small table, where he proceeded to point out a "beautiful woman" smoking a cigar: "That's the sexiest thing I've ever seen; look at the way she pulls that cigar out of her mouth." He then ordered two cigars and insisted that PJ smoke one. She felt violated, humiliated, and ashamed, "because he made me smoke a cigar so he could think about having oral sex with me."

Six PE sessions with the same upsetting scene yielded no symptom relief. PJ's failure to show any improvement after six exposure sessions marked a treatment roadblock. What was keeping PJ from habituating? Was exposure not being applied properly? (This seemed unlikely, as the treating clinician had had considerable success treating PTSD with exposure therapy for nearly 20 years.) Was PE not the right treatment for PJ? Were emotions other than fear more primary in maintaining her PTSD response? To be sure, *spontaneous restructuring*[2] of critical PTSD cognitions had not occurred during the six exposure sessions.

While grappling with such questions, the clinician noted that PJ had been dutifully doing her homework of daily listening to the audiotaped exposure sessions and did not appear to be engaging in avoidance behaviors. The clinician also reexamined PJ's specific cognitions relating to her perception of threat and concluded that her cognitions relating to *humiliation*, *embarrassment*, and *powerlessness* were more distressing than those relating to *fear*. In his reconceptualization the clinician hypothesized that: (1) the treatment roadblock had occurred because he (the clinician) had wrongly identified fear as the predominant PTSD emotion and had thus been employing the wrong cognitive-behavioral intervention (PE), (2) humiliation, embarrassment, and powerlessness were the predominant PTSD emotions, and (3) cognitive restructuring interventions would be a better treatment choice for the patient's PTSD.

Because PJ's most upsetting cognitions were visual in nature (recurring images of being harassed by her boss), interventions that focused on activating and modifying her upsetting imagery and associated beliefs seemed indicated (Beck et al., 1985; Smucker & Dancu, 1999). A clinical decision was made to employ IRRT—an integrative, cognitive restructuring treatment that employs *exposure* to activate the fear memory, *imagery modification* to replace traumatic imagery with mastery and coping imagery, and *linguistic processing* to promote cognitive shifts in trauma-related beliefs and schemas (Smucker & Dancu, 1999).

The initial IRRT cognitive restructuring session failed to result in any substantial change in either PJ's cognitions or her subjective units of discomfort (SUDS) self-report ratings. At the end of the session, however, PJ reported feeling just as she had at age 14. In the postimagery debriefing, PJ shared that she had been sexually assaulted as a teenager, though she was not comfortable revealing any further details at that time. (PJ had not disclosed this information at intake.) She did, however, acknowledge a possible connection between this earlier sexual trauma and her current thoughts and feelings about her

---

[2] Foa (personal communication, 2001) has noted that spontaneous cognitive restructuring sometimes occurs during exposure sessions with patients with PTSD. However, little is known about when, why, and how spontaneous cognitive restructuring occurs, or about why it often does not occur during exposure.

boss. At the next session, PJ consented to several IRRT cognitive restructuring sessions focusing on her earlier sexual trauma. During imaginal exposure, PJ described asking her parents for permission to go to the prom, being forbidden by her father, and then "sneaking out" with a friend after her mother had gone to work and her father to bed. Following a "wonderful time" at the prom, PJ returned home at 5:00 A.M. to "sneak back into the house." While opening the door, she saw a red glow in the living room and knew that her father was waiting for her. In the transcripts that follow, *humiliation* and *anger* emerged as the dominant trauma-related emotions:

CLIENT: He said, "Where have you been all night?" I said that I had snuck out and gone to the prom. He said, "You had sex with that boy, didn't you?"

THERAPIST: Can you describe this in the present tense, as if it were happening now?

CLIENT: I didn't have sex with him. He's a nice boy and wouldn't do that! He says, " I know you had sex with him. Come over here and stand in front of me!" I walk over and am standing in front of him. I'm really scared. Suddenly he grabs my pants and pulls them down and then he grabs my panties and pulls them down too. I cover up my genitals, but he slaps me and tells me he's going to prove that I had sex with my boyfriend. He hits me again and knocks me down. While I'm on the floor, he grabs my pants and panties and pulls them completely off. I'm just shaking! He says, "Now spread your legs. I have to check and see what you've been doing tonight." I say, "No, I can't." He says, "Oh yes you will!" He forces me back down and puts his legs between my legs and forces them apart. Then he takes his fingers and pushes them up into my vagina. I hate him, but I'm too scared to do anything!

THERAPIST: Can you now visualize yourself as an adult today entering the room? (PJ nods.) As an adult looking at PJ with her father forcing his hand into her vagina, is there anything that you, PJ today, would like to do or say?

CLIENT: I'd like to turn and walk out. It makes me sick to see what he is doing to her.

THERAPIST: So, you'd like to just let him continue to keep his hand in her vagina?

CLIENT: No! No! I want to scream at him to stop it and tell him to leave her alone!

THERAPIST: Can you say that to him directly?

CLIENT: Stop it you asshole! Get away from her!

THERAPIST: How does he respond?

CLIENT: He just looks at me and keeps feeling her genitals. I hate him. I yell at him again but he doesn't stop. So I run over and kick him in the crotch. He rolls away, but I kick him again. I say, "How do you like it you bastard?" He just rolls over and groans. I kick him again, and keep kicking him until he stops moving.

THERAPIST: What happens next?

CLIENT: I walk over to PJ, help her up and say, "He won't ever hurt you again." She starts to cry. I hold and comfort her, then take her to the bathroom and clean her up. We go upstairs and I help her get dressed. Then I get the other kids up and take them out to my red convertible. PJ doesn't come out, so I go back into the house. She's staring at him. I take her out to the car, then get some matches, go back in and light the house on fire. I go back out, start the car, and we all drive away singing while the house burns down.

THERAPIST: And how do you feel now?

CLIENT: I feel good. I feel like a huge weight has been taken off of my back.

During the preceding imagery session, PJ was able to activate, rescript, and reprocess the previously unprocessed cognitions of humiliation and anger associated with her earlier Type I trauma. After two subsequent IRRT sessions, PJ felt "resolved" about the work she had done on her father-perpetrated sexual assault trauma and indicated that she was ready to again focus on her recent traumatic harassment encounters with her boss.

Three additional IRRT sessions were needed to facilitate emotional processing of her current distressing cognitions vis-à-vis her boss. *Humiliation* and *anger* again emerged as the dominant trauma-related emotions. Having successfully processed her earlier sexual trauma, PJ was now able with relative ease to cognitively restructure and emotionally process her recent boss-related harassment, which led to a significant reduction in her intrusions and avoidance behaviors. After two additional maintenance sessions, PTSD treatment was terminated. PJ's clinical gains continued to improve posttreatment, and at 6-month follow-up she remained symptom free.

Case Example 2 (Oil Truck Accident and Explosion)

Sam, a 38-year-old, married truck driver, was referred for cognitive-behavioral therapy by his workers' compensation carrier 14 months after he experienced a dramatic vehicular accident. The large oil truck that Sam was driving collided with a car driven by an 85-year-old man while the car was backing onto a busy divided highway from an exit that the driver had taken in error. The truck went out of control, jackknifed, and minutes later exploded into flames. Sam managed to crawl out of the capsized cab, help the elderly couple from their car, and assist other bystanders who were in harm's way from the impending explosion of the oil truck. Shortly after the police, ambulance, and fire squad arrived, Sam felt "numb" while looking on in "a state of shock" as his truck went up in flames. Sam was taken to the hospital, treated for minor injuries, and released later that day. Several days later, Sam began to develop acute stress disorder symptoms, which subsequently developed into PTSD, chronic type.

Although Sam made several attempts to return to work in the weeks following the accident, he continued to struggle with flashbacks, nightmares, and startle responses relating to the accident and became increasingly upset with his employer of 18 years for not showing more understanding, flexibility, and support. Sam also developed a phobic fear of truck driving, which generalized to all freeway driving. Three months after the accident, Sam was placed on long-term medical leave. Although Sam received ongoing supportive therapy while on medical leave, he remained unable to return to work on a permanent basis, as his PTSD symptoms and driving phobia became more entrenched.

Fourteen months after the accident Sam's workers' compensation carrier requested that he be treated with cognitive-behavioral therapy. Evaluation data at intake confirmed the diagnosis of PTSD. Sam also reported struggling with chronic sleep disturbance. Because of recurring intrusive flashbacks of the accident, which Sam experienced nightly while falling asleep, he would "wake up in a daze" and feel like he was back in the truck at the scene of the accident trying to get out before it exploded. Sam shared how he continued to visually replay the entire accident scenario "thousands of times," hoping that he would someday "wake up" and find out that the accident had been only a bad dream.

The clinician used the PTSD algorithmic treatment model to complete the following conceptualization of Sam's specific trauma characteristics: (1) vehicular accident; (2) Type I trauma; (3) single event, short duration (minutes); (4) age 37; (5) human-perpetrated, unintentional; (6) no prior perpetrator–victim relationship; (7) high severity (life threatening); (8) low emotional upset, high emotional numbing (at time of trauma); (9) trauma coping responses: (a) peritrauma—emotional numbness, adaptive coping (climbed out of jackknifed cab himself, helped others to get out of harm's way before the truck exploded); (b) posttrauma—avoidance, denial; (10) PTSD symptoms: daily recurring flashbacks, nightmares, chronic sleep disturbance, hypervigilance, startle reaction, avoidance, and depression; (11) predominant PTSD emotion and related cognitions: *fear* ("I'm afraid of driving truck. . . . I'll lose control and have another accident," "I'm afraid of my feelings"); (12) other trauma-related emotions and cognitions: *guilt* and *self-blame* ("It's my fault, I shouldn't have gone to work that day. . . . I shouldn't have swerved my truck"), *anger at self* ("I shouldn't be so weak and wimpy . . . men don't cry like this"), *anger at boss* ("My boss should be more understanding and supportive"); (13) no previous traumas reported.

Because fear was identified as the predominant PTSD emotion and avoidance the primary coping strategy, exposure was deemed the treatment of choice. A treatment plan was developed that included: (1) *PE* for the intrusive flashbacks and related PTSD symptoms, including daily listening to the audiotaped exposure session and recording of SUDS levels; (2) *in vivo* exposure (later in treatment) involving: (a) a return to the site of the accident, (b) graded exposure to freeway driving, and (c) graded exposure to truck driving (initially as passenger then as driver). It was explained to Sam that compliance with all phases of exposure was essential to the success of treatment, especially the daily listening to the audiotaped exposure sessions.

PE was begun the following session. Sam's SUDS remained high (90–100) throughout most of the exposure session, as he visually and emotionally relived the accident. He reported feeling ashamed and "emotionally weak" because of the crying he exhibited during exposure: "I'm a 38-year-old truck driver and I shouldn't be crying like this." As the exposure session progressed, Sam remembered more details of the accident. Five additional PE sessions were conducted. Although Sam agreed to listen daily to the audiotaped PE sessions, he complained that listening to the tapes was very difficult for him and that he'd rather ignore the images and emotions relating to the accident.

As exposure treatment progressed, it became increasingly evident that Sam was not habituating. He continued to become extremely upset and agitated during the exposure sessions, as his SUDS remained consistently high. Sam's failure to show any improvement after six exposure sessions marked a significant treatment roadblock. While reflecting on this treatment impasse, the clinician reexamined the PTSD algorithmic treatment conceptualization of Sam. Was fear not the predominant PTSD emotion? Was there another PTSD emotion more primary than fear? Although Sam felt some anger toward his boss for not being more understanding and supportive, his anger clearly seemed to be a secondary trauma-related emotion. In addition, Sam did not appear to feel any resentment or anger toward the 85-year-old driver who had accidently backed into his path. It did appear, however, that avoidance and denial continued to be Sam's primary coping strategies during the 16 months since the trauma, as reflected in the ongoing difficulties he had listening to the audiotaped exposure sessions.

Sam's wife, who had grown increasingly impatient with his lack of progress, asked to be present at the next session. She reported that Sam seldom listened to the exposure tapes and, when he did, he was not really listening—that he was either asleep, watching TV, or "tinkering around" with projects in the garage. Sam acknowledged these avoidance behaviors. Thus it appeared that Sam's continued avoidance behaviors were preventing habituation and had become a significant roadblock in treatment.

In order to maximize homework compliance and reduce avoidance, a revised homework plan was put into action that involved Sam's wife being present while he listened (twice daily) to the audiotaped PE sessions. The homework intervention had a positive effect on Sam's treatment, as immediate improvement was noted in his mood and exposure SUDS ratings. Several sessions later, an *in vivo* exposure session was conducted that involved Sam going to the site of the accident with the therapist. In spite of his high anticipatory anxiety, Sam managed the *in vivo* exposure very well. He was surprised at the ease with which he was able to walk the therapist through the entire accident and describe in detail what, when, where, and how the events had occurred.

Following Sam's successful exposure to the accident site, treatment progressed relatively quickly. Ten additional therapy sessions were needed, as Sam's increased sense of mastery over his trauma-related fears showed marked improvement from one session to the next. PE to the traumatic memory was continued simultaneously with *in vivo* exposure to truck and freeway driving. Although Sam was able to quickly master his freeway-driving fears as soon as he stopped avoiding freeways, mastering his truck driving fears was more challenging—especially his anticipatory anxiety. Sam's father (also a truck driver) agreed to be part of Sam's graded exposure to truck driving, which involved Sam initially as passenger, then as driver. After several weeks of daily truck driving, Sam was also able to gain mastery over his truck driving fears and began to plan for his return to work.

Toward the end of treatment, a cognitive restructuring session was conducted that involved the development of adaptive imagery, in which Sam visualized himself assertively expressing his anger (a secondary trauma emotion) to his boss for not being more supportive of his postaccident adjustment difficulties. The cognitive rehearsal imagery session was followed by an actual meeting between Sam and his boss which, according to Sam, went very well. A few weeks later Sam returned to work half days, which gradually progressed to full days.

Following Sam's return to work, a termination plan was set up. Sam's flashbacks and nightmares had stopped altogether, his depression and anxiety levels had decreased significantly, and he once again felt hopeful and optimistic about his future. Although he still reported occasional intrusions of the accident, he no longer became upset by them or exhibited any avoidance behaviors. Two maintenance sessions were scheduled, the last of which Sam cancelled because, "there's no reason for me to come in any more." At 6-month follow-up, Sam maintained his treatment gains, while manifesting no further PTSD symptoms or avoidance behaviors. At 3-year follow-up, Sam not only remained completely symptom free but had become the proud owner of his own trucking business.

Case Example 3 (Work-Related/Life-Threatening Physical Assault)

FB, a 39-year-old female, was referred for psychological treatment 8 months after a traumatic incident in which a coworker had assaulted her with a 24-inch pipe wrench. During the 4½ years prior to the assault, FB had been subjected to ongoing sexual harassment while working in an all-male department: degrading comments about her gender, homosexual orientation, intellect, and work performance; verbal threats directed at FB and her family; and intimidating physical gestures. On numerous occasions she had reported the harassing incidents, but supervisors at various levels either ignored her complaints or were ineffective in rectifying the situation.

At intake, FB reported experiencing frequent nightmares and flashbacks of the traumatic assault. She continued to fear for her safety, was in a constant state of hypervigilance, and had a pronounced startle response. She reported difficulty sleeping and often got up to check doors and windows at night. Her inability to concentrate was exacerbated by ruminative thinking about the distressing events she experienced at work. FB also reported that she had received psychological treatment in her early twenties following another incident at work in which a bomb had exploded in her face. She felt that she had recovered from this earlier trauma, stating, "I just learned to deal with it," and had returned to work after recovering from her physical injuries.

The clinician's conceptualization of FB's specific trauma characteristics, in accordance with the PTSD algorithmic treatment model, was as follows: (1) physical assault; (2) Type I trauma; (3) single major traumatic event of short duration (less than a minute), multiple previous harassment events spanning a period of several years; (4) age 39; (5) human-perpetrated, intentional; (6) employee–employee relationship; (7) high severity (life threatening); (8) high emotional upset, no dissociation or emotional numbing at time of trauma; (9) trauma coping responses: (a) peritrauma—behavioral paralysis, passive endurance; (b) posttrauma—generalized avoidance, repetitive checking of doors and windows at night; (10) PTSD symptoms: daily recurring flashbacks, nightmares, chronic hypervigilance, startle response, loss of concentration, chronic sleep disturbance, depression; (11) predominant PTSD emotions and related cognitions: *vulnerability* ("I'm an open target"), *powerlessness* ("I'm helpless and unable to protect myself from attack"); (12) other trauma-related emotions and cognitions: *fear* ("He wants to kill me"); (13) Previous trauma experienced 15 years earlier involving a bomb exploding in her face.

According to the PTSD algorithm treatment model, PE by itself would *not* be indicated, as fear did not appear to be the primary PTSD emotion. The clinician thus decided to use a combined exposure–cognitive restructuring approach that employed: (1) imaginal exposure to activate the fear memory; (2) imagery modification to replace the recurring, traumatic imagery with mastery/coping imagery, and (3) cognitive restructuring to challenge, modify, and linguistically process cognitions of vulnerability and powerlessness. IRRT was deemed the cognitive restructuring treatment of choice.

During the *imaginal exposure* phase of treatment, FB described reporting for duty on the night of the assault and learning that her assigned coworker was the "ringleader" of the continuing harassment against her. Several hours into the job—following many degrading comments and threatening bodily gestures—the coworker threw a 24-inch pipe wrench at her while she was preparing the service van for departure from the job site. The wrench missed hitting her head by millimeters. FB believed at that moment that the perpetrator was going to kill her, as she felt completely vulnerable and powerless. During *mastery imagery*, FB was able to directly confront her cognitions of helplessness and vulnerability by visualizing her "survivor self" today confronting the perpetrator and rescuing her "traumatized self" from the threatening situation. FB appeared to experience an "empowering moment" vis-à-vis the perpetrator when she visualized herself today hurling the wrench at his head and "seeing" the surprised, shocked look in his eyes. During the subsequent *self-calming/self-nurturing imagery*, FB was able to visualize her "survivor self" nurturing and reassuring her "traumatized self." At the end of the session, FB appeared much calmer and relieved "because I was able to see myself dealing with the assault." PJ's homework assignment was to listen daily to the audiotape of the entire exposure–restructuring imagery session.

At her next appointment, however, FB appeared more distraught than at intake and was feeling quite hopeless and negative about her treatment. FB had not done her homework, her avoidance behaviors had increased, and she had stayed at home isolated in her bedroom for most of the week. She also reported an increase in nightmares and flashbacks. Although in the previous session FB had developed powerful mastery imagery vis-à-vis her assailant and was able to develop adaptive self-nurturing and self-reassuring imagery, her symptoms had nonetheless worsened. This dramatic escalation of symptoms after one cognitive restructuring session posed a significant roadblock in FB's treatment. Why was the CR session followed by an escalation of symptoms? Were the CR interventions ineffective, or perhaps even contraindicated with FB? Was fear the dominant PTSD emotion after all? Or was progress being thwarted by other, still unidentified trauma-related emotions and cognitions?

While pondering such questions, the clinician recalled FB's earlier reference to a bombing incident she had experienced years earlier, which she reportedly had "just learned to deal with." The clinician decided to inquire further about the bombing event, in order to ascertain whether unprocessed material from this earlier trauma was interfering with the emotional processing of her more recent traumatic assault. Further questioning revealed that FB had indeed become preoccupied with the earlier bombing incident since the CR session and was now experiencing frequent intrusive flashbacks of that trauma. FB acknowledged that coping with the bombing at that time had meant "putting it out of my mind as quickly as possible" whenever she experienced any related intrusions. FB further noted that her feelings about her recent assault were similar to those of the earlier bombing incident. It thus appeared that her earlier unprocessed trauma was presenting a significant treatment roadblock by impeding the processing of her most recent trauma.

In the clinician's reconceptualization, fear was hypothesized to be the predominant emotion and avoidance the primary coping strategy sustaining her PTSD symptoms. (FB noted that at the time of the explosion, she thought she was going to die). The clinician therefore decided to proceed with PE to the original trauma—the bombing. The subsequent exposure session revealed that during the bombing, FB had sustained considerable burns to her face, arms, and hands. Even though her hearing and balance were significantly impaired for some time thereafter, no one had informed her of the severity of her injuries or of what the expected course of recovery would be. In addition, FB had been held in protective custody immediately after the bombing, and she was unable to see her physical injuries because of extensive bandaging. The PE session further revealed that FB had not feared death at the time of the explosion as she had originally reported. On the contrary, she had been quite aware of being alive and had never felt that death was imminent. After the removal of her bandages, however, FB was horrified at how she looked. She believed that her body was permanently mutilated and that the body she had once known "was lost." Thus it appeared that unprocessed trauma-related *grief* (rather than fear) was FB's predominant PTSD emotion.

At this point, the clinician decided to reemploy IRRT as the CR treatment as a means of activating, modifying, and processing FB's cognitions related to her traumatic grief. The following are excerpts of the subsequent IRRT session:

THERAPIST: What do you think is happening to you?

CLIENT: I don't know. I'm really uncomfortable and something is burning me. It feels surreal, because I can't see and I can't hear anything, and I'm in a lot of pain.

THERAPIST: What do you think is going to happen to you?

CLIENT: Don't know. I feel like something really bad has happened to me. I'm not dead, but I'm freaked out because this doesn't seem real. I can't hear or see anyone.

In the mastery imagery that followed, FB was able to visualize her "survivor self" confronting the bomber and helping the police subdue him. The mastery imagery resulted in the correction of inaccurate appraisals of what had really happened to her body at the time of the trauma, which is reflected in the following excerpts:

THERAPIST: What do you, the survivor today, want to do or say to the traumatized you?

CLIENT: You're damned lucky. Your face isn't going to be trashed for life.

THERAPIST: How close are you when you tell her this?

CLIENT: I'm right there. I just keep running the water on that hand and arm and keep the towels on her face. I tell her what happened, that a pipe bomb blew up and that she's not going to be ugly, she's not going to be blind, she's not burned all over, she's not going to be deaf, and she's going to get through this.

THERAPIST: And as you say that to her, how does she respond now?

CLIENT: It makes her feel better. It would have been nice if she had known that then.

FB listened to the audiotaped IRRT session several times during the following week. At the next session (1 week later), she reported a complete absence of flashbacks and nightmares for both traumatic events. Her other PTSD symptoms also showed significant improvement, including her sleep and concentration. Two weeks following this IRRT session, her PTSD treatment was terminated. Her gains were maintained at 3-month and 6-month follow-up.

FB is an example of an individual victimized by two separate, unrelated, and unprocessed Type I traumas. Initially, treatment was sought for PTSD symptoms pertaining to the most recent human-perpetrated trauma of physical assault. A treatment roadblock emerged when the initial CR session resulted in an escalation of PTSD symptoms relating to an earlier traumatic event that FB had "just tried to forget." The clinician hypothesized that this earlier unprocessed trauma was interfering with treatment and would need to be processed (emotionally and cognitively) before progress with FB's more recent trauma could be achieved. Although fear was initially thought to be the predominant PTSD emotion of the original trauma, trauma-related *grief* emerged during PE as the most prominent and upsetting emotion maintaining her PTSD symptoms. In a single IRRT cognitive restructuring session, FB was able to remove the treatment roadblock of the earlier trauma by modifying and processing the trauma-related images and beliefs sustaining her grief, which in turn led to an immediate abatement of her PTSD symptoms.

SUMMARY

A variety of treatment techniques have been developed to address PTSD symptoms over the past 20 years. The best-documented outcomes have been from treatments incorporating cognitive restructuring and exposure-based interventions designed to enhance emotional processing of traumatic events. Yet, in spite of the reported efficacy of cognitive-behavioral therapies with PTSD, cognitive-behavioral therapy failures with this clinical population also exist. A deficiency in the PTSD outcome studies has been a failure to address treatment roadblocks and failures when they arise. Rather than directing the focus of outcome research toward empirically examining which specific trauma characteristics might be most amenable to which types of interventions, proponents of cognitive and exposure treatments have tended to argue that if their empirically supported treatment is not working with a particular patient, then the treatment is not being properly employed. Unfortunately, this approach to addressing treatment failures has left practicing clinicians little in the way of theoretical models or empirical guidelines on how to handle PTSD treatment roadblocks with individual patients when they arise.

In this chapter, we have emphasized that no empirically supported cognitive or exposure-based treatment is appropriate for all types of trauma or PTSD sufferers. Our own clinical data and observations of treating trauma victims over the past 20 years, together with a review of the current PTSD treatment outcome literature, has led us to advance an individualized PTSD algorithmic treatment model designed to aid the clinician in assessing which cognitive-behavioral interventions are most likely to be effective, depending on the specific trauma characteristics of the patient. Three case studies are presented that demonstrate how the clinician can apply the PTSD algorithmic treatment model to identify, conceptualize, and address specific obstacles and roadblocks as they arise. The case examples reveal the clinician's own thought processes and working hypotheses while addressing each treatment roadblock and illustrate how the clinician can (1) match treatment interventions with specific trauma characteristics and (2) methodically alter the specific cognitive-behavioral therapy interventions (when indicated) using clear and practical clinical guidelines.

REFERENCES

Beauregard, M., Lévesque, L., & Bourgouin, P. (2001). Neural correlates of conscious self-regulation of emotion. *Journal of Neuroscience, 21*, 1–6.

Beck, A. T., Emery, G., & Greenberg, R. L. (1985). *Anxiety disorders and phobias: A cognitive perspective*. New York: Basic Books.

Becker, C. B., & Zayfert, C. (2001). Integrating DBT-based techniques and concepts to facilitate exposure treatment for PTSD. *Cognitive and Behavioral Practice, 8*(2), 107–122.

Becker, C. B., Zayfert, C., & Anderson, E. (in press). A survey of psychologists' attitudes towards and utilization of exposure therapy for PTSD. *Behaviour Research and Therapy.*

Brewin, C. R. (2001). A cognitive neuroscience account of posttraumatic stress disorder and its treatment. *Behavior Research and Therapy, 39*(4), 373–393.

Brewin, C. R., Andrews, B., & Rose, S. (2000). Fear, helplessness and horror in posttraumatic stress disorder: Investigating DSM-IV Criterion 2A in victims of violent crime. *Journal of Traumatic Stress, 13,* 499–509.

Bryant, R. A. (2002, August). *CBT in the treatment of acute stress disorder.* Paper presented at the annual convention of the American Psychological Association.

Damasio, A. R. (1998). Emotion in the perspective of an integrated nervous system. *Brain Research Reviews, 26,* 83–86.

Dunmore, E., Clark, D. M., & Ehlers, A. (1999). Cognitive factors involved in the onset and maintenance of PTSD. *Behavior Research and Therapy, 37,* 809–827.

Ehlers, A., Mayou, R. A., & Bryant, B. (1998). Psychological predictors of posttraumatic stress disorder after motor vehicle accidents. *Journal of Abnormal Psychology, 107*(3), 508–519.

Foa, E. B., & Kozak, M. J. (1986). Emotional processing of fear: Exposure to corrective information. *Psychological Bulletin, 99*(1), 20–35.

Foa, E. B., & Meadows, E. A. (1997). Psychosocial treatments for posttraumatic stress disorder: A critical review. *Annual Review of Psychology, 48,* 449–480.

Foa, E. B., Riggs, D. S., & Massie, E. D. (1995). The impact of fear activation and anger on the efficacy of exposure treatment for posttraumatic stress disorder. *Behavior Therapy, 26,* 487–499.

Grey, N., Young, K., & Holmes, E. (2002). Cognitive restructuring within reliving: A treatment for peritraumatic emotional "hotspots" in posttraumatic stress disorder. *Behavioral and Cognitive Psychotherapy, 30*(1), 37–56.

Grunert, B. K., Devine, C. A., Matloub, H. S., Sanger, J. R., Yousif, N. J., Anderson, R. C., & Roell, S. M. (1992). Psychological adjustment following work-related hand injury: 18-month follow-up. *Annals of Plastic Surgery, 29*(6), 537–542.

Grunert, B. K., Devine, C. A., Smith, C. J., Matloub, H. S., Sanger, J. R., & Yousif, N. J. (1992). Graded work exposure to promote work return after severe hand trauma: A replicated study. *Annals of Plastic Surgery, 29*(6), 532–536.

Grunert, B. K., & Dzwierzynski, W. W. (1997). Prognostic factors for return to work following severe hand injuries. *Techniques in Hand and Upper Extremity Surgery, 1*(3), 213–218.

Grunert, B. K., & Grunert, S. (2003). *Exposure-based treatments for industrially injured workers: A 20-year retrospective analysis.* Manuscript in preparation.

Grunert, B. K., Matloub, H. S., Sanger, J. R., & Yousif, N. J. (1990). Treatment of posttraumatic stress disorder after work-related hand trauma. *Journal of Hand Surgery, 15A*(3), 511–515.

Grunert, B. K., Smucker, M. R., Weis, J. M., & Rusch, M. D. (2003). When prolonged exposure fails: Adding an imagery-based cognitive restructuring component in the treatment of industrial accident victims suffering from PTSD. *Cognitive and Behavioral Practice, (10)*4.

Grunert, B. K., Weis, J. M., & Rusch, M. D. (2000, March). *Imagery rescripting after failed imaginal exposure for PTSD following industrial injury.* Paper presented at the Third World Conference of the International Society for Traumatic Stress Studies, Melbourne, Australia.

Lee, D., Scragg, P., & Turner, S. (2001). The role of shame and guilt in traumatic events: A clinical model of shame-based and guilt-based PTSD. *British Journal of Medical Psychology, 74*(4), 451–466.

Leskela, J., Dieperink, M., & Thuras, P. (2002). Shame and posttraumatic disorder. *Journal of Traumatic Stress, 15*(3), 223–226.

Novaco, R. W., & Chemtob, C. M. (2002). Anger and combat-related posttraumatic stress disorder. *Journal of Traumatic Stress, 15*(2), 123–132.

Sherman, J. J. (1998). Effects of psychotherapeutic treatments of PTSD: A meta-analysis of controlled clinical trials. *Journal of Traumatic Stress, 11*(3), 413–433.

Smucker, M. R. (1997). Posttraumatic stress disorder. In R. L. Leahy (Ed.), *Practicing cognitive therapy* (pp. 193–220). Northvale, NJ: Aronson.

Smucker, M. R., & Dancu, C. (1999). *Cognitive-behavioral treatment for adult survivors of childhood trauma: Imagery rescripting and reprocessing.* Northvale, NJ: Aronson.

Smucker, M. R., Dancu, C., Foa, E. B., & Niederee, J. L. (1995). Imagery rescripting: A new treatment for survivors of childhood sexual abuse suffering from posttraumatic stress. *Journal of Cognitive Psychotherapy: An International Quarterly, 9*(1), 3–17.

Terr, L. C. (1991). Acute responses to external events and posttraumatic stress disorders. In L. Melvin (Ed.), *Child and adolescent psychiatry: A comprehensive textbook* (pp. 755–763). Baltimore: Williams & Wilkins.

Zayfert, C., Becker, C. B., Gillock, K., & Schnurr, P. (2001, July). Drop-out from exposure therapy for PTSD in clinical practice. In C. Zayfert (Chair), *Problems implementing exposure therapy for PTSD.* Symposium conducted at the World Congress of Behavioral and Cognitive Therapies, Vancouver, Canada.

10

Binge-Eating and Other Eating Disorders

Nicole A. Schaffer

Eating disorders affect approximately 5 million people in the United States annually (Becker, Grinspoon, Klibanski, & Herzog, 1999). Obesity, anorexia nervosa, bulimia nervosa, and binge-eating disorder have become increasingly more prevalent in industrialized Western societies (Polivy & Herman, 2002). Treating these disorders is of great concern to health professionals, and, although many different approaches have been developed, a clear understanding of the etiology, prevention, and treatment of eating disorders has remained elusive.

Bulimia nervosa (BN) is characterized by recurrent binge episodes in which an individual "eats an unusually large amount of food in a discrete period of time with an accompanied sense of loss of control," followed by inappropriate compensatory weight-control practices such as regular use of purging (vomiting, laxatives, diuretics), fasting, or excessive exercise (American Psychiatric Association, 1994). The binge-eating behavior seen in BN also characterizes about half of the patients with anorexia nervosa (AN; Becker et al., 1999).

Binge-eating disorder (BED) shares the same diagnostic criteria as BN, excluding the use of compensatory behaviors in preventing weight gain. Because individuals with binge-eating disorder do not compensate for their large intake of food, they are frequently obese, with estimates in this population ranging from 30–50% (Spitzer et al., 1992, 1993). To date, BED is included in the appendix of the DSM-IV and has only recently received recognition as a significant clinical problem (Grilo, 1996). Individuals with BED often report that in their past attempts to lose weight, they have tried every diet possible and have not been successful. There are two separate issues that must be delineated and emphasized to our patients—weight loss and reduction of binge-eating behavior.

Obesity is not just a clinical problem; it is also a public heath epidemic for the United States. Approximately 25% of Americans are obese, with rising prevalence rates (Leibbrand & Fichter, 2002). Obesity, as well as eating disorders, is associated with an increased risk for cardiovascular disease, diabetes mellitus, hypertension, medical complications, and other illnesses (Foreyt, Poston, & Goodrick, 1996; Leibbrand & Fichter, 2001). Interventions are vital, as a loss of 5–10% of a person's weight will reduce his or her health risks considerably (Leibbrand & Fichter, 2001).

Compared with their nonbingeing counterparts, obese binge eaters experience greater levels of psychopathology (i.e., depression, anxiety), excessive dieting and weight concerns, greater body dissatisfaction, preoccupation with thinness, and increased levels of cognitive distortions (Nauta, Hospers, Jansen, & Kok, 2000) . There is also a higher incidence of drug and alcohol abuse and personality disorders in obese binge eaters (Bruce & Wilfley, 1996; de Zwaan & Mitchell, 1992; Marcus, Wing, & Hopkins, 1988; Telch & Agras, 1994).

Treatment strategies for binge eating have evolved out of the work that is known to be efficacious for BN. Interpersonal psychotherapy (IPT) and cognitive-behavioral therapy have been the most extensively researched psychological treatments (Fairburn, Marcus, & Wilson, 1993; Fairburn, 1993). Cognitive-behavioral therapy has been shown to be superior to pharmacotherapy and has lower attrition rates (Agras et al., 1992). It is superior to alternative psychotherapies, with the exception of IPT, which has a similar long-term outcome (Agras, Walsh, Fairburn, Wilson, & Kraemer, 2000). Cognitive-behavioral therapy modified for the treatment of obese individuals with BED (Fairburn et al., 1993) has also shown superior results over a wait-list control group (Agras et al., 1995; Wilfley et al., 1993; Telch, Agras, Rossiter, Wilfley, & Kenardy, 1990). Typically, reductions in both the episodes of binge eating and eating-disordered symptoms have been demonstrated by participants in cognitive-behavioral therapy (Wilson & Pike, 2001).

The cognitive-behavioral model of BED describes a self-perpetuating cycle in which low self-esteem and feelings of worthlessness can lead to extreme concerns about shape and weight with a pursuit of thinness. Low self-worth based on appearance drives the individual to diet, restricting her food intake, which, for both psychological and physiological reasons, ultimately results in binge eating. The pattern repeats itself, and the cycle begins again (Fairburn, Cooper, & Cooper, 1986; Fairburn & Wilson, 1993).

Behavioral techniques are used to reduce binge eating by establishing stable eating patterns and decreasing rigid dieting. Cognitive techniques help eliminate dichotomous thinking and dysfunctional beliefs (see Fairburn & Wilson, 1993, for a more detailed description).

Although cognitive-behavioral therapy is regarded as the first line of treatment and considered the "gold standard," controlled treatment trials show that approximately 50% of patients do not respond (Agras et al., 1995; Telch et al., 1990). Why are these patients resistant to treatment, and why do they often terminate prematurely? Only by examining issues of noncompliance, attrition, and lack of treatment response can we propose new techniques and modify current treatment strategies. Critics of cognitive therapy propose that not enough attention is given to the emotional experience of the patient or to interpersonal issues and that the importance of the patient–therapist relationship is underestimated (Wonderlich, Mitchell, Peterson, & Crow, 2001).

Research on the efficacy of cognitive-behavioral therapy in treating BN and BED has been based solely on manual-driven protocols. These structured protocols leave little room for clinicians to individualize treatment. In clinical practice, therapists usually do not strictly abide by a manual-based treatment protocol. Although this allows for error and subjectivity, it enables clinicians to be creative in their therapeutic approach in order to overcome the difficulties they experience with eating-disordered patients. One of the initial obstacles therapists encounter is that when they ask binge eaters to establish regular eating patterns, an intense fear of gaining weight emerges. Interfering with the patient's attempts to change her eating patterns, this fear is often misconstrued as ambivalence or, even worse, resistance. Additional factors that clinicians may recognize as impeding standard interventions include: motivational issues, lack of self-control, a perfectionist belief system, dichotomous thinking, inability to self-regulate affective states, and a lack of interoceptive awareness. It is my goal to apply relevant and current research findings to the development of interventions used with this population with the aim of improving our individual techniques and furthering our patients' success.

Although this chapter focuses mainly on binge eating in obesity, considerable overlap exists among the features of eating disorders. As with the other eating disorders, the main symptoms of AN include a disturbance in eating; preoccupation with weight, shape, and food; body dissatisfaction; and low self-esteem based on the evaluation of weight and shape (Fairburn, Shafran, & Cooper, 1998; Polivy & Herman, 2002). Poor treatment outcome in AN has been shown to be correlated with increased severity of symptoms, deficient motivation in therapy, failure of previous treatments, duration of illness, and comorbid psychopathology (Towell, Woodford, Reid, Rooney, & Towell, 2001). Due to the paucity of empirical data on treatments for AN (Wilson & Pike, 2001) and space limitations, this chapter does not focus on therapeutic strategies in the treatment of AN (see

Fairburn, Shafran, & Cooper, 1998, for a comprehensive review on cognitive behavioral treatment for AN).

Finally, the assessment and management of disordered eating and obesity calls for a multidisciplinary approach. In addition to the psychological component, medical evaluation and nutritional counseling are important aspects of treating these illnesses.

MOTIVATIONAL ISSUES

Patients who agree to commit to therapy often experience a common source of frustration: losing motivation. Motivation has been clearly identified as a significant variable that predicts treatment outcome, and it must be addressed from the outset of therapy (Prochaska, DiClemente, & Norcross, 1992).

Prochaska and DiClemente (1982) have conceptualized a model of behavior change used to understand the therapeutic process and outcome in the treatment of addictive disorders. According to this transtheoretical model, there are five stages that reflect different levels of motivation and readiness to change. We can adapt this model to our understanding of BED. Prochaska and DiClemente's (1982) model emphasizes a nonlinear progression through efforts to change. Individuals can move forward to long-term change (i.e., maintenance), revert back to an earlier stage, or even relapse to maladaptive behaviors. Although five stages have been named—precontemplation, contemplation, preparation, action and maintenance (Prochaska, DiClemente, & Norcross, 1992)—for the sake of conceptual simplicity, I will use three stages: *contemplation, action,* and *maintenance.* The "stages of change" model provides a framework in which patients can take their own "motivational temperature." At each stage, the clinician can match the appropriate intervention with the individual's identified stage of change, refining treatment approaches accordingly. At any given point in the cyclical stages of change, ambivalence may need to be reassessed by the clinician (Miller & Rollnick, 1991).

CONTEMPLATION

During the contemplation stage, patients are aware that a problem exists but are unable to make a commitment for action. Often, the awareness that one needs to change his or her eating patterns comes from a personal trigger (e.g., health consequences, comments from family or friends, or seeing an old photograph). Patients are convinced that the amount of energy it would take to address the problem outweighs the potential benefits of implementing a solution. Clinicians need to elicit the feelings of fear linked with their beliefs about what is required to change behavior. Often patients are terrified of gaining weight if they change the way they eat. They will state adamantly that they are committed to treatment, yet if we ignore their associated fears, we may end up believing our patients are resistant and become frustrated.

Patients may be unable to articulate this internal conflict that prevents them from behavioral change. Close attention should be paid to the therapist–patient relationship, as therapists often experience a sense of helplessness and frustration. This may not be a function of the therapist's skills but rather a reflection of the patient's feelings of ineffectuality. This should be mirrored back to the patient so that she genuinely feels validated. The therapist may say, "It's occurred to me that I have been feeling frustrated and even somewhat helpless as I'm listening to you. If I'm feeling this way, I can only imagine what you must be feeling. You must really feel like you're stuck."

The clinician's task is to help tip the balance in favor of change. A decision matrix can illuminate the perceived negative and positive short- and long-term consequences. It clarifies unrealistic expectations, barriers to change, and distorted thinking.

Case Example

Jen is a 24-year-old, single, Caucasian woman who met full DSM-IV research criteria for BED. She initially began to worry about her weight in the ninth grade. She states, "In high school my mom would watch me eat and tell me what I should or shouldn't eat. I began to refrain from eating in front of her, and when she wasn't around I ate whatever I could get my hands on. In the eleventh grade, it got worse. I realized that when I didn't eat, I lost weight, and guys started paying attention to me."

Jen was asked to consider both short- and long-term negative and positive consequences of continuing her problem behavior versus changing her behavior. Her decision analysis is illustrated in Figure 10.1.

Jen's matrix highlights her perceived obstacles. She finds the idea of losing weight overwhelming. She believes that she will have to adhere to a strict diet, thus feeling deprived. She has negative cognitions pertaining to her physical appearance and self-worth. Food has become associated with two interpersonal extremes. She either isolates herself and binges, or she has a boyfriend and does not eat.

THERAPIST: What does it mean for you to feel out of control?

JEN: I will not be able to stop my eating.

THERAPIST: And then what?

JEN: I'll get fat, never have a good life and end up miserable.

	Perceived Short-Term Consequences		Perceived Long-Term Consequences	
	Negative	Positive	Negative	Positive
If I continue to binge eat (don't change) . . .	I will feel fat, disgusting, and out of control. I will have no social life because I isolate myself.	It's easier, less effort, feels better in the moment, and I don't have to confront feelings of failure.	I will be more depressed, continue gaining weight, and be unhappy. I may develop other health problems.	I won't have to deal with any of my issues and worry about the future or changing.
If I change my eating patterns (eat healthily) . . .	It will be too hard. I will feel deprived. I don't know how else to cope. I'm not going to succeed.	It will be a huge accomplishment. I will have more control over my eating. I will start to lose weight.	It requires too much of me to eat healthily.	My life will be more in control, being healthy and happy. I will get married and not have to deal with issues that I am struggling with now.

FIGURE 10.1. Decision analysis form for Jen. Adapted from Marlatt and Gordon (1985). Copyright 1985 by The Guilford Press. Adapted by permission.

To explore these dysfunctional thoughts, therapists can use the vertical descent technique (Beck, Wright, Newman, & Liese, 1993). After each thought is verbalized by the patient, she is asked what that particular cognition meant to her and what is the worst that could happen. Jen ultimately believes she will "never have a boyfriend and be happy," leaving her to feel worthless. She states, "When I'm heavy I isolate in my apartment, I don't like to get dressed, or go out, therefore I won't meet anyone. I will never get married. I will be miserable forever."

THERAPIST: What do you think is so difficult about changing your eating patterns?

JEN: I don't have the willpower. I have to be consistent. I can't do it and I don't know how. I'm going to have to exercise and I must be busy constantly so I can't focus on food.

THERAPIST: Is food the only way you know how to cope with your problems?

JEN: Yes! Food is the only thing that makes me feel better. I don't think about feeling sick afterwards. I just know it tastes good.

It is possible to reframe Jen's belief that she must have willpower, stating, "I don't believe this has to do with willpower. It's not a moral failure. I just think you haven't learned the appropriate coping skills. We have to teach you how to replace your unhealthy habits with more adaptive behaviors."

Jen continues to think she must deprive herself of food, and in her mind this requires that she must always be busy. Dietary management and adapting stable eating patterns must be discussed, for Jen has the black-or-white notion that either she indulges or restricts. She fears the lack of structure in her schedule, considering it to be a powerful trigger. Time-management skills can help Jen handle large chunks of time when she is bored or to be more aware of when she is overextended.

Factors that either help to motivate the patient or, on the contrary, attenuate motivation can be elucidated by asking the following questions: "Do you understand that your binge eating must be addressed first before we focus on weight loss? What are your expectations regarding binge eating and losing weight? Are they realistic?"

JEN: I expect that I will be able to lose weight consistently and somehow I will still be allowed to eat. I probably won't lose as much weight as I want. I understand that I have to stop binge eating first, but that makes me uneasy. I want the magic cure which I know is not realistic. Losing one to two pounds per week is not acceptable to me.

THERAPIST: What do you think it will take to meet your goals? How do you actually view the process of behavioral change (is it by luck, hard work, or fate)?

JEN: It's going to be one long struggle. Eventually I will able to change the way I think, hopefully. I always look at others and compare myself. I look at their body first, then, I look to see what they are eating, and if they are skinny I wonder, "why can't I eat that"? It enrages me when I see skinny people eat whatever they want.

THERAPIST: Do you have confidence in yourself that you will be able to plan ahead and think about the consequences of your overeating? Do you tend to take responsibility for your actions, or are you more likely to wait until things just happen?

JEN: I'm bad at planning. I'm more of the "whatever happens in the moment" type. But I do know that if I had a boyfriend it would be easier for me to lose weight.

THERAPIST: Why is that?

JEN: If there was someone to look good for, I would change. I would want to see him more so I would have to be skinny and eat less.

THERAPIST: Are you aware of your cognitive distortions? Do you use a lot of "all-or-nothing" thinking?

JEN: Yes! I'm a big, fat pig. I'm a failure. I'm never going to be happy. What's wrong with me?

THERAPIST: Are you able to keep a food journal consistently?

JEN: Sometimes. But I forget, or if I have a "bad food" day I won't want to write it down.

THERAPIST: Do you have other ways to reward yourself besides using food?

JEN: Umm . . . shopping . . . but I only do that when I'm skinny.

Jen's expectation of losing more than 1–2 pounds a week is unrealistic, and she is setting herself up for failure. Her belief that it is easy for others to "be skinny" leaves her feeling more like a victim. Jen must learn how to take responsibility for change and not blame it on fate or external factors. There is little intrinsic motivation for Jen to lose weight, because she connects weight loss with having a boyfriend. Jen needs to develop her own personal reasons for changing her behavior and must have the confidence in her ability to do so, without a boyfriend. Cognitive restructuring for her dichotomous thinking is also important so that she can motivate herself through reinforcing self-talk. Finally, Jen must learn how to choose small nonfood rewards.

Self-Efficacy

One of the theoretical frameworks applicable to weight management is Bandura's (1977) social learning theory (Dennis & Goldberg, 1996). Self-efficacy reflects an individual's belief that she is capable of performing a particular behavior that will lead to a desired outcome (Bandura, 1977). In this context, it refers to an individual's belief in her ability to initiate a distinct eating and/or exercise behavior or to cope with high-risk situations to prevent a relapse to maladaptive behaviors (Marlatt, 1985; Thomas, 1995). When faced with a high-risk situation, individuals with low self-efficacy are more likely to surrender to temptation, whereas those with high self-efficacy are able to cope effectively (Clark, Abrams, Niaura, Eaton, & Rossi, 1991).

Little empirical research exists on the role of self-efficacy in binge-eating disorder. Cargill, Clark, Pera, Niaura, and Abrams (1999) have found a negative correlation between self-efficacy and binge eating, identifying poor perception of body image and feelings of shame as integral components. Other intervention studies have shown that high ratings of self-efficacy prior to treatment were significantly associated with weight loss (Bernier & Avard, 1986), along with positive changes in physical activity (Sallis, Pinski, Grossman, Patterson, & Nader, 1988).

Our patients frequently have low levels of self-efficacy and hold a common perception that they will fail in their attempts to change their disordered eating. During the contemplation stage, it is important for clinicians to assess self-efficacy. By asking questions about patients' past attempts to change their behavior, factors that either contributed to success or impeded progress will be identified. For example, a patient may reveal that when she had lost weight at one time, she had been on an exercise program. The therapist will use this information to work with her on setting small goals to begin an exercise program now.

If the patient cannot identify successful factors, setting small concrete goals weekly is useful. Clinicians can tell their patients, "This week, all I want you to do is to take one day and see if you can eat every three to four hours. That's it. I just want you to focus on one day on which you will do this." Focusing on one day rather than seven is easier and usually can be met with success. Setting and meeting small goals will increase self-efficacy, which, in turn, will motive the patient to go ahead and try another goal.

ACTION STAGE

A favorable outcome of the contemplation stage is increased self-efficacy, preparing the patient to move to the action stage. Although patients have more confidence, we still must continue to remind them that change will not be immediate. Mistakes are inevitable and human. During the action stage, clinicians may witness patients' feelings of lack of control, perfectionistic beliefs, and dichotomous thinking. Patients frequently engage in this "all-or-nothing" thinking and interpret their mistakes as total failures, deciding "it's not worth it." If they slip one day (i.e., binge), they are more vulnerable to stating, "That's it. I blew it. I can't do this." Patients must be reminded about the changes they have made thus far and realize that change is not a matter of "being perfect" versus "being a failure."

Specific Roadblocks

Goal Setting

Setting reasonable goals is a critical factor in successfully changing behavior. Goals must be small, specific, and manageable. Have the patient focus on achieving a concrete, more proximal goal rather than a long-term outcome of weight loss. Our patients tend to say, "Tomorrow I'm going to be good, eat better and exercise more." Although commendable, it does not tell us exactly what the patient will do to achieve this; it is vague and abstract. What does "good" mean? What does "eating better" actually entail? *When* will the patient exercise? *What* will she do? *Where* will she do this? What if something prevents her from doing it? It is more effective to have your patient declare, "During this week I will choose three days in which I will concentrate on eating consistently every three to four hours. That means I will eat three meals (breakfast, lunch, and dinner) with two to three snacks in between. The other four days I will not be overly vigilant about my eating. My priority is to focus on *when* I eat, not what I eat." If the patient sees that she can stabilize her eating patterns for a few days, gradually she is able to shape her behavior to do this every day. By slowly and successfully integrating this defined goal into her behavioral repertoire, she will be more confident in her ability to change.

Appropriate goal setting in conjunction with contingency management helps maintain motivation (Grilo, Shiffman, & Wing, 1993). Each time the patient meets her designated goal, does she follow it with a nonfood reward? The concept of self-reward is often not familiar to patients with eating disorders. Therapists must elicit from their patients what they would consider a reward, something that is accessible and personally valuable (preferably not too expensive).

Jen had agreed to concentrate on 2 days during the week and 1 day on the weekend on which she would implement her changes. Taking into account her work, responsibilities, socializing, and other potential stressors, she chose these days accordingly. She thought about her week so that she could identify what could happen that would prevent her from following her plan. We discussed where she was going to be during each day and what times she would eat and focused on how she would make food readily accessible and available.

At first, Jen said that she would "make dinner when she got home." I asked her, "What if you have no food or you are too tired to cook?" She did not think this would be a problem. But in exploring this, I asked her, "What's in your kitchen now? Are you really going to go food shopping in the next couple of days—what if you don't? Are you going to pick up food somewhere, or will you order it in?" Jen realized she had to be practical and realistic about adopting this new behavior. In the past, she usually said, "I *should* go food shopping. I *should* cook healthy food. Why can't I get it together and not be so lazy?"

Patients may resist discussing the minutiae of their lives, believing that they already "know" what to do. It must be pointed out that the issue does not have to do with what they know but rather with what are they *willing* to do and what *can* they do, not what they "should" do. Often patients feel guilty when they do not have the time to go food shopping or cook. If cooking and shopping are not practical in someone's individual schedule, the therapist should help her develop an alternative plan. Many times patients hold the strict belief "I should have cooked my own food," rather than just buying prepared food or ordering it in.

Self-Monitoring

Self-monitoring via food journals helps to identify the antecedents and consequences surrounding binge episodes. Patients can ask themselves:

- Am I able to detect a pattern and frequency in my binges?
- Are there particular foods I crave when I binge?
- Am I aware of my emotions before, during, and/or after the binge?
- Are my triggers external (environmental) or internal (emotional, cognitive)?

In addition to observing daily food intake, self-monitoring enables patients to plan menus ahead of time and to track their own progress. Some patients balk at the idea of self-monitoring. As therapists, we know the importance of keeping a food journal. The clinician can inform the patient that completing food journals and self-monitoring is one of the strongest predictors of successful weight loss (Boutelle & Kirschenbaum, 1998). Agree with and validate your patient's feelings when she complains it is tough to keep a food journal. Do not hesitate to say, "Who wants to keep a food journal? It's a pain. However, it's important that we figure out what will help you to keep one." Until a patient can demonstrate that she is able to consistently keep a food journal, the therapist should not move on to another aspect of treatment.

Stimulus Control

Stimulus control and response prevention requires that patients learn to identify environmental cues associated with the binge episode. Instead of their normal response (bingeing), they modify their behavior by avoiding a specific trigger or by decreasing the situations in which they will be tempted to overeat. When the patient realizes what is associated with her undesired eating, she can change these cues. This may entail removing certain foods from her home, controlling her portions, throwing away food, or eating in a specific place. Breaking the associated cues is not easy for patients—especially when habits are deeply ingrained.

After work, Jen feels exhausted and starving. She heads straight for the refrigerator. By asking Jen to walk into her home and, instead, wait 10 minutes before she opens the refrigerator, we use the tactic of delaying time so that she is able to proactively make a choice rather than impulsively reacting. However, here is the caveat: Patients often believe that by asking them to delay their behavior, you are really using "reverse psychology" and that they are not supposed to eat after those 10 minutes. This could not be further from the truth. In fact, the patient must agree that after she waits 10 minutes, she will open the refrigerator and eat something. In doing this, the patient will avoid those little mind games she plays with herself to withhold eating and see if she has the willpower. Willpower is not the issue here. The patient must learn how to use delayed time as a means of slowing her behavior down. Gradually, with shaping, the association of immediately opening the refrigerator after a stressful day at work can be severed.

Cognitive Restructuring

Binge eaters are characterized by their perfectionistic attitudes and dichotomous thinking, especially with respect toward self, food, shape, and weight (Cargill et al., 1999; Spitzer et al., 1993). Fairburn, Welch, Doll, Davies, and O'Conner (1997) have researched the potential variables that place an individual at risk for BED and found that repeated exposure to negative comments from family members about weight and negative self-evaluation were two major risk factors. Additional studies have shown that binge eaters have self-schemas related to unworthiness and rejection (Nauta et al., 2000).

Binge eaters may attempt to escape the unpleasant feelings created by disparaging cognitions (Heatherton & Baumeister, 1991). By focusing on bingeing, negative self-awareness is reduced. Clinicians can examine how their patients developed and maintained these perceptions. Addressing negative self-schemas apart from the cognitive distortions regarding food, shape, and weight is also central.

Jen's mother made comments about what she ate while she was growing up. She would ask, "Are you sure you want to eat that? You know, it's very fattening." Also, Jen noticed that the slimmer she became, the more attention she received from boys. The feared-fantasy technique here was useful: "What would happen if you never achieve this ideal shape?" Jen responded, "If I don't lose weight, I will be fat, disgusting, and never have a boyfriend." She jumps to the most negative outcome and predicts that she will always be rejected. When asked about her emotions during a binge episode, this is how she replied:

THERAPIST: Do you know what you feel prior to a binge? Are you aware of your emotions?

JEN: Before I binge, I could care less about what I feel. I don't feel anything. I'm on a mission.

THERAPIST: What happens during the binge?

JEN: I don't know. I don't want to be interrupted. I just put my feelings aside. I'm numb.

THERAPIST: How about when you are finished?

JEN: I feel fat, gross, and miserable.

THERAPIST: What would happen if something interrupted your binge and you couldn't continue eating?

JEN: I'd feel annoyed . . . kind of weird. I'd find a way to continue.

THERAPIST: What would happen if you couldn't continue—and you *had* to deal with those feelings?

JEN: Well, this might sound strange but I think I would feel hopeless. I'd feel . . . empty.

THERAPIST: And what would happen if you just stayed with that uncomfortable feeling of emptiness?

JEN: I wouldn't be able to do that—I've never done that before.

Binge eaters are afraid of what will happen if they eat a "forbidden food." They fear that they may start bingeing and be unable to stop. Patients often describe food as being "good" or "bad." They tend to engage in emotional reasoning, stating "I *feel* disgusting, therefore I must be disgusting. I *feel* so bloated, I'm fat."

Patients frequently make another cognitive error by overgeneralizing, using terms such as "never," "always," "everyone," and "no one." With Jen, a common theme is that she "will never have a boyfriend and never get married." These distortions can be challenged by asking, "How do you know you will never have a boyfriend? Have you had relationships in the past? And what makes you think you won't have one in the future?"

MAINTENANCE STAGE

"Maintenance" is defined as the "active prevention of relapse" (Marlatt & Gordon, 1985). Educating patients in the self-management principles behind the cognitive-behavioral model of relapse prevention is necessary to consolidate and maintain behavioral change (Marlatt & Gordon, 1985). Patients are asked to consider all of the techniques that they have learned and to identify which ones they are willing to use and which ones they find effective. The concept of a healthy lifestyle (including nutritional eating and regular exercise) is incorporated into treatment, and other problematic areas may have to be addressed, such as, stress management, assertiveness training, and body image issues.

Changing one's eating patterns is a lifelong commitment. Patients need to fully grasp the notion that slips (i.e., reverting to an old behavioral pattern) are the rule, not the exception. The difference between the occasional slip and a complete relapse to old behaviors must be explained. Patients tend to overgeneralize their mistakes into complete failures. Slips can be reframed into a learning experience by asking, "What could I have done differently to prevent this slip from occurring?" Answering this question will illuminate their high-risk situations.

The stress-coping model discussed in the addiction process (Wills & Shiffman, 1985) can be useful for binge eaters. This model posits that substances used by the individual serve as a means of coping with life stressors. It functions to either lessen negative affect or induce positive feelings (Wills & Shiffman, 1985). Instead of drugs or alcohol, food can be thought of as the substance used. Relapse is believed to be a consequence of maladaptive coping (bingeing) when an individual is faced with a high-risk situation (Grilo, Shiffman, & Wing, 1989; Marlatt & Gordon, 1985). Clinicians can explain to patients that coping strategies are to be conceptualized in a temporal fashion. Patients are taught to be aware of the antecedents that lead up to the high-risk situation. If they cannot avert the high-risk situation and begin overeating, how could they handle their problematic behavior in that immediate moment? If they have succumbed to bingeing against their desire, how do they cope with the aftermath of the binge?

Anticipatory, immediate, and restorative coping has been described in previous research (Wills & Shiffman, 1985). It is a practical distinction when teaching patients how to cope. Stating "Without 'AIR' I cannot survive" reminds patients of what they need to do. "AIR" is an acronym that stands for Anticipatory coping, Immediate coping, and Restorative coping. Anticipatory coping entails having the patient learn how to plan, prepare ahead, and problem solve. Questions to ask are: "Can I predict ahead and think about potential stressors? Where will I be most vulnerable?"

Immediate coping occurs in the attempt to resist the urge to binge when faced with the actual situation. Can the patient appropriately restructure her cognitions and interrupt the binge? "If I eat this, how will I feel afterward? If I choose not to eat, how will I feel? Is it worth eating? What kind of emotions and sensations will I have to deal with if I don't eat this immediately?"

Have patients carry a 3 × 5 personal coping card. They can write down their individual reasons for not wanting to binge and include the positive consequences they envision if they stop bingeing. It may be as simple as, "If I stop bingeing and start to lose weight, I will be able to wear that dress in my closet." When confronted with a high-risk situation, patients can immediately read their coping cards to easily recall their personal reasons for not wanting to give in to the binge. Patients can also write down coping statements (e.g., "I know that I'm experiencing an intense urge to eat, but I can handle this craving"; "I've just never given myself a chance to tolerate these uncomfortable feelings"; "It's like a wave and I have to ride it out"; "This will pass and I will have greater control").

Restorative coping is taught to patients after a binge episode, when they are likely to fall into the abstinence violation effect ("the goal violation effect"). Patients ask, "What is the effect of violating my goal of moderate to healthy eating?" We want patients to learn to minimize feelings of self-reproach while challenging their maladaptive cognitions ("It's no use, I can't do this, I give up"). In restorative coping, it is how the patient handles the aftermath of the binge that is crucial. If she can learn from the situation and see what precipitated the binge without harsh judgment, it is more likely she will maintain feelings of self-efficacy.

AFFECT REGULATION

According to Heatherton and Baumeister's "escape theory" (1991), binge eating may serve as an avoidant coping strategy used to reduce negative affective states (Castonguay, Eldredge, & Agras, 1995). Binge eaters have higher levels of aversive self-awareness resulting in negative self-evaluation and distress (Heatherton & Baumeister, 1991). By using cognitive narrowing, individuals shift their attention from an abstract preoccupation with the self to the concrete behaviors and sensations surrounding an immediate binge. Negative emotional states are frequently reported as common high-risk situations (Marlatt & Gordon, 1985). After a binge episode, negative affect intensifies, accompanied by distorted cognitions, resulting in the abstinence violation effect (Marlatt & Gordon, 1985).

Negative emotions have often been ignored in standard cognitive-behavioral therapy for BED. Although cognitive-behavioral therapy and IPT are the most extensively researched and efficacious treatments, neither one of these therapies targets affect regulation (Telch, 1997). Binge eaters have difficulty managing their negative emotions, and bingeing may serve as a maladaptive coping strategy. This lack of attention given to teaching emotion regulation may account for some of the noncompliance and resistance clinicians encounter.

Dialectical behavior therapy (DBT; Linehan, 1993a, 1993b), originally developed for patients with borderline personality disorder, assumes that these individuals are unable to identify, express, and tolerate their emotional states. This treatment teaches emotion regulation in lieu of maladaptive behaviors. By referring to Linehan's *Skills Training Manual* (1993b) and incorporating this theoretical model into my work with binge eaters, I have found two components to be most useful: (1) mindfulness; that is, skills in observing, describing, and experiencing emotions from a nonjudgmental stance; (2) emotion regulation; that is, skills in identifying, expressing, and tolerating emotional states and learning how to modulate affect (Safer, Telch, & Agras, 2001).

Mindfulness is considered the core skill on which other skills are based. Teaching mindfulness requires the individual to actively observe the contents of her mind in the very present without trying to avoid distressing thoughts or feelings and without becoming too attached (Linehan,1993a, 1993b). Instead, she acts as an observer and describes her emotional experience without self-criticism. By paying attention to what is happening in the present, patients learn how to gain more control of their reactions. The patient starts by focusing on her breathing, noting whether it is too shallow or deep, and then begins diaphragmatic breathing. When she notices her mind drifting away and the negative self-talk returning, she is to come back to her breathing once again. Focusing on the sensation of breathing in the "here and now" starts to break down the cognitive rigid rules concerning food, shape, and weight (Kabatznick, 1998). Emotion regulation is concurrently practiced as the individual then learns how to identify, label, articulate, and tolerate her emotions.

Binge eaters often describe "numbing out" while eating. When Jen was discussing what she felt, she was only able to state, "I don't care. I don't feel. I'm on a mission." She believed she would be unable to tolerate her emotions during that moment, especially once she recognized that she may feel "empty." Learning the skills of mindfulness enables her to identify particular feeling states. She could observe the contents of her mind and participate in the experience without anesthetizing herself by eating compulsively.

INTEROCEPTIVE AWARENESS

Binge eaters have difficulty in identifying interoceptive states (i.e., internal states such as hunger and satiety), possibly resulting from a history of restrained eating (Lowe, 1993). They do not recognize actual hunger and are often triggered by other factors, such as distorted cognitions, emotions, intense cravings, and dietary restraint (Waters, Hill, & Waller, 2000). To address this issue, Allen and Craighead (1999) developed an intervention called appetite awareness training (AAT), which uses self-monitoring based on appetite ratings, not on recording food intake and content. Adapting their technique is helpful for patients learning how to minimize eating in response to nonappetite cues. Allen and Craighead (1999) distinguish between two separate behaviors: (1) eating in response to moderate hunger, and (2) terminating eating in response to moderate fullness.

Figure 10.2 is a Hunger–Fullness Monitoring Record, which uses a scale from 1 to 7 to rate intensity of hunger. Patients should focus on the range between 2.5 and 5.5. When they rate their hunger 2.5 or below, this is an indication that they have waited too long to eat and are restricting. If they assign a rating of 5.5 or above, they have eaten too much. Patients record their hunger rating before they begin the meal and on completion of the meal. With practice, they become more attuned to their internal physiological hunger cues. Patients should not be introduced to monitoring their

Hunger–Fullness Ratings:

1 2 3 4 5 6 7

≤ 2.5 Restriction of food intake ≥ 5.5 Overeating and being "stuffed"

B = Before eating
A = After eating

	Monday	Tuesday	Wednesday	Thursday	Friday	Saturday	Sunday
Breakfast	B__A__	B__A__	B__A__	B__A__	B__A__	B__A__	B__A__
Snack	B__A__	B__A__	B__A__	B__A__	B__A__	B__A__	B__A__
Lunch	B__A__	B__A__	B__A__	B__A__	B__A__	B__A__	B__A__
Snack	B__A__	B__A__	B__A__	B__A__	B__A__	B__A__	B__A__
Dinner	B__A__	B__A__	B__A__	B__A__	B__A__	B__A__	B__A__
Snack	B__A__	B__A__	B__A__	B__A__	B__A__	B__A__	B__A__

FIGURE 10.2. Hunger–Fullness Monitoring Record. Adapted from Wylie-Rosett and Segal-Isaacson (1999). Copyright 1999 by the American Diabetes Association. Adapted by permission from the American Diabetes Association.

appetites until they demonstrate they can successfully keep a food journal and eat consistently (Allen & Craighead, 1999).

CONCLUSION

By understanding the various theoretical models that have been proposed for disordered eating, clinicians can be more effective in matching treatment to the patient. The difficulty that arises with this population stems from high attrition rates, noncompliance issues, and treatment resistance. Rather than using one strict intervention that may inherently have limited applicability to clinical practice, I integrate techniques from different theoretical models. Indeed, this integration of strategies from different therapies has not been subject to rigorous empirical testing, yet it extends my conceptualization of working with this complicated population. It is hoped that theory-driven models developed to understand disordered eating will continue to generate future therapeutic interventions.

REFERENCES

Agras, W. S., Rossiter, E. M., Arnow, B., Schneider, J. A., Telch, C. F., Raeburn, S. D., et al. (1992). Pharmacologic and cognitive-behavioral treatment for bulimia nervosa: A controlled comparison. *American Journal of Psychiatry, 149,* 82–87.

Agras, W. S., Telch, C. F., Arnow, B., Eldredge, K., Detzer, M. J., Henderson, J., & Marnell, M. (1995). Does interpersonal therapy help patients with binge eating disorder who fail to respond to cognitive-behavioral therapy? *Journal of Consulting and Clinical Psychology, 63,* 356–360.

Agras, W. S., Walsh, B. T., Fairburn, C. G., Wilson, G. T., & Kraemer, H. C. (2000). A multi-center comparison of cognitive-behavioral therapy and interpersonal psychotherapy for bulimia nervosa. *Archives of General Psychiatry, 57,* 459–466.

Allen, H. N., & Craighead, L. W. (1999). Appetite monitoring in the treatment of binge eating disorder. *Behavior Therapy, 30,* 253–272.

American Psychiatric Association. (1994). *Diagnostic and statistical manual of mental disorders* (4th ed.). Washington, DC: Author.

Bandura, A. (1977). Self-efficacy: Toward a unifying theory of behavioral change. *Psychological Review, 84*(2), 191–215.

Beck, A. T., Wright, F. D., Newman, C. F., & Liese, B. S. (1993). *Cognitive therapy of substance abuse.* New York: Guilford Press.

Becker, A. E., Grinspoon, S. K., Klibanski, A., & Herzog, D. B. (1999). Eating disorders. *New England Journal of Medicine, 340,* 1092–1098.

Bernier, M., & Avard, J. (1986). Self-efficacy, outcome and attrition in a weight reduction program. *Cognitive Therapy and Research, 10,* 319–338.

Boutelle, K. N., & Kirschenbaum, D. S. (1998). Further support for consistent self-monitoring as a vital component of successful weight control. *Obesity Research, 6*(3), 219–224.

Bruce, B., & Wilfley, D. (1996). Binge eating among the overweight population: A serious and prevalent problem. *Journal of the American Dietetic Association, 96*(1), 58–61.

Cargill, B. R., Clark, M. M., Pera, V., Niaura, R. S., & Abrams, D. B. (1999). Binge eating, body image, depression, and self-efficacy in an obese clinical population. *Obesity Research, 7,* 379–386.

Castonguay, L. G., Eldredge, K. L., & Agras, W. S. (1995). Binge eating disorder: Current state and future directions. *Clinical Psychology Review, 15*(8), 865–890.

Clark, M. M., Abrams, D. B., Niaura, R. S., Eaton, C. A., & Rossi, J. S. (1991). Self-efficacy in weight management. *Journal of Consulting and Clinical Psychology, 59*(5), 739–744.

Dennis, K. E., & Goldberg, A. P. (1996). Weight control self-efficacy types and transitions affect weight-loss outcomes in obese women. *Addictive Behaviors, 21*(1), 103–116.

de Zwaan, M., & Mitchell, J. E. (1992). Binge eating in the obese. *Annals of Medicine, 24,* 303–308.

Fairburn, C. G. (1993). Interpersonal psychotherapy for bulimia nervosa. In G. L. Klerman & M. M. Weissman (Eds.), *New applications of interpersonal psychotherapy* (pp. 353–378). Washington, DC: American Psychiatric Association.

Fairburn, C. G., Cooper, Z., & Cooper, P. J. (1986). The clinical features and maintenance of bulimia nervosa. In K. D. Brownell & J. P. Foreyt (Eds.), *Handbook of eating disorders: Physiology, psychology and treatment of obesity, anorexia and bulimia* (pp. 389–404). New York: Basic Books.

Fairburn, C. G., Marcus, M. D., & Wilson, G. T. (1993). Cognitive behavior therapy for binge eating and bulimia nervosa: A comprehensive treatment manual. In C. G. Fairburn & G. T. Wilson (Eds.), *Binge eating: Nature, assessment and treatment* (pp. 361–404). New York: Guilford Press.

Fairburn, C. G., Shafran, R., & Cooper, Z. (1998). A cognitive behavioral theory of anorexia nervosa. *Behavior Research and Therapy, 37,* 1–13.

Fairburn, C. G., Welch, S. L., Doll, H. A., Davies, B. A., & O'Conner, M. E. (1997). Risk factors for binge eating disorder: A community-based, case-control study. *Archives of General Psychiatry, 55,* 425–432.

Fairburn, C. G., & Wilson, G. T. (Eds.) (1993). *Binge eating: Nature, assessment, and treatment.* New York: Guilford Press.

Foreyt, J. P., Poston, W. S. C., & Goodrick, G. K. (1996). Future directions in obesity and eating disorders. *Addictive Behaviors, 21*(6), 767–778.

Grilo, C. M. (1996). Treatment of obesity: An integrative model. In J. K. Thompson (Ed.), *Body image, eating disorders and obesity.* Washington, DC: American Psychiatric Association.

Grilo, C. M., Shiffman, S., & Wing, R. R. (1989). Relapse crises and coping among dieters. *Journal of Consulting and Clinical Psychology, 57*(4), 488–495.

Grilo, C. M., Shiffman, S., & Wing, R. R. (1993). Coping with dietary relapse crises and their aftermath. *Addictive Behaviors, 18,* 89–102.

Heatherton, T. F., & Baumeister, R. F. (1991). Binge eating as escape from self-awareness. *Psychological Bulletin, 110*(1), 86–108.

Kabatznick, R. (1998). *The zen of eating: Ancient answers to modern weight problems.* New York: Penguin Putnam.

Leibbrand, R., & Fichter, M. M. (2002). Maintenance of weight loss after obesity treatment: Is continuous support necessary? *Behavior Research and Therapy, 40*(11), 1275–1289.

Linehan, M. M. (1993a). *Cognitive-behavioral treatment of borderline personality disorder.* New York: Guilford Press.

Linehan, M. M. (1993b). *Skills training manual for treating borderline personality disorder.* New York: Guilford Press.

Lowe, M. R. (1993). The effects of dieting on eating behavior: A three-factor model. *Psychological Bulletin, 114,* 100–121.

Marcus, M. D., Wing, R. R., & Hopkins, J. (1988). Obese binge eaters: Affect, cognitions, and response to behavioral weight control. *Journal of Consulting and Clinical Psychology, 56*(3), 433–439.

Marlatt, G. A. (1985). Coping and substance abuse: Implications for research, prevention, and treatment. In S. Shiffman & T. A. Wills (Eds.), *Coping and substance use* (pp. 365–386). New York: Academic Press.

Marlatt, G. A., & Gordon, J. R. (Eds.). (1985). *Relapse prevention: Maintenance strategies in the treatment of addictive behaviors.* New York: Guilford Press.

Miller, W. R., & Rollnick, S. (1991). *Motivational interviewing: Preparing people to change addictive behavior.* New York: Guilford Press.

Nauta, H., Hospers, H. J., Jansen, A., & Kok, G. (2000). Cognitions in obese binge eaters and obese non-binge eaters. *Cognitive Therapy and Research, 24*(5), 521–531.

Polivy, J., & Herman, C. P. (2002). Causes of eating disorders. *Annual Review of Psychology, 53,* 187–213.

Prochaska, J. O., & DiClemente, C. C. (1982). Transtheoretical therapy: Toward a more integrative model of change. *Psychotherapy: Theory, Research and Practice, 20,* 161–173.

Prochaska, J. O., DiClemente, C. C., & Norcross, J. C. (1992). In search of how people change: Applications to addictive behaviors. *American Psychologist, 47,* 1102–1114.

Safer, D. L., Telch, C. F., & Agras, W. S. (2001). Dialectical behavior therapy adapted for bulimia: A case report. *International Journal of Eating Disorders, 30,* 101–106.

Sallis, J. F., Pinski, R. B., Grossman, R. M., Patterson, T. L., & Nader, P. R. (1988). The development of self-efficacy scales for health-related diet and exercise behaviors. *Health Education Research, 3*(3), 283–292.

Spitzer, R. L., Devlin, M., Walsh, B. T., Hasin, D., Wing, R., Marcus, M., et al. (1992). Binge eating disorder: A multisite field trial of the diagnostic criteria. *International Journal of Eating Disorders, 11,* 191–203.

Spitzer, R. L., Yanovski, S., Wadden, T., Wing, R., Marcus, M. D., Stunkard, A., et al. (1993). Binge eating disorder: Its further validation in a multisite study. *International Journal of Eating Disorders, 13*(2), 137–153.

Telch, C. F. (1997). Skills training treatment for adaptive affect regulation in a woman with binge-eating disorder. *International Journal of Eating Disorders, 22,* 77–81.

Telch, C. F., & Agras, W. S. (1994). Obesity, binge eating and psychopathology: Are they related? *International Journal of Eating Disorders, 15*(1), 53–61.

Telch, C. F., Agras, W. S., Rossiter, E. M., Wilfley, D., & Kenardy, J. (1990). Group cognitive-behavioral therapy for the nonpurging bulimic: An initial evaluation. *Journal of Consulting and Clinical Psychology, 58,* 629–635.

Thomas, P. R. (Ed.). (1995). *Weighing the options: Criteria for evaluating weight-management programs.* Washington, DC: National Academy Press.

Towell, D. B., Woodford, S., Reid, S., Rooney, B., & Towell, A. (2001). Compliance and outcome in treatment-resistant anorexia and bulimia: A restrospective study. *British Journal of Clinical Psychology, 40,* 189–195.

Waters, A., Hill, A., & Waller, G. (2000). Internal and external antecedents of binge eating episodes in a group of women with bulimia nervosa. *International Journal of Eating Disorders, 29,* 17–22.

Wilfley, D. E., Agras, W. S., Telch, C. F., Rossiter, E. M., Schneider, J. A., Cole, A. G., et al. (1993). Group cognitive-behavioral therapy and group interpersonal psychotherapy for the nonpurging bulimic individual: A controlled comparison. *Journal of Consulting and Clinical Psychology, 61,* 296–305.

Wills, T. A., & Shiffman, S. (1985). Coping and substance use: A conceptual framework. In S. Shiffman & T. A. Wills (Eds.), *Coping and substance use* (pp. 3–24). New York: Academic Press.

Wilson, G. T., & Pike, K. M. (2001). Eating disorders. In Barlow, D. H. (Ed.), *Clinical handbook of psychological disorders: A step-by-step treatment manual* (pp. 332–375). New York: Guilford Press.

Wonderlich, S. A., Mitchell, J. E., Peterson, C. B., & Crow, S. (2001). Integrative cognitive therapy for bulimic behavior. In R. H. Striegel-Moore & L. Smolak (Eds.), *Eating disorders: Innovative directions in research and practice* (pp. 173–195). Washington, DC: American Psychological Association.

Wylie-Rosett, J., & Segal-Isaacson, C. J. (Eds.). (1999). *The leader's guide to the complete weight loss workbook: Proven techniques for controlling weight related health problems.* Alexandria, VA: American Diabetes Association.

Part IV

Couples and Families

11

Couple Therapy

Norman B. Epstein
Donald H. Baucom

Cognitive-behavioral therapy with individual clients poses a number of challenges, which are discussed in the other chapters in this book. Motivating just one individual to examine long-standing ways of thinking about the self and the world and to experiment with new ways of thinking and behaving can be a significant challenge. Factors contributing to an individual exhibiting "resistance" to the process of therapy and to changing his or her life patterns may involve characteristics of the client, such as extreme beliefs about the way things "should" be in the world, and characteristics of the therapist, such as a failure to listen empathically to the client's concerns. Consequently, cognitive-behavioral therapists who work with individuals must try to identify how each client may respond in idiosyncratic ways to interventions, based on both the client's personal characteristics and the therapist's behavior toward the client. As other authors in this volume have illustrated, a therapist must pay attention to the quality of his or her relationship with an individual client, so that the relationship can facilitate rather than interfere with change.

The complexities of therapy increase considerably when one works jointly with both members of a couple. Not only does the therapist need to consider the dynamics of the relationship between the two partners but must also attend to his or her relationship with each member of the couple, as well as to how each member perceives the therapist's relationship with the other person. Each partner is likely to notice any imbalances in the degrees to which the therapist talks to, smiles at, agrees with, interrupts, challenges, or in any other way interacts with the two of them. In addition, an intervention that might feel comfortable and work well with one partner may make the other uncomfortable, defensive, and so forth. Thus couple therapists face the challenge of simultaneously developing rapport with two people who may have quite different personal styles and agendas for therapy.

In spite of the complexities of couple therapy, there are important reasons for conducting conjoint sessions with a couple, based on family systems, social learning, and cognitive therapy concepts that form the foundation of cognitive-behavioral couple therapy (Baucom & Epstein, 1990; Epstein & Baucom, 2002). Systems and social learning models both emphasize *circular causality* in couple relationships, in which two partners continually exert mutual influences on each other's cognitions, emotions, and behavior. One of the key tasks facing couple therapists is modifying distressed partners' tendency to think in linear causal terms and to hold each other responsible for relationship problems. For example, in the common demand–withdraw pattern that is associated with relationship distress (Christensen, 1988; Christensen & Heavey, 1990; Gottman, 1994), the individual who pursues the other in a demanding manner tends to explain the behavior as, "I need to pursue my partner to talk about issues because he or she keeps withdrawing," whereas the withdrawing individual explains his or her actions as, "I need to back off because my partner won't leave me alone." Elsewhere (Epstein & Baucom, 2002) we have described the importance of increasing *relational schematic thinking*, the person's tendency to think about relationship events in terms of dyadic interaction patterns rather than characteristics of each individual. Cognitive therapists are well aware that in individual therapy clients commonly present biased views of significant others who are not present. Consequently, conjoint sessions reduce the chance that a therapist will develop a distorted perception of a couple's problems, based on either the individual partners' own distorted views of their relationship or on their attempts to form an alliance with the therapist by portraying the other person in a negative light.

Couple therapists use a variety of interventions, described in this chapter, to draw partners' attention to ways in which each person contributes to a repetitive circular process in their interactions. Conjoint therapy sessions are invaluable because many of the interpersonal dynamics that occur during the couple's daily interactions outside the therapist's office also are exhibited during sessions. During conjoint sessions the therapist can draw the partners' attention to circular processes at the moment they occur. Conjoint sessions also allow the therapist to intervene directly to modify a couple's problematic behavioral patterns. Once a therapist has identified a particular negative behavior pattern, he or she can coach the couple in rehearsing more constructive ways of behaving toward each other, during sessions and as homework between sessions (Baucom & Epstein, 1990; Epstein & Baucom, 2002; Rathus & Sanderson, 1999).

Finally, mounting research evidence is showing that depression, anxiety disorders, substance abuse, and other disorders that traditionally have been assessed and treated on an individual basis are influenced by the person's significant relationships (e.g., Beach, 2000; Craske & Zoellner, 1995; Miklowitz & Goldstein, 1997; O'Farrell & Rotunda, 1997). Increasingly, couple and family therapy is being used either as an adjunctive treatment or as the primary treatment for many of these clinical problems (Baucom, Shoham, Mueser, Daiuto, & Stickle, 1998). If a therapist works solely with a member of a couple who is experiencing symptoms of psychopathology, opportunities may be missed to observe and intervene firsthand with couple interactions that exacerbate the individual's difficulties or to help the couple cope more effectively with the individual's symptoms. Thus there are compelling reasons for therapists who treat individual psychopathology to attend to couple dynamics as well, either in their own practice or by collaborating with couple therapists.

CHARACTERISTICS OF COUPLES THAT CAN CONTRIBUTE TO THERAPY ROADBLOCKS

Even though the members of a couple are sufficiently distressed about their relationship to seek help from a couple therapist, a variety of factors may still interfere with their levels of engagement and progress in therapy:

- Partners' negativity and hopelessness about change in their relationship.
- Discomfort about participating in joint therapy.
- Distress about changing current characteristics of the relationship.
- Failure to take personal responsibility for change.
- The therapist's ways of relating to the two partners and of conducting the therapy.

We describe each of these potential roadblocks to productive couple therapy and strategies for overcoming them in the following sections.

Partners' Negativity and Hopelessness about Change in Their Relationship

Couples who seek therapy commonly have a history together that includes memories of past hurts, disappointments, broken trust, and often past therapy experiences. Their memories of these events often are vivid and may override current positive behaviors of the other person, a process that Weiss (1980) has referred to as "sentiment override." Consequently, vivid memories of past negative events need to be discussed in therapy sessions, with the therapist supporting each person's natural inclination to want to feel safe from future recurrences (Epstein & Baucom, 2002). Memories of past hurts may produce overreactions to another person's relatively minor actions, and the therapist needs to guide the individual in challenging inferences that what is presently occurring is "the same old thing." It is important to guide each member of the couple in distinguishing his or her general views and feelings about the other member from the specific ways in which the person is behaving at the moment.

Thus individuals may have developed negative schemas about the characteristics of the partner, as well as about the ways in which the members of the couple interact (Dattilio, Epstein, & Baucom, 1998). Comments such as "We can't communicate" and "We are very different types of people" may reflect fixed negative views associated with a sense of hopelessness about the potential for the relationship to improve. Research studies have indicated that members of distressed couples are more likely than members of happy couples to attribute partners' negative behavior to stable, global traits (Bradbury & Fincham, 1990). Consequently, therapists need to guide partners in testing the validity of these fixed views and in considering information that suggests that patterns between members of the couple can be changed. One approach is to coach the individual in keeping track of situational variation in the other's behavior; that is, noting how the person behaves differently from one situation to another or from one time to another (Epstein & Baucom, 2002). This information counteracts the idea of an invariant trait, and it opens the door for exploration of what conditions (including the person's own behavior) tend to elicit the other's positive and negative responses.

Negative memories tend to be reinforced if an individual continues to perceive a similar pattern in a partner's behavior or if the partner is defensive and fails to take personal responsibility for his or her past actions. The therapist's challenge is to help members of a couple notice and give credit for even small positive changes, with each person taking personal responsibility for making changes (Baucom & Epstein, 1990; Epstein & Baucom, 2002). When possible, it is helpful to encourage an individual to express regret for his or her past actions that upset the partner, even if they were unintentional. The therapist can stress that this expression is not equivalent to taking the blame for a problem. Overall, the therapist needs to hear about each person's memories while attempting to keep the other person's defensiveness about the past incidents under control. As one approach to reducing partners' defensiveness, the therapist can state that he or she knows that the two people probably have different perspectives about an event and that the goal is merely to understand how each person perceives the event, rather than judging who is right or wrong.

Ultimately, reducing partners' hopelessness about the potential for improvement in their relationship depends on the therapist's ability to coach the couple in behaving more constructively with each other. Members of a couple need to observe that chronic negative interactions are decreasing and that they are behaving in more positive ways toward each other. Consequently, even though it is important to identify and modify individuals' distorted views of each other, it also is crucial to use behavioral interventions to improve the balance of positive to negative behavior that occurs in a couple's daily interactions. Elsewhere, we and others have provided detailed descriptions of methods for enhancing couples' communication skills, problem-solving skills, exchanges of social support, and other forms of positive behavior (Baucom & Epstein, 1990; Epstein & Baucom, 2002; Jacobson & Christensen, 1996; Jacobson & Margolin, 1979; Rathus & Sanderson, 1999; Stuart, 1980). We use the term "primary distress" to signify partners' distress over an unresolved core relationship issue, such as unmet intimacy needs, and the term "secondary distress" to describe the impact of negative interaction patterns (e.g., mutual criticism, demand–withdraw) that a couple has developed to cope with their unresolved concerns (Epstein & Baucom, 2002). The sooner the therapist is able to implement some change in the negative patterns that distressed couples bring to therapy, the lower the probability that hopelessness will act as a roadblock to the couple's working on key issues in their relationship.

Some couples experience hopelessness about overcoming their problems when ways of coping that worked for them in the past are ineffective with current issues or even exacerbate the problems. It is important for therapists to convey a *developmental perspective* to couples, noting that a relationship evolves over time rather than being static (Carter & McGoldrick, 1999). As time passes, the needs and challenges that the couple face change, and this requires changes in the approaches that will be successful in fulfilling those needs (Epstein & Baucom, 2002). For example, before having children a couple may have consistently had sufficient time to spend together, but after the birth of their first child they may find it very difficult to set aside enough time together. If they continue to rely on their usual strategy of spontaneously suggesting doing something together, they may find that they often must turn down each other's invitations due to competing responsibilities. This pattern may result in the couple developing a sense of hopelessness and a low level of motivation to try new approaches to their problem. A therapist may be able to counteract this hopelessness by discussing how the couple's relationship developed over time and by "normalizing" the challenges they are facing as their circumstances have changed. In particular, the therapist can note that the couple's usual approach to maintaining intimacy in their relationship was quite appropriate before they had children but that now they need to search for new approaches that provide a better match for these *normal* changes in their life.

Discomfort about Participating in Joint Therapy

Members of a couple may be concerned, often for good reason, that joint sessions will be aversive or otherwise unsafe. In addition, even when individuals are dissatisfied with some aspects of their relationship, they may fear that making particular types of changes will lead to negative consequences that they would rather avoid. Unless these concerns are addressed, partners are likely to resist participating in couple therapy at all or trying new ways of relating to each other.

Roadblocks Involving Individuals' Safety Concerns

Many individuals do not think of couple therapy as a safe setting in which they can improve their distressed relationships. It is important for the therapist to consider that members of unhappy relationships commonly have developed self-protective strategies to try to minimize their distress and that the prospect that a therapist may pressure them to abandon their defensive patterns can be threatening. Consequently, the therapist must explore whether each member of a couple is concerned about particular aspects of therapy and must address those concerns explicitly. For example, the close proximity of joint sessions, particularly when the therapist is focusing on communication skills, reduces partners' options for avoiding or withdrawing from each other, as they might typically do in daily life. Individuals who find these conditions distressing may avoid participating in communication exercises within and between sessions or may even drop out of therapy. The therapist should allow individuals to engage in some distancing during sessions when they are feeling significant distress; for example, by asking for a temporary "time out" for an agreed-on amount of time from a particularly distressing discussion.

Although it is important for the therapist to obtain a sample of a couple's typical interaction patterns, it is crucial to impose control over destructive interactions to protect partners from abuse and to reduce their avoidance of further therapy. We find it helpful to explain to couples initially that we would like to get a sample of how they communicate but that we will intervene to limit aversive interactions so that sessions will be constructive and both individuals can feel safe participating in therapy.

When working with individuals who have difficulty regulating high levels of emotion and negative behavior during conjoint therapy sessions, the therapist can impose structure by stating specific ground rules (e.g., no yelling, no verbal threats) and by interrupting the couple's interaction whenever a ground rule is violated. Occasionally a therapist may need to end a session if the members of the couple refuse to comply with such limits. The therapist then can request separate sessions with each partner, focused on preparing each person to moderate emotional expression and aversive behavior in subsequent conjoint sessions. Individual sessions establish the therapist's control of the therapy process and help each individual explore personal responses that interfere with his or her ability to behave constructively with the partner. This structure may reassure the couple that therapy will be a safe environment for working on relationship concerns.

When a therapist blocks partners' attempts to criticize and punish each other during sessions, it is important that the therapist convey empathy for each person's dissatisfaction with their relationship. The therapist can emphasize that a primary goal of therapy is to help the couple find effective ways to develop a more satisfying relationship and that the punitive approaches that they have been using have not led to improvements they desire. Instead, the therapist wants to help the partners develop new approaches that will work better.

Some individuals agree with the concept that it is important to control one's strong emotional reactions to a partner but have difficulty doing so. They may need assistance in reducing or coping with anxiety, anger, and other negative emotions that occur when they interact with their partners. Stress inoculation and anger management training procedures can be used to help individuals regulate strong emotion in the presence of significant others (Deffenbacher, 1996; Meichenbaum, 1985; Neidig & Friedman, 1984). For example, a therapist can inquire about partners' "hot" cognitions that tend to be associated with their strong emotions (e.g., "She has no right to treat me that way! I'll teach her a lesson!"). The therapist can discuss ways in which such thoughts fuel negative emotions and can coach each person in devising self-statements that may reduce his or her own strong emotions or control how they are expressed. For example, the preceding "hot cognitions" might be counteracted by thoughts such as, "She has a right to her opinion, just as I have a right to mine, and it won't change her mind if I attack her." Other useful therapeutic interventions include relaxation training, cognitive and behavioral distraction techniques (shifting attention toward thoughts and activities that are interesting and enjoyable), physical exercise, and other self-soothing activities (Bourne, 1995; Deffenbacher, 1996; Linehan, 1993).

Much of the work in couple therapy takes place between sessions, as the partners carry out various homework assignments designed to modify the ways in which they interact with each other on a daily basis. Consequently, the therapist needs to create structure to give the partners a sense of safety outside the office, as well as within sessions. It is important that the therapist and couple make explicit plans concerning specific actions that the partners can take to control abusive experiences at home. For example, if the couple has had a conflictual discussion during a session, at the end of the session the therapist can coach the couple in devising specific plans to prevent their feelings from erupting later into aversive interactions at home. Similarly, when a couple has been practicing communication skills during sessions, the therapist has opportunities to monitor and intervene with negative behavior. However, when the couple's homework involves further practice at home, the therapist and couple need to plan ways that the partners can monitor their own interactions and interrupt negative responses. If members of a couple doubt that they will experience problems with aversive interactions at home, the therapist can suggest that the couple can never be sure that all will go well and can challenge them to devise "contingency plans" in the event of unanticipated problems.

When there appears to be danger of physical abuse, it is crucial that the therapist not conduct any interventions that could place any individual at risk of harm between sessions. The therapist should interview each partner separately to determine whether the individual fears for his or her safety or whether past abusive incidents suggest that events during therapy sessions could lead to future abuse. Couple therapy should be suspended if it appears that it may elicit violence. A detailed discussion of the assessment and clinical management of abuse is beyond the scope of this chapter, but readers can consult sources such as Heyman and Neidig (1997) and Holtzworth-Munroe, Beatty, and Anglin (1995).

Personal Standards Regarding Expression of Conflict in Close Relationships

Individuals vary in their beliefs regarding "normal" and "proper" ways in which members of close relationships should handle areas of conflict (Epstein & Baucom, 2002). These beliefs commonly have been shaped by each person's earlier relationship experiences, such as the degree to which he or she was exposed to open expression of conflict in the family of origin. On the one hand, an individual may use the earlier experience as a model to be emulated (e.g., "My parents never raised their voices to each other, and that's the way couples should behave"), but on the other hand a person may view the past experiences as undesirable (e.g., "The yelling in our house was awful, so I'm going to live in a calm household"). These personal standards may act as a roadblock to progress in couple therapy by contributing to partners' being excessively or inadequately expressive with each other in sessions and at home.

For example, a therapist's goal of facilitating open communication between partners may conflict with an individual's goal of avoiding open expressiveness that he or she considers distasteful or even damaging to the couple's relationship. In such cases it is important for the therapist to explore the person's belief and its origin in prior relationship experiences. While communicating respect for the person's concerns about expressiveness, the therapist can guide him or her in identifying disadvantages of withholding feelings within the relationship. The therapist also can coach the person in planning small behavioral experiments in which he or she tries low levels of expressiveness and observes its effects.

In contrast, when an individual believes that it is appropriate to "let all of your feelings out, and not hold anything back," the therapist needs to explore the bases for the belief, as well as advantages and disadvantages of unbridled expressiveness. The individual's belief may act as a roadblock to couple therapy, limiting his or her awareness of negative effects that the behavior is having on the relationship (e.g., the partner finds the behavior aversive and either withdraws or retaliates). Sometimes it is helpful if the therapist elicits feedback from the person's partner that indicates that the individual's excessive expressiveness has not had the impact that he or she desires. For example, Jim believed that Hannah would pay more attention and respect his opinions if he expressed himself aggressively, but Hannah told him in therapy that his yelling "turns me off and reduces my respect for you."

Differences in Partners' Agendas for Their Relationship and for Therapy

Couple therapists must consider the possibility that the two members of a couple have different agendas for being in the therapist's office together. Often one person is more highly motivated than the other to participate in therapy, and at times one individual is opposed to the idea of joint therapy.

Some individuals tend to view couple therapy as a setting in which they can express their distress about a partner's problems and try to enlist the therapist's assistance as leverage for pressuring the partner to change (i.e., the partner is viewed as the source of the couple's problems). Other individuals view therapy as an opportunity to obtain an expert outsider's feedback about ways in which the couple can work together to solve problems (i.e., the person views both members of the couple as responsible for relationship problems). In addition, the members of a couple may have very different beliefs about the types of changes that are needed to create a more satisfying relationship. For example, one member of a couple may believe that increased togetherness and sharing will make them a happier couple. In contrast, the other member may believe that the couple's conflicts will decrease if his or her partner can become more accepting of differences in their preferences for autonomy versus togetherness.

Furthermore, some couples include one member who is highly motivated to make the relationship succeed and another member who has become disengaged emotionally and may desire to end the relationship. Sometimes the latter individual initially has an unstated goal of telling the partner during therapy about his or her decision to leave the relationship and may even want the therapist to take on the role of helping the distraught partner cope with the breakup.

Such discrepancies in partners' agendas for therapy tend to reflect differences in their goals for their relationship. Consequently, the roadblock of conflicting agendas in therapy can be a window into the struggles that the couple is experiencing in their daily life together. For example, the therapist might point out how one person's pressuring the other to participate in couple therapy and the other person's resistance to participating seems to reflect a broader problematic demand–withdraw pattern in the couple's relationship that the partners need to alter in some way. The therapist can explore the pursuing individual's standards for how they believe the withdrawing partner should behave. Thus Ken believed that Sarah should be interested in a high level of togetherness and sharing of personal feelings. The therapist guided Ken in considering whether his standard that his partner must share his personal preference for a high level of togetherness versus autonomy was unrealistic. Similarly, the therapist may guide the withdrawing partner in considering the validity of his or her own standards; in this case the therapist coached Sarah in evaluating the advantages and disadvantages of her belief that members of a couple should not constrain each other's activities at all. The therapist also can point out how each member of the couple contributes to the circular process of their demand–withdraw pattern and can stress that the best opportunity for change may involve each person's making an effort to change his or her part of the cycle. For example, Ken might decrease requests that Sarah spend all of her free time with him and continuously talk with him. In turn, Sarah might initiate a joint activity with Ken from time to time, as well as agreeing to join him in some of the activities he suggests.

When it becomes clear that one member of a couple wants to continue their relationship but the other member wants to end it, the therapist needs to help the couple redefine goals for therapy, or the conflicting goals will be a roadblock to further work together in therapy. The therapist may focus the couple on a *shared* goal of determining how the partners can relate in constructive rather than destructive ways in dealing with their different *individual* goals for their relationship. How can they manage their negative emotions, such as anger, so they can collaborate in finding reasonable solutions to important issues such as division of property and custody of children? How can they avoid drawing their children into their couple conflicts? If the therapist redefines the purpose of therapy as helping the couple accept the need to collaborate on minimizing damage to themselves and others who are affected by their conflicts, it may be easier to engage both partners in therapeutic work.

Distress about Changing Current Characteristics of the Relationship

Discomfort with Changing Self-Protective Strategies

As noted earlier, it is normal for each member of a distressed couple to develop self-protective strategies to avoid being hurt, disappointed, or angered further by the other person. Some self-protective strategies involve avoidance of the partner; for example, some individuals increase their involvement in activities such as jobs, household tasks, and leisure activities with friends in order to reduce overall time spent with the partner. Other individuals may avoid only particular situations in which they expect that problems will occur. For example, some individuals avoid discussions of finances because past discussions of finances led to upsetting arguments with their partner, but they talk relatively openly about some other topics. Although the avoidance pattern may reduce the person's distress in the short run, it typically fails to resolve important relationship issues. Partners who are used to avoiding each other are likely to find conjoint couple therapy threatening and avoid it as well, so therapists need to create conditions in sessions in which avoidance is less attractive.

Other individuals tend to protect themselves through aggressive means, criticizing, threatening, and blaming the partner for their relationship problems. As a result, the partner is too busy defending him- or herself or withdrawing from the individual's aggressive behavior to present much of a threat to the individual. An individual's aggressive approach to self-protection may have been learned earlier in life, as a relatively effective way of coping with aggression from significant others. Such a pattern also may have been reinforced in the person's current relationship if it was at least periodically successful in "backing off" a demanding partner. We have found that individuals often are less defensive about considering changes in their self-protective strategies if the therapist acknowledges the advantages that the strategies have produced, as well as emphasizing the negative consequences and suggesting advantages of experimenting with new approaches. It may be helpful for the therapist to turn to a person's partner and say something such as, "Sarah, Ken seems to be concerned that if he backs off from his usual style of pursuing you for togetherness, you won't do much of anything with him. What are some things you might say or do to demonstrate to Ken that he doesn't have to be so concerned about that and that you are willing to share aspects of life with him?" In order to reduce the therapy roadblock of problematic self-protective responses, often "behavioral experiments" are needed, in which the person is able to see firsthand that alternative responses work well.

Some individuals feel threatened by the possibility that therapy will promote changes that will expose an area of personal vulnerability. For example, if an individual feels insecure about his or her ability to please a partner sexually, it may be convenient that the couple has developed a pattern in which their busy schedules result in little time for sex. Consequently, if a therapist identifies that the couple is suffering from an overall lack of intimacy and suggests setting a goal of increasing their time together, that individual may find the prospect of such a change distressing. Often the other member of the couple is aware of the person's avoidance pattern but may not know the underlying reasons for it; and instead of revealing the vulnerability to the therapist, the individual may fail to carry out homework involving increased "couple time." Thus it is important for the therapist to explore each partner's thoughts and emotions about proposed changes in the couple's interactions and to probe for underlying concerns (in individual sessions if necessary) when one or both members of a couple fail to comply with homework (Epstein & Baucom, 2002).

Discomfort with Changes That May Reduce Individuals' Power/Control

A therapist must respect the existing distribution of power in a couple, even when he or she believes that shifting it is appropriate; for example, when one member's depression appears to be influenced by the other's controlling behavior. An individual who holds more power is likely to become uncomfortable if he or she perceives that changes in the couple's relationship will reduce that power, because the status quo is reinforcing for that individual.

Similarly, therapists commonly focus on the disadvantages of partners' negative behaviors, such as criticisms, venting of anger, and so forth, but individuals have continued to behave in these ways because they have experienced reinforcing consequences for the actions. For example, Doris described how venting her anger toward Sid felt good, and she enjoyed seeing how it made Sid more subdued when they were having a disagreement. When a therapist asks a client to moderate expression of anger toward a partner, the individual may experience it as a request to stop responding in a way that makes him or her feel strong, self-righteous, and invulnerable. Unless the therapist can demonstrate to the individual that these losses will be balanced by significant gains, including new ways to feel strong and safe, the reinforcing quality of the aggressive expression will continue to be a roadblock in therapy. It is important for a therapist to acknowledge payoffs of current aggressive behavior and to guide the person to weigh these advantages against the disadvantages of behaving in that manner (Neidig & Friedman, 1984). This procedure can highlight negative consequences that the person may have overlooked or minimized, such as losing the partner's love and respect.

Another aspect of couple therapy that has the potential to create a roadblock to progress based on power issues involves the therapist's challenging of each individual's cognitions. In individual cognitive therapy, many clients are open to input from a therapist regarding information that suggests that their cognitions may be inappropriate or invalid in some respects. Although other chapters in this book discuss instances in which an individual resists such input from a therapist, the fact that the therapist is an outsider whom the client commonly views as supportive often results in the client being fairly open to the therapist's input. In contrast, during joint couple therapy sessions, it is very common that individuals are uncomfortable having the therapist challenge their thinking in front of their partners who have a history of trying to invalidate their views. Therapists need to be aware that many individuals who are open to examining their unrealistic beliefs and cognitive distortions in one-to-one sessions are much less receptive to the same types of therapist input during joint sessions. They perceive the cognitive restructuring interventions as making them lose face or as giving their partners greater power in ongoing debates over who is right or wrong. Consequently, we tend to avoid using terms such as "distortion" and "invalid cognition" in couple sessions because they can be perceived as evaluative, and we consistently try to express empathy for both partners' experiences of distress in their relationship. It generally is helpful for the therapist to emphasize during the initial session that he or she considers it very important to have a balanced relationship with the two people and that if either individual perceives any bias or lack of balance, he or she should discuss it in the session. Concerning the challenging of partners' cognitions, the therapist can note that it is his or her role to help *both* individuals be aware that people's perceptions and interpretations of events in close relationships can be subjective and that it is important to check the appropriateness of one's thinking. Once partners come to view their couple therapist as fair-minded and supportive, they tend to be more open to cognitive restructuring interventions (Epstein & Baucom, 2002).

Reluctance to Change Other Aspects of the Current Relationship Patterns That Are Reinforcing

As already described, individuals who have greater power within their relationship are likely to resist changing the status quo in ways that might decrease the payoffs from their position. Therapists need to consider a variety of other aspects of a couple's current relationship patterns that may be reinforcing, because individuals may not be motivated to make changes unless the new patterns involve sources of reinforcement that are comparable to the old ones.

An individual's *avoidance or withdrawal from conditions that he or she experiences as aversive* can be maintained by powerful negative reinforcement processes. Consequently, individual cognitive-behavioral therapy for anxiety disorders includes strategies to reduce clients' avoidance of feared stimuli. Similarly, in the absence of a risk for abuse, therapists need to help members of couples reduce their avoidance of each other, so they can learn that problems can be solved through active collaboration. Therapists can guide the members of a couple in devising a hierarchy of threatening situations involving interaction with each other and can set up exposure experiments during and between sessions. For example, Beth and Jack avoided spending time together based on their fear of aversive arguments. After ruling out the potential for physically and psychologically abusive behavior, their therapist coached them in devising a hierarchy of shared activities with increasing degrees of interaction, starting with renting a movie to watch together. Once the couple had success with this relatively safe interaction, they moved on to types of interaction that involved more sharing of thoughts and emotions.

Failure to Take Personal Responsibility for Change

The members of distressed couples commonly blame each other more than themselves for relationship problems (Baucom & Epstein, 1990; Bradbury & Fincham, 1990; Epstein & Baucom, 2002). Some possible functions of blaming a partner include protection of one's self-esteem and reduced pressure to change one's behavior patterns (Baucom, 1987). In addition, it may be easier for an individual to monitor a partner's behavior than to observe his or her own actions objectively. As we noted earlier, individuals commonly think about events in their relationship in linear causal terms, rather than with circular causal concepts that involve the two individuals' influences on each other. Because members of a couple may be too defensive to accept feedback from each other about the effects of their behavior, feedback from a therapist whom the individuals believe has no vested interest in proving that anyone is at fault may be more effective. The therapist also can videotape therapy sessions and play back portions for the couple that illustrate the partners' mutual influences. It is important to distinguish between *blaming* an individual for a problem and identifying how he or she *contributes* to a negative pattern and can contribute to a solution.

The members of a couple often look to a therapist for help in getting the other person to change, and they may exhibit ingratiating or seductive behavior intended to enlist the therapist as an ally. The therapist can explicitly state that his or her goals are to avoid taking sides and to help the members of the couple find ways to get along better and resolve issues in their relationship. It is important that the therapist explicitly balance supporting and challenging both members of the couple. The therapist can preface such interventions with a comment such as, "I wouldn't be helpful to you as a couple if I tended to side with one of you, because the other person probably would feel misunderstood and would become angry and defensive. It's my job to notice and help you be aware of ways that both of you can contribute to solving the difficulties that you have been experiencing as a couple. Sometimes I'll point out something to one of you, and sometimes to the other. Often I'll point out a circular pattern that both of you participate in."

When a therapist notices that the members of a couple are "standing on ceremony," waiting for the other person to make changes first, the therapist can focus their attention on the negative consequences of that approach, in particular a frustrating stalemate. The therapist can commend each individual for past effort that he or she has put into the relationship but also can stress that whenever a person chooses to wait for another person to act, he or she is at the mercy of what the other person does or does not do. The therapist also can state that initiating change is not equivalent to taking the blame or all of the responsibility for solving the couple's problems. There is value in knowing that one is making a positive effort to improve the relationship.

The Therapist's Ways of Relating to the Two Partners and of Conducting the Therapy

Although many roadblocks to effective cognitive-behavioral therapy involve characteristics of the couple, the ways in which the therapist conducts the therapy also can interfere with progress. In particular, the therapist needs to anticipate potential roadblocks and to intervene in ways that minimize the risks.

For example, the therapist may identify or feel sympathetic with one member of a couple more than with the other, creating the potential for an alliance with that person and negative responses from the other. During sessions, a therapist who is more sympathetic to the views or circumstances of one individual may look at and speak to that person more often than the other, a pattern that both partners are likely to notice. Similarly, the therapist might consider one person's agenda for therapy more appropriate or desirable than the other's agenda and thus express more agreement with that individual. The other partner may then resist the therapist's interventions. Consequently, the therapist must get a sense of each person's agenda, convey understanding of it, and emphasize that in order for therapy to be successful both members of the couple need to perceive that the therapy is benefiting them.

Couple therapy has great potential to elicit the therapist's personal schemas related to experiences in his or her own couple and family relationships. For example, if a therapist has experienced his or her own partner as inappropriately controlling, the therapist may be sensitive to perceiving a member of a client couple as overly controlling with the partner. In order to minimize such "countertransference" reactions, it is important that couple therapists think about ways in which clients remind them of their own relationships and monitor personal reactions. Consultation from professional peers may help reduce negative responses to clients that reduce one's rapport and effectiveness with them.

A therapist also can elicit resistance from members of a couple if he or she attempts to push the pace of change faster than they can tolerate. Individuals who have become accustomed to particular interaction patterns will likely experience discomfort when attempting to relate to each other in new ways, particularly if they are uncertain that the outcomes will be positive. Each person may be wary of taking the risk of changing in case the other person fails to change. Consequently, therapists who encourage members of a couple to open themselves to potential hurt and disappointment need to empathize with each person's concerns about doing so. As described earlier, it is helpful to create conditions in which the members of the couple can "test the waters" by making changes gradually.

In contrast to roadblocks created when a therapist seems to intervene too fast, members of some couples may lose confidence in a therapist who seems to be intervening too slowly to reduce their relationship distress. For example, it is common for therapists to coach couples in practicing expressive and listening communication skills by discussing relatively low-conflict topics before attempting to deal with core relationship issues (Baucom & Epstein, 1990; Epstein & Baucom, 2002). The rationale for beginning with benign topics is that "hot" topics often elicit intense emotions and negative cognitions that interfere with the partners' ability to use the constructive communication guidelines. In order to maximize the couple's early successes, the therapist asks them to avoid discussions of their most significant concerns. This approach sometimes leads one or both members of a couple to be concerned that the therapy is "superficial" and that the therapist is ignoring the issues of greatest concern to them. The risk of losing rapport with the couple can be reduced if the therapist provides a convincing rationale for the gradual approach to discussing presenting problems.

As noted earlier, it is important that the therapist respect a couple's values, traditions, and power hierarchy. Thus, if a therapist believes that one member of a couple is too controlling and quickly attempts to increase the less powerful member's role in the couple's decision making, the controlling partner may take offense and resist the therapist's input. In some cases the therapist's efforts also will alienate the less powerful partner, who may value the other's leadership in their relationship and may view the therapist as disrespectful. It often helps for the therapist to validate a controlling individual's concerns; for example, "Lenny, it seems very appropriate for you to have a goal of raising children who are cooperative and respectful." Then the therapist can point out that the *methods* by which the person is attempting to achieve these worthwhile goals seem to have had negative effects. Thus the therapist could say to Lenny, "I have noticed that because you feel that Denise is too lenient with the children, you criticize her parenting, especially in front of the children. Denise has described how your criticism feels harsh and degrading, and it hurts and angers her. The two of you end up arguing about who is right or wrong rather than cooperating in providing a consistent approach with your kids. In therapy we can focus on exploring alternative ways to deal with your different parenting approaches, to find a way to avoid power struggles and to develop cooperation with each other." The therapist would help the couple use decision-making communication skills to identify alternative responses that each person could try in their new efforts to collaborate in raising their children (Epstein & Baucom, 2002).

SUMMARY

Couple therapy forces members of a distressed couple to engage with each other in a confining setting, in which each person is, at a minimum, likely to be confronted with the other's complaints and, in some cases, may be subjected to a partner's abusive behavior. In addition, members of a couple may have developed a strong sense of hopelessness about the potential for improving the problems in their relationship, and therapy sessions may remind them of this seemingly hopeless situation. Furthermore, in some couples one member has accrued particular benefits from the status quo, and he or she perceives the prospect that changes created by therapy will result in a loss of those benefits. Consequently, on the one hand partners may have little hope that therapy can improve their relationship, but on the other hand they may fear that participation in therapy might produce unwelcome changes.

Each partner's self-protective strategies are likely to operate in couple therapy, serving to minimize personal hurt, threats to self-esteem, and loss of power. These self-protective strategies, which may involve avoidance, withdrawal, or aggressive behavior, themselves commonly become major sources of "secondary distress" in a couple's relationship (Epstein &

Baucom, 2002). Consequently, couple therapists need to be aware of partners' self-protective strategies that involve resistance to conjoint therapy, increase partners' awareness of the drawbacks of resistance to change, increase their confidence that therapy can lead to more mutually satisfying couple interactions, and promote more satisfying interactions.

REFERENCES

Baucom, D. H. (1987). Attributions in distressed relations: How can we explain them? In S. Duck & D. Perlman (Eds.), *Heterosexual relations, marriage and divorce* (pp. 177–206). London: Sage.

Baucom, D. H., & Epstein, N. (1990). *Cognitive-behavioral marital therapy.* New York: Brunner/Mazel.

Baucom, D. H., Shoham, V., Mueser, K. T., Daiuto, A. D., & Stickle, T. R. (1998). Empirically supported couples and family therapies for adult problems. *Journal of Consulting and Clinical Psychology, 66,* 53–88.

Beach, S. R. H. (Ed.). (2000). *Marital and family processes in depression: A scientific foundation for clinical practice.* Washington, DC: American Psychological Association.

Bourne, E. J. (1995). *The anxiety and phobia workbook* (2nd ed.). Oakland, CA: New Harbinger.

Bradbury, T. N., & Fincham, F. D. (1990). Attributions in marriage: Review and critique. *Psychological Bulletin, 107,* 3–33.

Carter, B., & McGoldrick, M. (Eds.). (1999). *The expanded family life cycle: Individual, family, and social perspectives* (3rd ed.). Boston: Allyn & Bacon.

Christensen, A. (1988). Dysfunctional interaction patterns in couples. In P. Noller & M. A. Fitzpatrick (Eds.), *Monographs in social psychology of language: No. 1. Perspectives on marital interaction* (pp. 31–52). Clevedon, UK: Multilingual Matters.

Christensen, A., & Heavey, C. L. (1990). Gender and social structure in the demand/withdraw pattern of marital conflict. *Journal of Personality and Social Psychology, 59,* 73–81.

Craske, M. G., & Zoellner, L. A. (1995). Anxiety disorders: The role of marital therapy. In N. S. Jacobson & A. S. Gurman (Eds.), *Clinical handbook of couple therapy* (pp. 394–410). New York: Guilford Press.

Dattilio, F. D., Epstein, N. B., & Baucom, D. H. (1998). An introduction to cognitive-behavioral therapy with couples and families. In F. M. Dattilio (Ed.), *Case studies in couple and family therapy: Systemic and cognitive perspectives* (pp. 1–36). New York: Guilford Press.

Deffenbacher, J. L. (1996). Cognitive–behavioral approaches to anger reduction. In K. S. Dobson & K. D. Craig (Eds.), *Advances in cognitive-behavioral therapy* (pp. 31–62). Thousand Oaks, CA: Sage.

Epstein, N. B., & Baucom, D. H. (2002). *Enhanced cognitive-behavioral therapy for couples: A contextual approach.* Washington, DC: American Psychological Association.

Gottman, J. M. (1994). *What predicts divorce?* Hillsdale, NJ: Erlbaum.

Heyman, R. E., & Neidig, P. H. (1997). Physical aggression couples treatment. In W. K. Halford & H. J. Markman (Eds.), *Clinical handbook of marriage and couples intervention* (pp. 589–617). Chichester, UK: Wiley.

Holtzworth-Munroe, A., Beatty, S. B., & Anglin, K. (1995). The assessment and treatment of marital violence: An introduction for the marital therapist. In N. S. Jacobson & A. S. Gurman (Eds.), *Clinical handbook of couple therapy* (pp. 317–349). New York: Guilford Press.

Jacobson, N. S., & Christensen, A. (1996). *Integrative couple therapy: Promoting acceptance and change.* New York: Norton.

Jacobson, N. S., & Margolin, G. (1979). *Marital therapy: Strategies based on social learning and behavior exchange principles.* New York: Brunner/Mazel.

Linehan, M. M. (1993). *Cognitive–behavioral treatment of borderline personality disorder.* New York: Guilford Press.

Meichenbaum, D. (1985). *Stress inoculation training.* New York: Pergamon Press.

Miklowitz, D. J., & Goldstein, M. J. (1997). *Bipolar disorder: A family-focused treatment approach.* New York: Guilford Press.

Neidig, P. H., & Friedman, D. H. (1984). *Spouse abuse: A treatment program for couples.* Champaign, IL: Research Press.

O'Farrell, T. J., & Rotunda, R. (1997). Couples interventions and alcohol abuse. In W. K. Halford & H. J. Markman (Eds.), *Clinical handbook of marriage and couples intervention* (pp. 555–588). Chichester, UK: Wiley.

Rathus, J. H., & Sanderson, W. C. (1999). *Marital distress: Cognitive behavioral interventions for couples.* Northvale, NJ: Aronson.

Stuart, R. B. (1980). *Helping couples change: A social learning approach to marital therapy.* New York: Guilford Press.

Weiss, R. L. (1980). Strategic behavioral marital therapy: Toward a model for assessment and intervention. In J. P. Vincent (Ed.), *Advances in family intervention, assessment and theory* (Vol. 1, pp. 229–271). Greenwich, CT: JAI Press.

12

Family Therapy

Frank M. Dattilio

The cognitive-behavioral approach to family therapy posits that members of a family simultaneously influence and are influenced by each other (Dattilio, 2001a; Leslie, 1988). Consequently, a behavior of one family member affects the behaviors, cognitions, and emotions of other members, which, in turn, elicit an entire set of cognitions, behaviors, and emotions in response (Dattilio, Epstein, & Baucom, 1998). As this cycle progresses, the volatility of the family dynamics can sometimes escalate, rendering family members vulnerable to a negative spiral of conflict, depending on the situation. With an increase in the number of family members involved, the dynamics become more complex (Dattilio, 2000). If serious psychopathology exists with one or more family members, then the treatment challenges become even more compounded.

Cognitive therapy, as originally set forth by Beck (1967), places a heavy emphasis on "schemas" or what have otherwise been defined as "core beliefs" (Beck, Rush, Shaw & Emery, 1979; Beck, 1967). Various authors have proposed different versions of schema theory to account for the processing of information in one's life. Most theoretical perspectives contend that individuals develop knowledge structures through interactions with their environment. These cognitive structures may be generically referred to as schemas. They serve an adaptive function by organizing experience into meaningful patterns and reducing the complexity of the environment. Through a mechanism of selectively limiting, guiding, and organizing information, processing activity of the person's schemas renders efficient thinking and action more likely to occur. As this concept is applied to family treatment, the therapeutic intervention is based on the assumptions with which family members interpret and evaluate one another and the emotions and behaviors that are generated in response to these cognitions. Although cognitive-behavioral theory does not suggest that cognitive processes cause all family behavior, it does stress that cognitive appraisal plays a significant role in the interrelationships existing among events, cognitions, emotions, and behaviors (Wright & Beck, 1993; Epstein, Schlesinger, & Dryden, 1988). During the therapeutic process, restructuring distorted beliefs has a pivotal impact on changing dysfunctional behaviors.

Schemas are also very important in the application of cognitive-behavioral therapy with families. Just as individuals maintain their own basic schemas about themselves, their world, and their future, they maintain a schema about their family's functioning as well. Some therapists believe that greater emphasis should be placed on examining cognitions among individual family members, as well as on what is termed by Dattilio (1993) "family schemata." Family schemas are jointly held beliefs about the family that have formed as a result of years of integrated interaction among members of the family unit. Elsewhere (Dattilio, 1993a, 1998b), I have suggested that individuals basically maintain two separate sets of schemas about families. These consist of family schemas related to the parents' family of origin and schemas related to families in general, or what Schwebel and Fine (1994) refer to as a "personal theory of family life." It is the experiences and perceptions from the family of origin that shape schemas about both the immediate family and families in general.

These schemas have a major impact on how the individual thinks, feels, and behaves within the family setting. Epstein et al. (1988) propose that schemas are "the longstanding and relatively stable basic assumptions that one holds about how the world works and his or her place in it" (p. 13). Schwebel and Fine (1992) elaborate on the term "family schemata" as used in the family model by describing it as:

> All of the cognitions that individuals hold about their own family life and about family life in general. Included in this set of cognitions are an individual's schema about family life, attributions about why events occur in the family, and beliefs about why events occur in the family, and beliefs about what should exist within the family unit (Baucom & Epstein, 1990). The family schema also contains ideas about how spousal relationships should work, what different types of problems should be expected in marriage and how they should be handled, what is involved in building and maintaining a healthy family, what responsibilities each family member should have, what consequences should be associated with failure to meet responsibilities or to fulfill roles, and what costs and benefits each individual should expect to have as a consequence of being in a marriage. (p. 50)

I have also suggested (Dattilio, 1993, 1998a, 2001a) that the family of origin of each partner in a relationship plays a crucial role in the shaping of

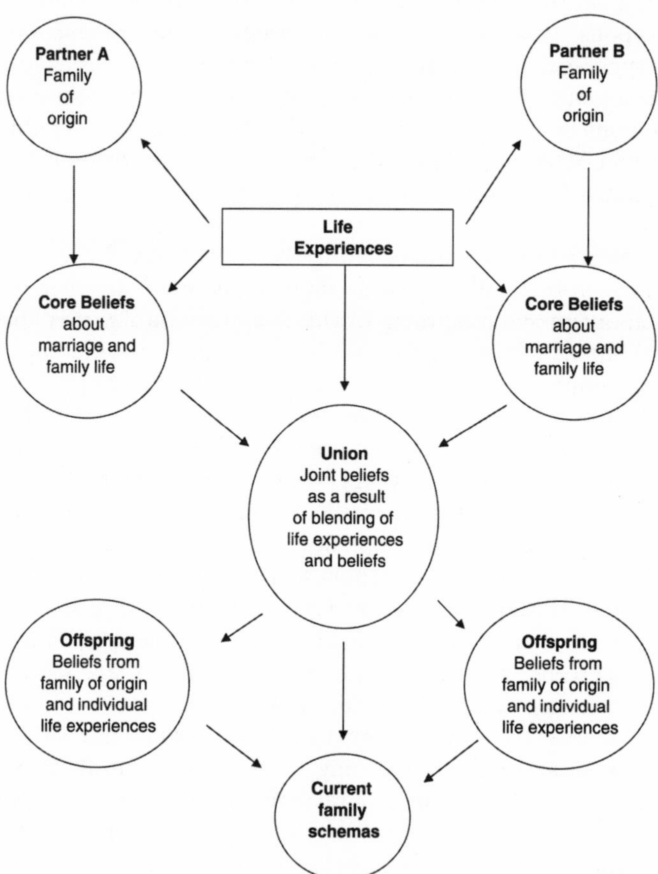

FIGURE 12.1. The development of family schemas.

immediate family schemas. Beliefs funneled from the family of origin may be both conscious and unconscious and contribute to a joint or blended schema that leads to the development of the current family schema (see Figure 12.1).

This family schema is then disseminated and applied in the rearing of the children, and, when integrated with their individual thoughts and perceptions of their environment and life experiences, contributes to the further development of the family schema. The family schemas are subject to change as major events occur during the course of family life (e.g., death, divorce), and they also continue to evolve over the course of ordinary day-to-day experience.

Consequently, the family schema is a very important area to address in cognitive-behavioral family therapy, one in which the greatest area of change usually occurs. This is accomplished by a series of cognitive and behavioral strategies used in restructuring the basic or core beliefs of the family and altering or modifying behavioral patterns. The behavioral component of cognitive-behavioral family therapy focuses on several aspects of family members' actions. These include (1) excess negative interaction and deficits in pleasing behaviors exchanged by family members; (2) expressive and listening skills used in communication; (3) problem-solving skills; and (4) negotiation and behavior-change skills. The theoretical models underlying behavioral approaches to family therapy are social learning theory (e.g., Bandura, 1977) and social exchange theory (e.g., Thibaut & Kelley, 1959).

DEVELOPMENT OF FAMILY SCHEMAS

The notion of schema as applied to families may explain some of the dynamics that constitute thinking styles and how these styles of thought affect emotional and behavioral patterns in family interaction (Dattilio, 1993). The term "family schema" is highlighted more clearly in the recent works by Dattilio (1998a, 2001a).

Family schemas originally develop from individual and conjoint belief systems that evolved from what the parents bring to the family relationship. Figure 12.1 provides an outline of the dynamics of how schemas evolve in a marital relationship and contributes to what Dattilio (1993, 1998a) refers to as a joint family schema. It is these schemas that serve as a template for family members in their functioning within the family dynamics. Schemas are also responsible for shaping perceptions, thoughts, reactions, feelings, and behaviors and guiding individuals through the many hurdles and challenges that are encountered in family life. A main grid for family schemas involves the family constitution. This evolving set of rules and standards govern family life and contribute to the balance of family functioning.

As with an individual's set of dynamics, schemas can become dysfunctional or maladaptive and can involve a root cause of distortion. A perfect example of such is the case, described later, in which the family jointly viewed me as "shifty and manipulative" simply because I functioned in the role of a "shrink," or someone who is in control of the situation. Sometimes schemas evolve and are never verbally discussed among family members but become innately understood. Family members may never speak to each other directly about certain beliefs but may make certain assumptions. For example, a family may view family therapy as a waste of time without ever discussing it among themselves. A second type of schema is the more overt family schema, which is something that every family member is aware of and that is talked about freely. This schema may typically involve rules and regulations that family members abide by (i.e., family business is never discussed outside of the home). In the aforementioned case, to discuss feelings was "taboo," and everyone knew it and abided by this belief.

It is hypothesized that it is the silent, unspoken family schemas that tend to contribute to more dysfunction in the family process. These are covert dynamics that may not always be clearly conceptualized by family members; for example, family members' denial of the father's problem with alcohol. The belief that it is awkward to speak directly to one another or with the family as a whole is steadfastly maintained. Therefore, the understanding or core belief is that it is easier to simply avoid confrontation and "let sleeping dogs lie" or, better yet, to engage in the same denial in order to mask father's problem with alcohol. This, obviously, is something that can cause difficulties with alienation and rejection and may also place specific family members, who serve as the conduit, in a precarious position with others or may even empower them (Dattilio, 1998c).

In addressing family schemas from a cognitive-behavioral perspective, it is important to follow a series of steps that can facilitate the process of schema analysis and restructuring:

- *Step 1.* Uncover and identify family schemas and highlight those areas of conflict and dysfunction that are fueled by the schemas. Schemas can be uncovered by probing automatic thoughts and using techniques such as downward arrow and Socratic questioning (Dattilio, 1998b). Once these schemas are identified, then verification should be made by obtaining some measure of agreement from family members.
- *Step 2.* Trace the origin of family schemas and how they have evolved to become an ingrained mechanism in the family process. This is done by probing into the parents' background and the parenting styles that their parents used during their upbringing. Similarities and differences should be delineated between parents to portray how they have contributed to their immediate family schemas.
- *Step 3.* Point out the need for modification or change, indicating how the restructuring of a schema may facilitate more adaptive functioning and harmonize interaction. At this stage, it is essential to convince the family that modification or change will ease the tension and level of conflict in the family atmosphere.
- *Step 4.* Elicit acknowledgment and cooperation from the family as a whole with the need to change or modify existing dysfunctional schemas. This step is imperative in order for change to actually oc-

cur. It paves the way for a collaborative effort between the therapist and the family members.

- *Step 5.* Assess the family's ability to make changes and plan strategies for facilitating them. It is important to determine how capable a family is of making changes. Contingencies may involve levels of intelligence, coping skills, and the level of resistance that exists within the family that can maintain a level of homeostasis.
- *Step 6.* Implement the change through the use of collaborative experiences, brainstorming ideas for modifying beliefs, and weighing the effects of the modifications to existing beliefs.
- *Step 7.* Enact the change and feel the fit. The use of family exercises and assignments is imperative in enacting permanent change (Dattilio, 2002).
- *Step 8.* Solidify the change as a permanent fixture through practice and remaining flexible to future modification.

ROADBLOCKS

These steps are sometimes very difficult to follow, depending on the family that one is dealing with.

The Shims, for example, were an inner-city family who were ordered to treatment by the court. A major problem from the beginning was that they detested the sentence. Slovenly dressed, with poor hygiene, most of them had rotted or missing teeth, including several of the teenagers. They all showed up for the initial visit, albeit begrudgingly. I had to wonder who was being sentenced, them or me.

Mr. Shim, the father and "head of household," often arrived for therapy with the smell of alcohol on his breath and his silver whiskers corkscrewing in different directions. He usually sat through the sessions with a sardonic smile on his face, saying very little. His wife compensated for his indifference and the children's recalcitrance by talking incessantly. The rest of the family sat disengaged and completely uninterested in what was going on in the room, unless, of course, one of the kids belched or passed gas, thus setting off an avalanche of laughter among the others. I dreaded working with this family. They made no bones about sharing their disdain for me, either. Certainly, this was not a good "therapeutic fit." The roadblocks were not *between* us, they *were* us. But the Shims had little choice and neither did I, as they had been remanded and I was specifically appointed by a high-powered judge to work with them as a "favor" to the court.

The family had been sentenced in response to charges of theft and receiving stolen property. It was said that the entire family was involved in a sort of "theft ring," something the Shims vehemently denied. Aside from our mutual disenchantment, there were plenty of other barriers to the treatment with the Shims, obstacles that gave the term "roadblock" new meaning. There was the father's alcoholism and unemployment and what appeared to be an underlying depression and possible early onset of dementia. Cannabis abuse was rampant among the children. And then there was the mother's denial of everything, particularly of her teenage son's criminal behavior and of her husband's chronic substance abuse. To complete the picture, this family was functioning at a very low intellectual level, probably in the borderline retarded range. Needless to say, all of this made me uncertain about whether or not I could really do anything for the Shims.

Unfortunately, for therapists who work with families who are forced into treatment, these challenges are not unusual. The major focus in working from a cognitive-behavioral perspective is to effect change through restructuring thoughts and modifying behaviors—that is, if change is viable.

The term "roadblock" is defined by *Webster's New World Dictionary* as a barricade or anything that interferes with progress. Most roadblocks or barricades in life interfere with progress on both sides of the obstacle. In family therapy, as with any form of treatment, roadblocks may occur on both sides of the therapist's desk, as is so poignantly portrayed in the case of the Shims. That is, blocks occur on the part of the therapist as well as the client. Therefore, roadblocks may entail the resistance of both clients and therapist, a situation that can seriously impede the progress of treatment and sometimes bring therapy to a halt.

In his recent work on resistance, Leahy (2001) discusses the concept of resistance in cognitive therapy and essentially defines it as anything that impedes the treatment process by either the patient or the therapist. In the next section, several roadblocks are outlined that can often impede the progress of family therapy from both standpoints. Certain steps are discussed regarding what may be done to counteract roadblocks.

Therapist Roadblocks

Many roadblocks develop on the part of a therapist when working with particularly difficult families. These blocks may include the therapist's own resistance or defense mechanisms that may surface during the course of treatment. The aforementioned case is an excellent example of how resistance occurred on both sides of the fence, particularly the therapist's reaction to the family's behavior. Sometimes, it is not even necessary for a case to be as difficult as the one mentioned here in order for roadblocks to develop. The therapist's failure to work through his or her own issues from his or her family of origin is one of the less recognized roadblocks that occur in family therapy. A perfect example of this situation would be a therapist who never worked through conflict with his or her own parents and who may be blinded from recognizing to what extent a youth is engaging in distortions in his or her thinking regarding his or her parents. Therefore, because of the therapist's own unresolved conflicts, the course of treatment may be affected. In addition, the situation may become further diluted and transferences may occur. In another type of roadblock, the therapist may feel overwhelmed or helpless in the face of a difficult case due to insufficient training or supervision. Such an impediment can often segue into failure. It may also contribute to burnout or stalled movement, thus hindering the therapeutic process. In working with the Shims, it was essential for me to reevaluate my own cognitions about working with such an arduous situation and to address my own distortions regarding my effectiveness as a therapist.

I later realized that I had been sabotaging myself from the start of treatment by engaging in catastrophic thoughts about what a disaster therapy would be prior to even beginning. In a sense, I was resisting having to deal with what I erroneously perceived as "the bottom of the barrel" after having the luxury of dealing with educated, high-functioning families in the past. What is more, I was personalizing the Shims's dysfunction and viewing it as a "failure waiting to happen."

In such cases, it is recommended that individual therapists seek peer review or consultation or even supervision during periods in which such conflicts may arise. This is usually an indication that the therapist may have lost his or her objectivity and needs to regain some sense of balance. In the case of the Shims, I felt the need to confer with a colleague who had worked with families that came from similar socioeconomic backgrounds. This particular mentor was very skillful in helping me reframe my thinking by suggesting that I not take offense at this family's behavior and recalcitrance to treatment. In short, I learned to distance myself appropriately and to view their behavior as a result of their problems. I had to face the fact that I was personalizing and pressuring myself to be successful with a very difficult situation. This family presented with such an arduous front that I viewed myself as being destined to fail. Restructuring my thinking and belief system about success in treatment was an important issue for me; at the same time, getting back on track and dealing with this damaged family system was the best thing I could do. Once I was able to overcome this roadblock for myself, I was able to advance and be more successful in helping this family through their own roadblocks in the treatment process.

Unrealistic Expectations

Setting realistic expectations is a very important part of family therapy, or of any type of treatment for that matter. Being overzealous about what one is able to accomplish in treatment is a very common pitfall of novice therapists, which may cause stress for the therapist and may set him or her and the family up for failure. For example, attempting to help Mr. Shim rehabilitate from his alcohol dependence without inpatient detoxification and family support might be considered "magical thinking." Such an ingrained pattern would certainly not change unless a number of key dynamics in the family changed. This is something that requires time and much prodding and may not be very viable, particularly with a family such as this one. Being able to size up a family situation is essential for all parties involved so that realistic expectations can be set. Sometimes, expectations may even need to be reset throughout the course of therapy. Therefore, one way of overcoming the obstacle is to be as realistic and flexible as possible as to what can be accomplished in treatment and when.

There were a myriad of issues to be addressed with the Shims, and it was unlikely that the majority of them would ever be achieved. I knew somewhere in my mind that the family would not likely remain in treatment. Therefore, to establish a realistic expectation of getting them to show up for therapy was a major accomplishment and obviously a first step.

Cultural Obstacles

Cultural issues are certainly an aspect of treatment that need to be considered when working with families. Currently, the United States has experienced the greatest influx of immigrants since the early 19th century. It is estimated that more than 1 million legal and undocumented immigrants arrive annually (McGoldrick, Giordano, & Pearce, 1996).

Although many immigrant families in the United States become acculturated, households still honor certain customs based on their cultural heritage. Many of these cultural and environmental aspects can be deeply ingrained in the family and may be perceived by someone unfamiliar with that culture as deliberate resistance to change. A classic example involves a Polish family that I worked with several years ago who had migrated from Krakow. Upon introducing a homework assignment for which I requested family members to gather information, I perceived the father's noncompliance as a major resistance to treatment. It was not until speaking with a colleague, a Polish psychiatrist working in Warsaw, that I learned that such resistance was not an uncommon factor found among Polish males, particularly those who were a product of former Soviet bloc nations. He explained to me that, as a result of the Nazi occupation in Poland and the subsequent presence of Communism, many individuals, particularly males, had difficulty with being told what to do. This was not only a cultural characteristic but also a remnant of years of oppression. Once I understood this collective concept more clearly, I was then able to restructure my approach and implement it in a more collaborative vein, making it appealing to the father of this family. I essentially asked the father for permission to work through him, which he willingly granted. This example is not unusual, particularly with offspring of families who have been subjected to oppression in various nations (Dattilio, 2001b).

Individuals conducting family therapy should familiarize themselves with various cultural aspects in the literature, as well as with the environments from which individuals hail, in order to avoid roadblocks. One excellent and comprehensive text on this topic is the book *Ethnicity and Family Therapy* (McGoldrick et al., 1996). This work offers family therapists a great deal of insight into how families of various cultures operate. It may also provide therapists with enough information to determine whether or not a family is operating from a rigidly held belief due to their culture or whether it is more reflective of a personality trait, or possibly both.

Racial Issues

Sometimes, the fact that family therapists might be of a different race from that of the family they are working with could become a problem. In the aforementioned case, the fact that I was of a different socioeconomic status surfaced as an issue later in treatment with the Shims, when the topic of dealing with racial issues among families was discussed. Many of the Shim children had difficulty understanding how I could possibly comprehend the struggles that they faced, having been reared in an upper-middle-class Caucasian neighborhood. This was clearly an issue that I needed to sort out. I had to decide whether or not this objection was a smoke screen for them to sidestep the salient issues in therapy. I decided to confront them on this matter and induce them to consider that, even though I was not African American and did not live in a lower socioeconomic environment, I was willing to listen and try to learn to expand my knowledge base of their struggles.

Environmental Forces

Another roadblock to treatment may involve families who are exposed to environments that inhibit or impede change incurred during the course of therapy. (Obviously, for a family who meets in therapy for 90 minutes each week, returning to an environment that lures them away from the direction of treatment will no doubt be counterproductive to everything that is achieved during the course of therapy.) In this particular case with the Shims, therapeutic interventions had very little power against the strong environmental forces that created a need for them to survive via a life of crime and sometimes violence. From a behavioral standpoint, the mere notion of constant reinforcement in the home environment was a great antagonist to any therapeutic change, unless of course the family was willing to adopt wholeheartedly the desire to change and, therefore, make their best attempt to transform in the face of those environmental forces. Unfortunately, a goal of changing motivation is sometimes very difficult to achieve and reverts to the earlier issue about setting realistic expectations. I was successful with the Shims in inducing them eventually to consider relocating in order to make a fresh start with their lives. Sometimes, changing behaviors entails changing the environmental surroundings, if possible.

Psychopathology

Psychopathology is clearly one of the major hurdles in treatment with families, particularly when significant psychopathology exists with one or more family members.

Axis II disorders typically raise challenging roadblocks during the course of treatment, particularly when they exist in one of the parents. Certain personality disorders may impede the process to the point at which progress comes to a screeching halt. In most cases, individuals with severe Axis II disorders resist being referred for individual therapy; however, when the disorder is less severe, certain aspects may be addressed directly in the family therapy process. This, of course, depends largely on the cooperation of the family member diagnosed with the disorder. For example, in the aforementioned case, it was determined during the course of treatment that Mr. Shim had a substantial amount of narcissism with strong passive–aggressive features. His heavy substance abuse made it extremely difficult to address his personality issues without his agreement to submit for detoxification and treatment. The fact that he was also nonverbal during the course of treatment was a major problem, particularly because his wife tended to compensate by speaking incessantly, making it easier for him to remain taciturn and to keep his individual issues covert.

In this particular case, I requested that the parents sit next to each other, and I addressed them as a united front. I then attempted to accentuate the mother's power in the hopes that it might draw the father's feelings to the surface. I viewed him as being the one who actually had the real power in the family, even though he seldomly spoke. He operated behind the scenes, whereas the mother was the front person. In essence, I tried to capitalize on the father's narcissism. Unfortunately, this blew up in my face after Mr. Shim failed to show up for several appointments because of "fatigue." I then decided to switch gears and stroke him by telling him that I needed him to help me address important issues in the family and that I could not do it without him. Taking him off the hot seat and putting his wife in the spotlight was appealing to him. This seemed to peak his interest, and he began to cooperate and show up for visits more regularly, albeit still slightly intoxicated. It would be much later in treatment that I would gradually work my way to addressing his personal issues.

Other psychopathology that may be less severe than Axis II disorders but nonetheless just as challenging concerns some of the Axis I disorders. For example, in cases in which a parent may be agoraphobic, this diagnosis may have a profound effect on rerouting distribution of power in the family. There are cases in which children are "parentified," which also can be a major obstacle that must be addressed, not only in family therapy but also individually.

Low Intellectual and Cognitive Functioning

Insight is one of the hallmarks of cognitive-behavior therapy. Historically, it has been stated that, when individuals lack significant insight, they may respond more favorably to pure behavioral interventions. This is certainly the case with the family in this chapter, who were all functioning at a very low intellectual level. In contrast, however, they were very high functioning when it came to "street smarts" and, in many respects, I was no match for them. I did use metaphors as much as possible, however, to help them to expand their thinking. They seemed to respond well to concrete metaphors, as well as to straight behavioral interventions. For example, I had them make a list of the qualities that contributed to their forming together in order to work cohesively in their circles of crime. Even though the behavioral act was not condoned, I stressed the concept of cohesiveness and how the family pulled together in order to engage in such covert acts as unlawfully entering a home. We then talked about how some of these same skills could be turned around to be used in a more productive fashion that would not get them involved with the law. During the course of these discussions, we used language that they were familiar with, such as "staying thick" and not "ratting each other out," and so forth. I then attempted to transfer this measure of cohesion by urging them to support each other in the same fashion in order to remain clean and abide by the law. We brainstormed about ways to earn money and deal with authority conflicts. In essence, we began to include a change of behavior by restructuring schemas indirectly.

Effects of Previous Treatment

Progress in family therapy may be impeded by experiences that the family may have had with previous therapists. In this particular case, the Shims had never set foot in a therapist's office previously, and, as far as they were concerned, they "wouldn't be caught dead with a shrink." In other cases, however, a specific roadblock may involve treatment with previous therapists who work differently and who may have had a negative effect on the family's ability to benefit from treatment. Trust is one of the important factors in therapy. Consequently, if a family came to distrust a previous therapist, establishing a line of trust will require a longer period of time and cause the therapist to proceed cautiously.

Sometimes, previous therapy may have been halted by a family because that therapist was being effective or touched on a sensitive issue with the family. The family may tend to use the former therapist as a scapegoat and "trash" him or her. It is essential that a therapist not play into or support the denigration of a former therapist but instead to direct his or her energy toward exploring alternative ways to help the family.

Applying Pressure at the Wrong Time

It has been my experience that sometimes you have to push during the course of therapy in order to facilitate change. At times when movement is stalled, you need to nudge a family to elicit change.

For example, at one point in therapy with the Shims, the children had ganged up on the mother about her incessant nagging. The father refused to take a stand, and I decided to nudge him to respond.

DATTILIO: What do you think about what's going on between your wife and kids right now?

FATHER: Don't know. What do you want me to say?

DATTILIO: Say what you think or what you feel.

FATHER: Don't feel nottin! Don't think nottin!

DATTILIO: Well, you must feel or think something.

FATHER: Nope, nottin.

DATTILIO: Why not?

FATHER: I don't know, I don't much listen I guess.

DATTILIO: So you tune them out?

FATHER: I guess.

This transaction was clearly stalled, particularly because the father did not want to commit himself. My suspicion was that he had lots of thoughts and feelings about what was going on but that he maintained a certain power in his neutrality. I decided to step in and help the mother deal with her children's criticism by exploring alternatives with her. I then asked the father to deliberately side with the kids against the mother, to join them in criticizing her nagging. He did not like this at all.

DATTILIO: Don't you want to bash your wife for nagging all of the time?

FATHER: You're trying to make a "dick" out of me, ain't ya?

DATTILIO: A dick? Why no, what gives you that impression?

FATHER: Bullshit—you's psychiatrizing with me.

DATTILIO: No, I am just trying to get you to 'fess up to your feelings, that's all.

FATHER: Shit. . . .

DATTILIO: Try to understand that, when you sit there all quiet and stuff, you give everyone in the family a very powerful message.

FATHER: What . . . .what message?

DATTILIO: A silent message that you support them.

FATHER: So, what if I do?

DATTILIO: Then be a man and say so.

FATHER: Up yours!

DATTILIO: Whatever—think about it.

I heard more from this father during the preceding exchange than I had in the previous six sessions. Even though the exchange at this point was rather negative and heated, it produced some movement and got us "unstuck" from our gridlock. From this point in treatment, we were able to move in a direction toward change, just in the sense that father was now verbalizing his thoughts and feelings, which shifted the dynamics of treatment.

Inadequate Use of Homework Assignments

Homework assignments, sometimes referred to as "out-of-session assignments," are an extremely important aspect of treatment and are often an integral part of a therapist's leverage in overcoming roadblocks (Dattilio, 2002). Cognitive-behavioral therapists are recognized more prominently than those in any other modality for emphasizing homework assignments as a key aspect of treatment. Due to the multiple dynamics among family members, structure is an important part of therapy. The systematic use of homework assignments transforms the therapeutic process into a 24-hour experience. Because the majority of time occurs outside of the therapy session, such assignments serve to keep the context of therapy fresh during the interim periods between sessions and promotes a transfer from the therapy session to the environment.

Homework assignments may be particularly helpful, thrusting a family into active involvement, signifying that they have already acknowledged the notion that change is beneficial at both the personal and interpersonal levels (Prochaska, DiClemente, & Norcross, 1992).

In the particular case of the Shims, I needed to develop a homework strategy that would facilitate their joint participation and would encourage a positive cohesiveness and some empirical coping strategies. For homework, I decided to assign the task of having them look for new housing together as a family unit. They all agreed that part of their problem was their living environment, so I urged them to each take a part in gathering information on a new home location. This facilitated them in working cohesively toward a common cause that was productive. It was the first step toward working in a positive vein. This also served as a new activity for the Shims to try out together, and I also had them tack on a pleasure task of going out to eat afterward—something that they had avoided for years.

In our subsequent visit, we discussed everyone's feelings about the experience.

Inoculation against Backsliding

Another very common roadblock in treatment is backsliding. It is easy to fall back into previous behaviors, particularly when the propensity is strong. Therefore, an effective strategy may involve the therapist inoculating both him- or herself and the family against the propensity to backslide and to discuss how this should be handled. For example, it was obvious that the Shims might be extremely tempted to become involved again with theft or receiving stolen property. We discussed a mechanism for them to use to cope with the temptation of taking something that did not belong to them. This procedure included following a number of steps in order to break the cycle of regression.

1. They were advised that, if a friend called who was notorious for trouble, they should not accept the telephone call right away but call him or her back. In the interim, they should think about what to say if he or she proposed something illegal. They should think about the choices they had at their disposal and the power to choose. Because power was one of the major issues in this family, we spoke about how to exercise that strength by successfully avoiding trouble. I also suggested that the family members might be afraid to ask each other for support.

2. Two of the triggers that led to stealing were boredom and anger. Some of the kids reported that they usually committed a theft during periods in which they were bored and had little to do or when they were angry

about something. Therefore, we developed a list of alternative behaviors for them to consider, which involved more productive activities and facilitative methods for expressing their anger.

3. Avoiding the pitfall of negative self-image was another area to highlight in order to prevent backsliding. Whenever the family got down on themselves, they tended to backslide into old patterns. This pattern is typical for many. Consequently, the Shims were prompted to monitor each other's negative or unflattering self-talk as a means to promote morale.

4. Restructuring their thoughts about the need to act on impulse provided another major coping skill. Teaching family members to delay acting on their impulses via thought stopping or diversion of activity was extremely effective.

DISCUSSION

Conducting any type of psychotherapy is often difficult regardless of the population. If it were not for the existence of roadblocks in treatment, self-help would occur more successfully, and the need for this book would be nonexistent. Therapists will encounter endless roadblocks during the course of their careers in working with individuals, couples, and families. Learning to use various tools and techniques and to maintain a steady stream of patience is probably the greatest asset that any therapist can acquire. The most important roadblock for therapists to overcome is to accept the notion that roadblocks are a necessary part of the therapeutic process and an eternal challenge to endure.

REFERENCES

Bandura, A. (1977). *Social learning theory.* Englewood Cliffs, NJ: Prentice-Hall.

Baucom, D. H., & Epstein, N. B. (1990). *Cognitive-behavioral marital therapy.* New York: Brunner/Mazel.

Beck, A. T. (1967). *Depression: Clinical, experimental and theoretical aspects.* New York: Hoeber.

Beck, A. T., Rush, J. A., Shaw, B. F., & Emery, G. (1979). *Cognitive therapy of depression,* New York: Guilford Press.

Dattilio, F. M. (1993). Cognitive techniques with couples and families. *Family Journal, 1*(1), 51–65.

Dattilio, F. M. (Ed.). (1998a). *Case studies in couple and family therapy: Systemic and cognitive perspectives.* New York: Guilford Press.

Dattilio, F. M. (1998b). Cognitive-behavior family therapy. In F. M. Dattilio (Ed.), *Case studies in couple and family therapy: Systemic and cognitive perspectives* (pp. 62–84). New York: Guilford Press.

Dattilio, F. M. (1998c). Finding the fit between cognitive-behavioral and family therapy. *Family Therapy Networker, 22*(4), 63–73.

Dattilio, F. M. (2000). Families in crisis. In F. M. Dattilio & A. Freeman (Eds.), *Cognitive-behavioral strategies in crisis intervention* (2nd ed., pp. 316–338). New York: Guilford Press.

Dattilio, F. M. (2001a). Cognitive-behavioral family therapy: Contemporary myths and misconceptions. *Contemporary Family Therapy, 23*(1), 3–18.

Dattilio, F. M. (2001b). The ripple effects of depressive schemas on psychiatric patients [Letter to the editor]. *Archives of Psychiatry and Psychotherapy, 3*(2), 90–91.

Dattilio, F. M. (2002). Using homework assignments in couple and family therapy. *Journal of Clinical Psychology, 58*(5), 570–583.

Dattilio, F. M., Epstein, N. B., & Baucom, D. H. (1998). An introduction to cognitive-behavioral therapy with couples and families. In F. M. Dattilio (Ed.), *Case studies in couple and family therapy: Systemic and cognitive perspectives* (pp. 1–36). New York: Guilford Press.

Epstein, N., Schlesinger, S., & Dryden, W. (1988). Concepts and methods of cognitive-behavioral family treatment. In N. Epstein, S. Schlesinger, & W. Dryden (Eds.), *Cognitive-behavior therapy with families* (pp. 5–48). New York: Brunner/Mazel.

Leahy, R. L. (2001). *Overcoming resistance in cognitive therapy.* New York: Guilford Press.

Leslie, L. A. (1988). Cognitive-behavioral and systems models of family therapy: How compatible are they? In N. Epstein, S. E. Schlesinger, & W. Dryden (Eds.), *Cognitive-behavioral therapy with families* (pp. 49–83). New York: Brunner/Mazel.

McGoldrick, M., Giordano, J., & Pearce, J. K. (Eds.). (1996). *Ethnicity and family therapy* (2nd ed.). New York: Guilford Press.

Minuchin, S. (1997). *Dialogue for the millennium.* New York: New York University.

Prochaska, J. O., DiClemente, C. C., & Norcross, J. C. (1992). In search of how people change: Applications for addictive behaviors. *American Psychologist, 47,* 1102–1114.

Schwebel, A. I., & Fine, M. A. (1992). Cognitive-behavior family therapy. *Journal of Family Psychotherapy, 3,* 73–91.

Schwebel, A. I., & Fine, M. A. (1994). *Understanding and helping families: A cognitive-behavioral approach.* Hillsdale, NJ: Erlbaum.

Thibaut, J., & Kelley, H. H. (1959). *The social psychology of groups.* New York: Wiley.

Wright, J. H., & Beck, A. T. (1993). Family cognitive therapy with inpatients. In J. H. Wright, M. E. Thase, A. T. Beck, & J. W. Ludgate (Eds.), *Cognitive therapy with inpatients* (pp. 176–190). New York: Guilford Press.

Part V

Psychotherapy Process

13

Difficult-to-Treat Patients: The Approach from Dialectical Behavior Therapy

Christine Foertsch
Sharon Y. Manning
Linda Dimeff

WHAT IS A "ROADBLOCK"?

"Roadblock" is a good term for the process of getting stuck with a patient in psychotherapy, insofar as it is broad, descriptive, and nonjudgmental. When the roadblock is attributed directly to the patient's behavior, comparable descriptors include "resistant," "unmotivated," "oppositional," "uncooperative and noncollaborative," "stuck," or "haven't hit bottom." As a class of behaviors, they represent some of the most difficult problems faced by psychotherapists, particularly when working with difficult and challenging patients such as those with borderline personality disorder (BPD).

This chapter approaches the definition and treatment of roadblocks from the perspective of dialectical behavior therapy (DBT; Linehan, 1993a, 1993b). DBT is a comprehensive, empirically supported behavioral treatment for BPD that integrates Eastern and Western philosophies, including Zen, behaviorism, and dialectics. The main dialectic in DBT is balancing change (through standard problem-solving procedures) with radical acceptance. Unlike many other behavioral approaches, DBT is a team-provided treatment composed of several modes of treatment. Standard DBT modes include weekly individual psychotherapy, weekly group skills training, as-needed phone consultation (to facilitate skills generalization), and a therapist consultation team (to enhance therapist motivation and capability to treat patients with BPD). Consistent with other behavioral approaches, the focus of treatment follows a set of hierarchically arranged behavioral targets to decrease the most severe and life-threatening behaviors first, followed by behaviors that interfere with the treatment and behaviors that interfere with the patient's quality of life (e.g., homelessness, Axis I disorders, etc.) while increasing behavioral skills.

In DBT, a therapeutic "roadblock" is conceptualized as any behavioral or interpersonal event that leads to the momentary or protracted derailment of the process of therapy and the patient's progress. Derailment can occur inside the session or outside, whenever the patient is attempting to implement behavioral change. We begin this discussion of roadblocks by looking through the lens of the DBT biosocial theory of borderline personality disorder. The elements of this theory (emotion dysregulation and invalidation) provide a broad base from which to understand why patients and therapists get stuck in treatment. Next we describe how DBT addresses and treats therapeutic roadblocks. The remaining portion of the chapter is organized according to specific behavioral roadblocks that commonly occur in treating patients with BPD and the major DBT strategies designed to treat them. These strategies include skills training, motivation and commitment strategies, validation, and dialectical strategies. Finally, we focus on therapist treatment-interfering behaviors and use of the DBT consultation team as the solution to this roadblock.

BORDERLINE PERSONALITY DISORDER AND THE STRUGGLE TO CHANGE

Designed specifically for notoriously difficult-to-treat individuals with BPD, DBT has always been at home with identifying and removing roadblocks to therapeutic progress. Indeed, many clinicians have come to equate BPD with the interpersonal and emotional obstacles that interfere with treatment from the start; having BPD means that one struggles with treatment. Many aspects of DBT are geared to treating these roadblocks in an effective and compassionate fashion that simultaneously acknowledges "how can it be otherwise" while insisting on change.

Linehan (1993a) hypothesizes that two factors, emotional vulnerability and invalidation, are central in the development and maintenance of BPD and are also generally responsible for the slow process of behavioral change. Emotional vulnerability refers to the tendency for individuals with BPD to be highly emotionally sensitive to stimuli, to react with intense and extreme emotional arousal to these cues, and to equilibrate slowly. It is posited that these patterns are visible in childhood and persist throughout adulthood, and it is frequently the case that this vulnerability affects the process of psychotherapy. Simply, exposure to a small "dose" of a particular stimuli is all that is needed to generate an extreme or intense emotional response. In comparison with other people, patients with BPD require more time to return to a relaxed physiological and emotional state. For example, a patient with BPD might be acutely aware of minor fluctuations in her therapist's mood from session to session and become intensely worried and fearful in response to the therapist having an "off" day. Although many patients may think, "My therapist is having an 'off' day," patients with BPD may become extremely emotionally dysregulated during session, so much so that they are unable to work on their life problems and unable to describe their emotion. Out of session, the patient's tendency toward intense emotion is in turn disruptive of other important spheres of life (e.g., overt behavior, interpersonal relationships, cognitive functioning). For example, behavioral control is often erratic or limited, and impulsive, self-destructive behavior frequently functions as an emotion regulation device. In the face of persistent and high emotional states, cognitive functioning is severely disrupted, characterized by polarized thinking, excessive worry, racing thoughts, dissociation, and cognitive rigidity. Occasionally, psychosis is present.

Emotion dysregulation and the previously described sequelae are clearly related to the process of therapeutic change and regularly impede it in the treatment of the individual with BPD. The essence of behavior therapy is acquiring new learning; however, basic learning processes (attention, reflection, memory, problem solving) are dramatically interrupted by strong emotion. Furthermore, emotion dysregulation can also interrupt collaboration and lead to "tug-of-war" or impasses. For example, behavioral analysis and other problem-solving strategies regularly grind to a halt as patients dissociate, stop talking, attack the therapist, or become willful in a nonconscious effort to avoid or escape the stimuli evoking strong emotions (e.g., repeat the response "I don't know"). Out of session, solutions become difficult if not impossible to implement in the face of strong emotion, leading to frustration and hopelessness in patient and therapist alike.

Pervasive invalidation by the environment, the second dimension in Linehan's (1993a) biosocial theory of BPD, is characterized by dismissive, pathologizing, critical, or punitive communication by the environment in response to the individual's report of private experience. Examples of invalidating environments run the gamut from extreme abuse (e.g., parent who blames or beats a child for accusing a relative of sexual abuse) to a poorness of fit between the child's special needs and temperament and his or her environment (e.g., a socially shy and awkward child within a family of extroverts who repeatedly dismiss the child's expressions of extreme anxiety or offer insufficient help in solving it). Not surprisingly, over the course of time, invalidation leads to moderate to severe emotional arousal, and the individual with BPD vacillates between assuming the stance of the invalidating environment (experiencing self-hatred, perfectionistic standards, oversimplifying the ease of problem solving) and her own (more natural) stance of intense emotionality and self-expression. Over countless conflictual transactions, invalidation becomes a loathsome, albeit familiar, experience to which the individual is highly sensitized. A sense of desperation and feelings of rage often surround issues of who is wrong and who is right, issues that figuratively and literally become life and death for the person with BPD. Importantly, this desperation and rage can become attached to *all* processes directed at change, associated as they are with early (and current) life experiences of being changed, controlled, or ignored in highly punitive or egregious ways. This situation obviously bodes poorly for therapies whose mission and process is explicitly change oriented, and the expected arousal, intense emotionality, and therapeutic stalls regularly characterize the treatments of individuals with BPD.

THERAPY ROADBLOCKS DEFINED: TREATMENT-INTERFERING BEHAVIORS

The first step in resolving therapeutic roadblocks in DBT is to clearly and nonjudgmentally define them as such and to include them in a matter-of-fact way in patients' lists of target behaviors. DBT defines these roadblocks as "treatment-interfering behaviors" (TIBs), a target second only to threats to the very life or physical safety of the patient. Patients are oriented to these events early on in treatment, and commitment to decrease them is elicited. Importantly, DBT recognizes explicitly that not only do patients engage in emotion-based behaviors that impede the progress of therapy but therapists do as well. It is expected that caregivers responsible for the safety and well-being of highly distressed and frequently suicidal patients will themselves become emotionally dysregulated during session or when responding to a patient crisis outside of session resulting in therapist-generated TIBs. Careful behavioral analysis frequently reveals that many treatment impasses described by therapists are in fact due to patient *and* therapist TIBs in combination and in transaction with one another.

Treatment-Interfering Behaviors by Patients

In DBT, patient-generated TIBs are primarily addressed within the context of individual psychotherapy. Patient-generated TIBs in DBT include those behaviors that compromise the effectiveness of the treatment or decrease the therapist's motivation to treat the patient and lead to therapist burnout. Categories of patient-generated TIBs include nonattendance (e.g., missing therapy or group, coming late, or dissociating during session), noncompliance (e.g., failing to do or forgetting to bring to session one's homework from the preceding week, refusing to record or monitor targeted behaviors on a diary card, refusing to get rid of lethal means "just in case" she decides to take her life in the future), and noncollaborative behaviors (e.g., becoming mute during a chain analysis of a recent self-harm episode, verbally attacking or personally criticizing the therapist during his or her efforts to help a patient solve a problem), and other behaviors that "push therapists' limits," such as frequently calling the psychotherapist during a crisis in the middle of the night, verbally or physically attacking the therapist, or repeatedly making threats to file a lawsuit against the therapist. Behaviors that push therapists' limits are expected to differ from therapist to therapist, even within a given DBT team. For example, one of our patients had wanted to do psychotherapy while sitting on her therapist's office floor. Although sitting on the floor during therapy had been an acceptable behavior to many other therapists on the team, it nonetheless was extremely distracting to the primary therapist.

Within the DBT skills training mode, a distinction is made between extreme behaviors that threaten to destroy therapy (e.g., burning the clinic down, physically assaulting another group member) and those that interfere with it (e.g., coming late, leaving early, missing sessions, not doing assigned homework, etc.). In general, the primary emphasis in the skills group is on skills acquisition and strengthening, and attention is diverted from these tasks only when therapy-destroying behavior emerges. Treatment-interfering behavior of lesser intensity is generally ignored or briefly highlighted as a way to demonstrate use of a specific skill (see example on p. 263). Persistent TIBs occurring in skills training group are referred back to the individual therapist and treated within that mode.

Importantly, DBT therapists approach all patient-generated TIBs just as they do other problems presented by the patient—in a matter-of-fact and straightforward problem-solving fashion that simultaneously conveys acceptance and compassion for the patient with a minimum of emotion-laden terminology (e.g., "manipulative," "naïve"), and that is genuinely nonjudgmental. With its roots in mindfulness and other contemplative practices, this acceptance-based approach in DBT emphasizes how every event or behavior is "just as it should be," in that every behavior is caused (either by one's biology or learning history). Having conceptualized the problem in nonjudgmental and behaviorally specific terms, the DBT therapist then moves to solving whatever problem is identified through a thorough analysis of the TIB. In our experience, most therapists are generally capable of remaining nonjudgmental and compassionate unless the TIB is such that it triggers a high degree of emotion dysregulation in the therapist (e.g., patient destroys the therapist's waiting room, attacks the therapist in a very hurtful fashion, etc). Interestingly, what is required of the therapist in these moments of high emotional arousal is the same set of DBT skills (Linehan,

1993b) taught to patients in the DBT skills training group (e.g., skills to tolerate a crisis without making it worse and to observe and describe emotions without acting on them or acting opposite to emotions).

Treatment-Interfering Behavior by Therapists

As stated previously, DBT recognizes that therapists are vulnerable to emotion dysregulation and that this vulnerability can and does lead to therapeutic stalls and impasses. In fact, DBT takes the position that many roadblocks could not occur without some type of transaction between both parties, as opposed to seating the difficulty in one or the other camp.

In general, therapist TIBs take the form of failing to synthesize the "extremes" of treatment, for example, becoming too rigid, too flexible, too change oriented, or too accepting. For example, a therapist might "fall into the pool" of hopelessness and behavioral passivity with the patient; he or she believes too much in the patient's conceptualization of his or her own helplessness to end suffering. This stance might result in the therapist attempting to control other caregivers or the environment in order to protect the patient from stress. This behavior in turn might reinforce the patient for helpless behaviors, leading to passivity, help rejection, and unrealistic expectations of others. Therapists can also become too invalidating or judgmental in sessions, and this is often accompanied by subtle or clear expressions of frustration or anger with the patient, with the therapist's emotion fueling an impasse.

TIBs by therapist also take the form of disrespectful or other "unmindful" behaviors, for example, chronically being late, taking phone calls or pages during sessions, becoming judgmental or harsh toward the patient, chewing gum in sessions, or forgetting important material the patient has described. These behaviors may be particularly difficult to address, as they may be quite subtle and may or may not have an acute impact but rather may exert a more protracted influence. Further, they may be considered "routine" by some therapists and will not even be brought before the team for discussion. It is likely that patients will notice and be affected by these behaviors over time, experiencing the therapist as uncaring and becoming emotionally dysregulated or uncollaborative in response.

Another common TIB involves the therapist's inattention to his or her own personal limits in treating patients with BPD or the therapist's failure to inform the patient when limits are being crossed. Consider the classic example of a patient with BPD who frequently calls the DBT therapist during crises but is unwilling to practice any new skills to solve the problem. The patient meets each suggestion by the therapist with a passive, helpless response. The therapist's problem with the phone calls is not that the patient is calling but how the patient behaves during the calls. Over time, the therapist becomes increasingly annoyed and frustrated by the calls but does not communicate the problem to the patient for fear that he or she will stop calling altogether and will instead resort to dysfunctional rather than skillful behavior to solve the crisis. If left unaddressed, it is easy to see how the therapist would increasingly feel generally annoyed by the patient and less eager to engage wholeheartedly in the treatment.

COMMON ROADBLOCKS RESOLVED: PROBLEM SOLVING, VALIDATION, AND DIALECTICS IN DIALECTICAL BEHAVIOR THERAPY

We now turn to several common roadblocks in treating severely disordered individuals with BPD: emotion dysregulation interfering with progress, change focus being experienced as invalidation, protracted tug-of-war, and therapist emotion dysregulation decreasing usual competence.

Roadblock 1: Emotion Dysregulation Interfering with Implementing Steps toward Change

This roadblock occurs whenever strong and unmodulated emotions arise in or outside therapy and compromise the ability of the patient with BPD to generate a skillful response when a skillful response is needed. In fact, most treatment noncompliance among patients with BPD occurs within a context of emotion dysregulation or out of fear of becoming emotionally dysregulated. It is not hard to find a plethora of examples of treatment noncompliance resulting from patients' emotion dysregulation or the threat of landing in a bottomless, inescapable abyss should they engage in the necessary therapeutic task. The socially anxious patient repeatedly misses the group sessions or leaves the group before he or she is called on to review the homework; another patient dissociates during a behavioral chain analysis of events leading up to a recent suicide attempt.

Problem-Solving Strategies: Skills Training

Like many other behavior therapies, DBT emphasizes teaching and strengthening new behavioral skills by acquiring and strengthening new skills to regulate emotions (emotion regulation skills), to tolerate emotional distress when change is slow or unlikely (distress tolerance skills), to be more effective in interpersonal conflicts (interpersonal effectiveness skills), and to control attention in order to skillfully participate in the moment (mindfulness skills). *Emotion regulation* training teaches a range of behavioral and cognitive strategies for reducing unwanted emotional responses, as well as impulsive dysfunctional behaviors, by teaching how to identify and describe emotions, how to stop avoiding negative emotions, and how to increase positive emotions. *Distress tolerance* training teaches a number of impulse control and self-soothing techniques aimed at surviving crises without using drugs, attempting suicide, or engaging in other dysfunctional behavior. *Interpersonal effectiveness* teaches a variety of assertiveness skills to achieve one's objective while maintaining relationships and one's self-respect. *Mindfulness skills* include focusing attention on observing oneself or one's immediate context, describing observations, participating (spontaneously), being nonjudgmental, focusing awareness, and becoming more effective (focusing on what works).

Whether analyzing a behavior that occurred outside of session or targeting a problematic in-session behavior, the DBT individual therapist will first highlight the dysfunctional behavior, then ask the patient to identify an alternative, skillful behavior. If the patient is successful in generating a skillful behavior, the DBT therapist will typically move to having the patient rehearse the skill to help strengthen and generalize use of the skill to the relevant context. If the patient is unable to generate a skill, then the therapist will teach the patient a new skill, followed by rehearsal of its use.

THERAPIST: Let's see, last week you agreed to actually go to skills training group despite the fact that you hate going because you're really shy. Did you go?

PATIENT: (*Looks down, shakes her foot rapidly, balls each fist as if to strike her legs; is silent.*)

THERAPIST: What just happened? I asked you about group and you became silent and you look really upset.

PATIENT: I suck! I'm such a loser!

THERAPIST: You can be so harsh and judgmental toward yourself, Casey. Did you happen to observe the judgments fly by there? How about starting over without the judgment and self-invalidation?

PATIENT: What do you mean? I am a loser!

THERAPIST: Saying you're a loser is shorthand for a description of characteristics about yourself that you don't like and find distasteful. The problem with the shorthand version is that it simultaneously conveys, "I am bad." You can always spot a judgment when descriptions of reality get abridged into "good/bad" or "should/shouldn't." The way out of the judgment is the skill of describing, just the facts. You don't have to give up your preferences, just the judgment. So try it. When you said "I'm a loser" in response to me asking about group, what did you mean?

PATIENT: I meant that I am fed up and frustrated with myself for not doing what I need to. It's hard to be a person who has so many problems. I really get tired of being so shy.

THERAPIST: That was a perfect reframe of the judgment and a crystal clear description of what you meant and what gets in your way of going to group. Let's get working on what would be helpful to help you be able to go.

When the TIB arises in skills training group, the skills trainer will treat it as an opportunity to teach or strengthen a new or existing skill. For example, a patient begins crying during homework review as she describes a painful and difficult situation she faced during the week in which she applied skills. As she continues further, she has more and more difficulty speaking, and she is becoming overwhelmed by intense negative emotions. The therapist scans the room and realizes that other group members are also appearing agitated and overwhelmed by their emotions in response: One member is doodling and appearing completely disengaged from the group, another has her head down on the table and is covering her face, another begins crying. In response, the DBT group leader would likely suggest the practice of a skill from the distress tolerance crisis survival strategies that is intended to help tolerate a difficult situation: "Hey, listen, group. I'd like to suggest that we pause for a moment and practice a crisis survival skill. Let's focus on the skill of relaxation—relaxing our bodies so our minds also relax. So sit back in your chair and find a comfortable position. It may be helpful to scan your body for any tension and, as you find tension, gently release those muscles. Very nice. Focus on calm, gentle breaths, breathing gently in and out. We're going to keep going here with the homework review, but should you notice yourself becoming emotionally dysregulated, return to your breath, focus on calming and relaxing your body. All right?"

Roadblock 2: Decreased Motivation to Implement the Skillful Behavior

Oftentimes, the problem causing the roadblock does not result from a skills deficit but is one of insufficient motivation to engage in the skillful behavioral response. Although patients may at one moment commit to a particular course of action, they frequently "lose steam" during the crisis. It is as if their previous resolve to give up the dysfunctional behavior drifted quietly and unceremoniously away. By motivation, we are referring to conditions (whether antecedents, consequences, or intrapersonal variables) that are sufficient to support the commission of a behavior. Motivation can be said to exist when variables necessary to elicit and maintain a behavior in a particular context exist. Given the availability of a particular behavior within the individual's repertoire (i.e., adequate skills), sufficient motivation is presumed if a particular behavior is performed. Insufficient motivation is presumed if a particular behavior is not performed.

Increasing the patient's motivation to emit functional behaviors, to inhibit dysfunctional responses, and to remain engaged in the treatment are central to DBT and are woven seamlessly throughout the treatment. Strategies that pertain to increasing motivation include behavioral analysis, contingency clarification, metaphors, cognitive restructuring, and emphasis on the relationship. Indeed, all DBT strategies not designed to teach skills are designed to enhance motivation.

A particular subset of motivation-enhancing strategies is the *commitment* strategies. These strategies serve to orient the individual toward a particular goal (short term or long term) and to clarify the contingencies that support behavior. Commitment strategies elicit a verbal agreement to engage in a particular behavior, as there is evidence that such verbal agreements, although not providing a guarantee, increase the probability of the patient engaging in the targeted behavior (Wang & Katsev, 1990; Hall, Havassy, & Wasserman, 1990). For example, a therapist might ask, "Do you promise not to harm yourself tonight even if your urges skyrocket?" or "For how long will you absolutely commit to not drinking, come hell or high water? Thirty minutes? Until 10 o'clock?" or "You will throw away your razor blades [used to harm oneself] after you get home, won't you?"

Commitment is generally manifested as both a "wanting" and a "willingness" to do something, as well as the actual commission of the planned behavior. The therapist frequently assesses the patient's commitment to work on a task or problem by asking directly and, in most circumstances, taking "yes" for an answer. It is assumed that commitment will wax and wane over the course of a week, if not over the course of minutes, and therefore must be strengthened, as would any adaptive behavior. The therapist simultaneously works with the patient to both increase both commitment and emotion regulation skills, again with the purpose of paving the way for more consistent behavioral change.

Significantly, DBT deems commitments to caring others as more compelling and motivating in the lives of individuals with BPD than are commitments to themselves or other, more abstract values in life. The treatment seeks to harness the power of these interpersonal commitments to connect the patient more and more meaningfully to his or her own goals, linking commitment to treatment targets with his or her own "wise mind" version of a life worth living. For example, imagine a therapist asking a question that hits a sensitive nerve with the patient. In response, the patient raises her voice and describes past mistakes of the therapist in a loud and pressured manner.

THERAPIST: Are you aware of how this extreme thinking and criticism of me [a treatment target or TIB] interferes with my getting to know you [the patient's personal goal]? It's like a barrier. I don't think you schlepped all the way here to leave not being understood. True?

PATIENT: True.

THERAPIST: Do you see that, as a consequence to having all these extreme, critical thoughts about yourself and me, I don't really get to see the problem? It's like a storm between us. Would you be willing to use other ways to express yourself, right now? Could we make this a target, for you to decrease this type of thinking and speaking so that I can understand you better?

In this case, the therapist attempts to motivate the patient by tapping into her interest in being understood and connected. This type of relationship contingency clarification is frequently used.

Roadblock 3: Change-Oriented Strategies as Invalidation

Insofar as efforts to change the patient have been associated with a history of criticism, blame, and even verbal abuse, problem-solving and other change-oriented strategies in behavior therapy are likely to cause arousal, aversion, and ultimately resistance. Change is tantamount to being "wrong," to surrendering an identity, to giving up a claim one has gone to great lengths to stake. Akin to the experience of "losing face" described in Eastern cultures, tremendous shame can surround such life changes, shame that the individual with BPD may regulate with a variety of self-destructive or maladaptive interpersonal behaviors (e.g., refusing to speak, blaming the therapist, quitting therapy). Further, as mentioned previously, therapists may become out of balance and too change oriented, failing to validate patient behavior that is actually valid with respect to short- or long-term goals. As the therapist pushes for more change, the patient with BPD further attempts to escape the change-focused cues through either retreating or attacking. It was this observation that led Linehan (1993a) to actively build validation into DBT as a counterbalance to problem solving.

Validation Strategies: Soothing the Road to Problem Solving

No therapeutic strategy cuts through the pain of this dilemma as cleanly and readily as does the therapist's liberal use of validation. Paradoxically, in adopting these strategies the therapist actually stops attempting to change the patient at all, standing very still, as it were, without any attempts at all toward movement or growth. In DBT, the essence of validation is the therapist's verbal or behavioral agreement with or confirmation of the patient's requests, feelings, or point of view. The frequency of validation in a DBT session is in itself so shocking to some people with BPD that it is enough to throw them off balance and prompt behavioral change. Some frequently observed therapist in-session examples of this strategy might be:

"It makes sense how you are angry now. Most people get angry when they can't get what they want."

"It's true, I am feeling frustrated right now. You are reading me correctly."

The patient requests that the therapist do something differently. The therapist does it differently.

Linehan (1997) has conceptualized validation according to six levels that increase in specificity to DBT (in comparison with other psychosocial treatments). Validation Level 1 (V1) refers to the therapist's mindful listening to and tracking of the patient's verbal and nonverbal communications. Validation Level 2 (V2) involves an accurate reflection of the patient's communication or expressions, frequently taking the form of a summary comment or an emotion-focused statement (e.g., "So I see the tears starting now and I hear you saying you were extremely hurt by this"). Validation Level 3 (V3) involves verbalizing that which is unarticulated or "reading between the lines," conveying an understanding of emotions or experiences based on knowledge of the patient and the antecedent circumstances. It communicates powerfully that one is known and knowable. For example, knowing that a patient regularly feels "in a double bind" when her husband does certain behaviors, a therapist, upon hearing of these behaviors of the husband, might say, "I bet this is when you started to feel really caught, like that 'double bind' you've described for me."

Validation Level 4 (V4) validates the patient's behavior with respect to past events or disordered biology. For example, during the first therapy session, the patient indicates that she is extremely anxious talking with the therapist about her problems. A V4 response might be, "In light of what I know about you so far, it makes perfect sense that you might find it extremely painful to talk openly about your feelings, given how you were punished for doing so as a child." In contrast to a V4 response, Validation Level 5 (V5) validates the patient's behavior with respect to the current circumstances or as a "normal," commonly seen behavior. A V5 response in the previous example might be, "It makes perfect sense that you're anxious talking with me. You've just met me. Most people do find it really hard to bare their souls to a stranger."

Finally, Validation Level 6 (V6; radical genuineness) validates the patient in total as an equal human being (as opposed to a fragile invalid). This level of validation takes the form of certain therapist behaviors, as well as the therapist's style. For example, speaking to the patient in an overly cautious, solicitous manner or using an unnatural (to the therapist) voice tone, language, or body posture would violate this strategy. Again, the implicit communication is that the patient is somehow not capable of tolerating the usual expectations, changes, or demands that characterize normal life. V6 interventions wherein the therapist acts in a natural manner or applies normal contingencies validate the patient as a competent individual.

Adopting a validating stance provides a helpful platform on which the therapist can meet the patient in the attempt to make behavioral change and therapeutic progress. Seeing the landscape wholly from the patient's view inherently provides an atmosphere of a team struggling with a problem as opposed to two people struggling with each other. It is usually only after adopting the patient's perspective as thoroughly as the validation strategies demand that the therapist can begin to offer relevant solutions. Once the therapist has fully entered the patient's world, the way out often becomes clear. For example, one of us (C.F.) treated a patient with severe mood dysregulation and self-injury, a psychotic disorder (paranoid beliefs), and bulimia. The patient would commonly experience extreme periods of emotion dysregulation prior to upcoming family gatherings or public events. Because the patient was also intelligent and articulate, her husband (understandably) expected her to be able to travel to these events without incident and to stay for the entire time required. Feeling that it was all "too much," the patient usually responded by lying in bed, drinking alcohol, and injuring herself for days prior to the event. Assuming the perspective of the patient with respect to the difficulty of this task, the therapist was easily able to generate alternative viable solutions (e.g., go to the gathering but for a briefer period, and bring a friend of the family who often stayed at their home). These solutions often validate both the patient's vulnerability and long-term goals (e.g., maintaining good relations with her husband) and are counter to the self-invalidating and perfectionistic solutions often arrived at by the patient. Solutions such as this powerfully overcome roadblocks, as they tend to minimize or eliminate the emotional vulnerability that is usually standing in the way of behavioral change.

Validation of the patient in some way is also an exceedingly powerful tool with which to manage in-session emotion dysregulation. If the therapist can offer a heartfelt description of the patient's experience (using V2 or V3), particularly elaborated by compassionate metaphors, it can often be sufficient to decrease the pain, shame, or defensiveness of the moment and to move the patient back toward problem solving or other helpful behavior. For example, a therapist might say, "You are like a person with a severe allergy to bee stings becoming panicked and unable to breathe, and when I ask you to try something different, that is like the bee sting." Most of us have experienced the decreased defensiveness and increased willingness that comes along with some important other firmly agreeing with or corroborating some portion of our experience; the patient's experience is no different.

Finally, validation, especially V5 and V6, is essential when the roadblock in therapy is due to a problematic transaction between therapist and patient. The typical scenario usually involves some amount of emotion dysregulation and complaining from both partners. A V5 intervention demands that the therapist nondefensively search for the patient's grain of truth with respect to the therapist's behavior and to acknowledge this verbally or to institute some type of self-change. Consider, for example, a patient who seldom asks for help outside of her weekly sessions and who telephones her therapist for help. Despite the patient's sense of urgency about the situation, the therapist forgets to return her call. The patient is "furious" at the scheduled appointment the next day, mincing no words in describing the therapist's transgression. A V5 response would acknowledge the validity of the patient's response (e.g., anger regarding the therapists' transgression): "Listen, it makes perfect sense that you're mad and frustrated. I completely agree that forgetting to call you back, particularly on the one occasion when you call looking for help, is tacky and a real mess up on my part." Typically, this kind of response will quickly function to diffuse the patient's anger. The genuineness, authenticity, and nonfragilizing style of communication by the therapist, characteristic of a V6 response, can further function to significantly strengthen the therapeutic relationship and significantly minimize obstacles in addressing in-session TIBs for most patients with BPD.

Roadblock 4: Protracted "Tug of War"

Many of the difficulties described so far also fall into this category, in which therapists and patients fall into polarized standoffs on highly charged topics. Examples include a patient refusing to give up access to lethal medications and the therapist refusing to see her until she does. Another patient refuses to attend skills training group on a regular basis, and the therapist refuses to continue seeing him beyond the initial treatment agreement unless he attends the groups. A therapist insists on one solution to a problem (e.g., gaining weight, AA meetings, antipsychotic medications), and the patient repeatedly refuses this solution. Both parties think that they are "right" and that the other is pathological or invalidating.

Dialectics in Dialectical Behavior Therapy

Dialectics in DBT refers to both a worldview informing the treatment as a whole and a strategy for logical argumentation. Both are extremely useful during a therapeutic impasse in helping to shift the balance in an unproductive tug-of-war, to show the well-worn battleground in a new light, and to reconstruct a source of conflict into a source of wisdom. As a worldview, DBT is always asking the therapist to be aware of and to work toward a synthesis between two polar opposites (thesis and antithesis) or extreme positions. The entire treatment seeks to continuously balance treatment strategies, that is, to balance both acceptance and change at all times, as if in a dance, both moving and standing still. Like in a dance, the blend is rarely 50:50 and requires an amount of "movement, speed, and flow" between the poles one is attempting to synthesize. It is this flow among strategies that is most helpful in getting patients and the therapy unstuck. For example, just as a patient reaches a frustration point in the effort toward self-change, the therapist may drop the change agenda entirely, focusing on how things are acceptable just as they are (validating the patient) or even suggesting a reversal of activity in the opposite direction ("extending").

The dialectical strategies used in DBT exemplify this process in that they inherently synthesize opposing positions. For example, an important and frequently used dialectical strategy is that of using metaphors. *Metaphors* generally depict a situation using imagery, thereby bypassing the usual verbal–logical analyses, as well as questions of right and wrong, that logic usually implies. Metaphor depicts the whole of the situation, shining new light on the interrelatedness of parts. Importantly, once the dilemma is framed metaphorically, resolutions are indicated as well. Consider a patient who appears to refuse all help when she is most in need of assistance. Metaphorically, the patient may be described as a panicked drowning swimmer who keeps flailing at the efforts of her rescue team. This alternative image provides a compassionate view of the patient's experience, as well as of the possible ways out (e.g., "stop flailing those arms and grab the life raft"). The best metaphors combine a stance of acceptance with that of change, fundamentally interrelating the two.

Another dialectical strategy involves looking at a particular problem from the vantage point of *wise mind.* Wise mind is a mindfulness skill that synthesizes the extremes of "emotion mind" (when behavior is under the control of emotions) and "rational mind" (when behavior is under the control of facts and logic). It is a way of apprehending a situation in total, relying on intuition, emotion, logic, and past experience. It is particularly helpful when a patient seems to be responding rigidly due to strong emotions or out of habit. One of our patients, for example, was recently struggling with the decision of whether to give up alcohol. With a history of striving for perfection to avert excessive criticism and invalidation by her father throughout her early years, in therapy this patient would rigidly defend her excessive use of alcohol, as if anticipating the same kind of attack and criticism from the therapist over her use of alcohol. This pattern of rigidly defending her use of alcohol interfered with her ability to stand back from the situation and evaluate her use of alcohol with respect to whether it was interfering with her long-term goals. The therapist instructed her to go within her wise mind and ask what she knew to be true about her use of alcohol and what was needed to achieve her long-term goals.

Roadblock 5: Therapist Emotion and Extreme Behaviors

As we have illustrated throughout, when roadblocks do emerge in DBT, an interplay or transaction between the patient's and therapist's behavior is typically evident, either in the development of a particular roadblock or in its maintenance. It is not uncommon, particularly in working with severely disordered and difficult-to-treat patients, for the therapist's own emotions to interfere with his or her ability and motivation to, in essence, adhere to the principles of the treatment and follow the manual. For example, a therapist stops pushing for change with a highly suicidal patient, fearing that any effort to get the patient to emit a new behavior will push him or her over the edge. Another therapist avoids discussing ongoing heroin use with a heroin-addicted patient, knowing that the patient will verbally attack him in highly personal ways should he raise the topic. Still another therapist is repulsed by the appearance of a particular patient and "can't stand" the patient's "meek, childish presentation." Fearing that her judgment and disgust will seep out into the session, she overcompensates by never mentioning or addressing treatment-relevant topics that are essential to the overall well-being of the patient and of the therapeutic relationship (e.g., the patient's extreme body odor or significantly delinquent payment). What is the emotionally dysregulated therapist who has stopped applying good treatment to do once this pattern has emerged? The frequent occurrence of problems like these in the treatment of multiply diagnosed patients indicates the necessity of ongoing peer supervision, which, in DBT, occurs in the consultation team.

In a nutshell, the DBT consultation team is a weekly meeting (typically 1 to 2 hours) made up of DBT therapists providing DBT modes to the patient (e.g., DBT skills trainer, pharmacotherapist, etc.). The functions of the consultation team are clearly defined and circumscribed—to enhance the DBT therapists' capabilities and motivation to treat their patients with BPD. The DBT consultation is not an administrative or chart-review meeting, nor is it solely a social support group intended to help the clinician feel better in the absence of improving the quality of care received by the patient. Linehan (1993a) has described a set of therapist agreements that function to set the tone for the DBT team meeting. Included among them are agreements to search for phenomenologically empathic interpretations of patients' behaviors, to accept that therapists are fallible and will make mistakes, to search for a dialectical synthesis when conflict arises by searching for the "both/and" position and by asking such questions as, "What is being left out?" and agreement to acknowledge and accept diversity (rather than consistency) in how patients are treated. In our own weekly consultation, therapists will divide up the available time between those people who require assistance. To ensure that solutions are generated from a thorough assessment of the problem behavior, only a handful of (typically no more than four) cases are discussed, following the DBT hierarchy of primary targets. This focus on depth (vs. breadth) becomes a crucial difference between the consultation group functioning as it is intended (i.e., with the purpose of enhancing therapists' skills and motivation) rather than as an administrative meeting at which cases are "staffed." Therapists on the consultation team are expected to maintain the DBT consultation team agreements and practice the DBT mindfulness skills throughout their participation in the team (e.g., observing and describing the process between a therapist and patient nonjudgmentally).

At its essence, the DBT consultation team can be thought of as "therapy for the therapist," at least with respect to the therapist's problems that arise in the context of the treatment. From this perspective, it is assumed that the very same therapeutic procedures and strategies used to treat patients may be required with the DBT therapist who is treating a multidisordered, difficult-to-treat patient with BPD. To illustrate, take the scenario of the therapist who would become emotionally dysregulated in response to her patient's very personal verbal attacks that followed any attempt on the therapist's part to address the patient's ongoing drug use. Historically, the therapist, like others before her, would inadvertently avoid or significantly curtail discussion of the patient's drug use in order to avoid the personal attacks. Rather than escaping from the verbal attack, what was required was for the therapist to persist in the discussion of the patient's ongoing drug use and to regulate her emotions in the face of the attacks. The team recognized what was required—preparing the therapist for the session by exposing her to the relevant cues (personal verbal attacks) until the therapist's intense arousal was extinguished. Indeed, the team-administered exposure procedure worked, and the therapist was able to remain effective with the patient, allowing for a frank conversation about the factors maintaining the patient's persistent use of drugs without becoming cognitively dysregulated in the face of the personal attacks.

We have discovered over the years that the set of treatment principles and strategies needed to remove the therapists' roadblocks to effective treatment is in many respects no different from the set of principles and strategies applied by DBT individual therapists in treating their patients. At times, what is required is a rigorous behavioral assessment of the factors inhibiting a more effective response from the therapist; at other times, validation of the difficulty in treating a particular patient is all that is required.

SUMMARY

Throughout this chapter, we have sought to emphasize the complex process of both defining and overcoming roadblocks in the treatment of difficult patients. We have highlighted the transactional nature of these phenomena, both in terms of the patient-centered variables that constitute roadblocks (e.g., a history of invalidation transacting with emotional dysregulation), as well as the interpersonal transaction between patient and therapist, which also may involve invalidation and intense emotional dysregulation. Similarly, the treatment of these impasses requires a complex interweaving of strategies, flexibly implementing them according to the needs of the moment but basing therapeutic choices on well-developed principles. DBT is well suited to this task, in that it is principle driven, composed of multiple strategies, and well versed in the treatment of therapeutic struggles in its emphasis on the treatment of BPD.

We began with a description of the variables constituting the DBT biosocial theory, demonstrating how both emotionality and invalidation contribute to roadblocks in therapy, particularly in therapies that are as oriented toward change as are most behavior therapies. Emotion dysregulation can naturally lead to interruptions in attention, reflection, learning, and collaboration, and experiences with invalidating histories can further the impasse in the context of the therapist's efforts to change the patient. Next, we described the DBT approach to treatment-interfering behaviors, which involves both a matter-of- fact (nonjudgmental) description of them and a regular focus on them over the course of treatment. Defining these problem behaviors (coming from both patient and therapist) ahead of time assists the patient, therapist, and DBT team in observing these behaviors when they occur and in treating them in an effectively compassionate manner. Finally, we described five common types of roadblocks, those due to intense emotionality, motivational deficits, change-oriented strategies, protracted "tugs of war," and therapist emotion and behavior. Indeed, any of the DBT strategies might have been used to treat any of these roadblocks, but we hoped to emphasize those treatment strategies that seemed to naturally correspond to the particular difficulty described. Again, it is often the moment-to-moment interweaving of multiple strategies that is the most effective.

Having the comfort and power of many roadblock-solving strategies in one's armamentarium is truly valuable in the therapy of difficult-to-treat patients. Surely, one of the aims of all effective treatments is to turn what can be a protracted, confusing, and painful struggle over movement and progress into a challenging but ultimately fulfilling dance, one that strengthens the relationship between the dancers and brings the patient closer to his or her ultimate goals.

REFERENCES

Hall, S. M., Havassy, B. E., & Wasserman, D. A. (1990). Commitment to abstinence and acute stress in relapse in alcohol, opiates and nicotine. *Journal of Consulting and Clinical Psychology, 58,* 175–181.

Linehan, M. M. (1993a). *Cognitive-behavioral therapy of borderline personality disorder.* New York: Guilford Press.

Linehan, M. M. (1993b). *Skills training manual for treating borderline personality disorder.* New York: Guilford Press.

Linehan, M. M. (1997). Validation and psychotherapy. In A. Bohart & L. S. Greenberg (Eds.), *Empathy and psychotherapy: New directions to theory, research, and practice.* Washington, DC: American Psychological Association.

Wang, T. H., & Katsev, R. D. (1990). Group commitment and resource conservation: Two field experiments on promoting recycling. *Journal of Applied Psychology, 20,* 265–275.

14

Obstacles or Opportunities?: A Relational Approach to Negotiating Alliance Ruptures

Christopher L. Stevens
J. Christopher Muran
Jeremy D. Safran

Few therapists, regardless of their orientation, would argue with the contention that a strong therapeutic alliance is important to successful therapy. One of the most consistent findings in psychotherapy research over the past 20 years has been that, regardless of other factors, the strength of the therapeutic alliance has a strong impact on outcome (Horvath & Symonds, 1991; Martin, Garske, & Davis, 2000). Following their meta-analysis of 79 studies, Martin et al. (2000) concluded that the empirical research to date supported the hypothesis that a strong alliance is beneficial in and of itself and that a patient may find a well-established alliance therapeutic regardless of other psychological interventions. Although they did not rule out the possibility that the alliance may have an indirect impact on outcome or may interact with other interventions, they concluded, "the strength of the alliance is predictive of outcome, whatever the mechanism underlying the relation" (Discussion section, ¶2). Similarly, there is ample evidence that weakened or poor alliance is a good predictor of early, unilateral termination (Ford, 1978; Shick-Tyron & Kane, 1990, 1993, 1995; Yeomans et al., 1994).

However, although there is general agreement that a strong therapeutic alliance is predictive of improved outcome and that a weakened alliance can lead to poor outcome or even termination, there is less agreement about how it functions as an agent of change. Traditionally, cognitive-behavioral therapy has separated the so-called "nonspecific" factors, such as the alliance, from technique, which has been considered the primary agent of change. Cognitive-behavioral therapy's greatest strength has been its consistent focus on clearly defined, easily operationalized techniques. Thus cognitive-behavioral therapy has a clear advantage in training, research, and practice over other therapeutic approaches. Having a clearly defined set of techniques with a strong theoretical underpinning has allowed researchers and practitioners alike to maintain a consistency in training and practice that is unusual in other models and has also provided a strong basis for empirical validation. This focus on technique has led cognitive-behavioral theorists and practitioners to deemphasize the so-called "nonspecific factors" such as the alliance.

This is not to say that cognitive-behavioral theorists have ignored or belittled the importance of the alliance. From the start, cognitive-behavioral therapy has emphasized the importance of establishing a strong collaborative relationship with patients. Therapists are encouraged to approach patients with genuine warmth and empathy, to work collaboratively to develop homework assignments, and to encourage patient feedback (Beck, Rush, Shaw, & Emery, 1979). Nevertheless, even while acknowledging the importance of the initial building of a strong alliance, many cognitive-behavioral thinkers have seen it as a prerequisite for therapy rather than an active part of the change process. In their article on the therapeutic alliance in cognitive-behavioral therapy, Raue and Goldfried (1994) compare the alliance's role in therapy to the use of anesthesia to prepare a patient for surgery. "Once surgery is underway, the primary concern is with the effective implementation of the surgical procedures—the primary reason the patient entered the treatment setting" (p. 135). Viewed this way, the alliance is seen as extremely important but no more responsible for change itself than anesthesia is for removing a tumor. If a strong alliance is absent, therapeutic work is impossible; but once established, the alliance is seen as a stable, static construct that moves into the background to allow for the smooth and effective application of technique.

Although Raue and Goldfried note that the alliance needs to be monitored for breakdowns, they, like many other cognitive-behavioral theorists (e.g., Goldfried, 1982; Beck, 1995), view ruptures in the alliance or patient resistance in terms of noncompliance: something to be overcome so that treatment can continue. According to Leahy (2001), cognitive and behavioral approaches have traditionally paid little attention to patient resistance. He notes that therapists faced with resistance have often been encouraged to continue to apply standard cognitive-behavioral techniques such as confronting irrational beliefs (Ellis, 1983, 1985) or cognitive distortions (Burns, 1989). Similarly, Raue and Goldfried suggest that when patients express reluctance to participate in certain techniques or to complete homework assignments, the therapist's job is to convince them that complying is in their best interest and to foster an attitude of friendly submission. "Therapy progresses smoothly when patients give up their preferred actions in return for the satisfaction arising from the therapy process (e.g., pleasing the therapist and avoiding confrontation)" (1994, p. 136). To do this, cognitive-behavioral therapists attempt to provide their patients with a clear rationalization for their approach, to work collaboratively to anticipate difficulties the patient might have, and to strategize with them about ways to overcome these problems. Raue and Goldfried (1994), for example, encourage therapists to be flexible in selecting tasks, even if that means choosing a task that they believe is less effective if it is more acceptable to the patient and therefore helps to reduce resistance. Unlike other approaches that see working with patient resistance as a central part of the change process, a traditional cognitive-behavioral approach views patient resistance as something to be overcome, so that proven techniques can once again be brought to bear on the patient's presenting problems.

Although the notion that the therapeutic relationship is primarily a foundation to support technique is not dissimilar to the way early psychodynamic thinkers approached the alliance (Zetzel, 1956, 1965), our investigations, based on Bordin's 1979 reconceptualization of the alliance (described in detail in the next section), have led us to view the alliance as a process of ongoing negotiation rather than a static backdrop to therapy and to see dealing with ruptures as a pivotal part of the treatment process (Safran & Segal, 1996; Safran, 1998; Safran & Muran, 1996, 1998, 2000; Muran, 2001, 2002; Safran, Muran, Samstag, & Stevens, 2002). Reconceptualizing the alliance in this way makes it possible to see how many traditional cognitive-behavioral interventions and assumptions work to promote change through the alliance, as well as to examine ways in which they may hinder treatment under some circumstances.

THE ALLIANCE AS PROCESS

Bordin, whose 1979 reformulation of the alliance as a transtheoretical concept has, in a large part, been responsible for its current central place in psychotherapy research, came to increasingly view ongoing negotiation as critical to the alliance's place in the change process (Bordin, 1979, 1980, 1994). Bordin suggests that all therapies, regardless of orientation, include some form of therapeutic alliance. The type of alliance varies depending on the type of therapy practiced and the demands placed on both the therapist and the patient, but all consist of agreement between the patient and therapist on three primary elements of therapeutic work: the goals and tasks of therapy and the emotional bond.

Briefly stated, the goals and tasks of therapy are the aims that patient and therapist are working toward and the methods they use to reach them. The tasks include such explicit techniques as examining automatic thoughts, as well as the more implicit factors, such as the direction of attention (internal vs. external) and the degree of direction or advice provided by the therapist. The third element, the bond, is the quality of the emotional connection between the patient and the therapist.

These three factors, the tasks, goals, and bond, function interdependently and influence one another in an ongoing fashion. The strength of the bond influences the degree to which patient and therapist are able to negotiate the tasks and goals of therapy. Conversely, the ability to negotiate tasks and goals will affect the strength of the bond.

Both patient and therapist start therapy with many preexisting characteristics and attitudes. The therapist comes from a particular theoretical orientation, with its implicit and explicit goals, methods, and biases, which he or she has chosen at least in part because of his or her own personality, background, needs, and strengths. Patients not only bring personality characteristics, preconceptions about therapy, and precipitating causes but are also shaped by the social and environmental stresses and supports in their lives. A strong working alliance depends on the ability of both parties to negotiate a good fit between these two sets of expectations and needs. According to this conceptualization of the alliance, technique cannot be seen as separate from the particular interpersonal dyad in which it is applied.

Bordin's (1979) formulation helps to provide a theoretical framework for clarifying how and why the negotiation of ruptures in the alliance is at the heart of the change process. More traditional conceptualizations of the alliance assume that there is only one therapeutic goal or task, or at least privilege one type of goal or task over others. In contrast to cognitive-behavioral therapy's assumption that technique lies at the heart of the change process whereas the alliance forms a static, stable base, Bordin's conceptualization is more process oriented. It assumes that the negotiation between therapist and patient of the tasks and goals of therapy is an ongoing process that takes place both implicitly and explicitly and that it is this process of negotiation that both provides the underlying conditions that are necessary for change to take place and forms an essential part of the change process in itself.

> The person who has collaborated in the building of a strong working alliance and in its repair, rebuilding and strengthening in the face of disruptive experiences, has in that process modified those ways of feeling thinking and

> acting that have contributed to inadequacy, unhappiness, and self-defeat and has acquired reactions useful for greater self-realization...the treatment resides in the alliance itself. The work of the alliance is the work of therapy. (Bordin, 1980, p. 63)

As discussed, both the therapist and patient bring into the therapeutic process a host of preexisting characteristics, beliefs, attitudes, and expectations. In this way, we believe, the therapeutic encounter is not unlike any other encounter between two people. For therapy to be successful, both parties need to be able to negotiate the needs of the self and the needs of others to form a working relationship. When things are running smoothly, much of this negotiating process takes place out of awareness. Therapists make decisions about what techniques to use and the timing of their application based on an implicit understanding of what the patient needs. Similarly, patients who are new to therapy may accept much of what seems strange or unusual about the therapeutic process based on the assumption that the therapist is a professional with their best interests at heart. Even slight or moderate disagreements are often addressed in a fairly simple and straightforward fashion (Safran, 1998; Safran & Muran, 1996, 1998, 2000; Muran, 2001, 2002; Safran et al., 2002). In these situations, the collaborative approach emphasized in cognitive-behavioral therapy is quite effective. By assuming that patients' reservations should be addressed and that patients deserve a clear explanation of the therapeutic process, cognitive-behavioral therapists address not only the patient's explicit need for understanding but also the underlying need to have his or her concerns and needs taken seriously. In this way, the cognitive-behavioral approach does much to contribute to the alliance's ability to promote change.

In other instances, however, the negotiation process itself breaks down. When such significant ruptures in the alliance occur, the faith that cognitive-behavioral therapists have in technique and the belief that ruptures in the alliance are roadblocks to be overcome can work to the detriment of the treatment. The study of common and specific factors in a cognitive-behavioral therapy-based treatment for depression conducted by Castonguay and his colleagues (Castonguay, Goldfried, Wiser, Raue, & Hays, 1996) provides a good example. In this case, both of the common factors under investigation, the alliance and the clients' emotional involvement in the treatment, were found to be predictive of improvement. Contrary to expectations, however, the therapist's focus on the impact of distorted cognitions on the symptoms of depression, a standard cognitive-behavioral intervention, was found to be correlated with poorer outcome. After analyzing the results, Castonguay and his colleagues concluded that when confronted with strains in the alliance, therapists sometimes increased their adherence to cognitive rationales and techniques, which appears to have worsened alliance ruptures. In this treatment, the therapists were instructed to follow Beck et al.'s (1979) injunction to address patients' opposition to treatment by challenging their distorted beliefs about cognitive-behavioral therapy, which, according to Castonguay and his colleagues, seemed to prove particularly problematic when patients were discussing emotionally laden interpersonal problems (Castonguay et al., 1996). Under such circumstances a different approach is required to understand the source of the breakdown in treatment. Given his or her beliefs about the role of the alliance, a cognitive-behavioral therapist's natural tendency is to attempt to return to the "real business" of therapy. To do so without understanding the nature of the rupture and how it reflects the patient's difficulties may, at best, ignore important issues and at worst lead to further problems with the alliance.

Although the ability to negotiate differences between the needs of the self and the needs of others is a basic developmental task that all humans must face, for some patients, at least, difficulties in doing so in a constructive fashion lie at the heart of the problems that bring them to therapy. For these patients, breaches in the therapeutic alliance are not obstacles to be smoothed over but represent the core of their difficulties in the world. In these cases, viewing problems in the relationship as an issue of noncompliance can prevent the therapist from recognizing an opportunity to gain access to and work with the patient's characteristic way of construing events and relationships and the problematic patterns of interpersonal behavior that emerge from this construal.

In these situations, being sensitive to moment-to-moment fluctuations in the ongoing negotiations that form the basis of the therapeutic alliance can allow the therapist to begin to identify the interpersonal patterns that form the basis of what have been called vicious cycles (Wachtel, 1993), cognitive interpersonal cycles (Safran & Segal, 1996), or the relational matrix (Mitchell, 1988). These cycles, in which the therapist will inevitably become embedded, are the core elements of the patient's difficulties in the world. They are central to understanding how working with breaches in the alliance can contribute to positive change.

RELATIONAL SCHEMAS AND COGNITIVE INTERPERSONAL CYCLES

Many developmental and relational theorists have come to believe that our need to maintain relationships is a basic human need (Bowlby, 1969, 1973, 1980; Stern, 1985; Sullivan, 1953, 1956). Like everything else, however, the manner in which we go about getting that need met depends on the context in which we develop. As we grow, we learn from our interactions with important attachment figures which behaviors and emotions lead to stronger attachments and which can lead to disruptions or breakdowns.

Healthy individuals develop a relatively flexible ability to express a wide range of feeling states and behaviors while preserving a reasonable expectation of establishing and maintaining significant relationships. In others, however, early learning experiences interfere with the development of a full range of emotional responses. Some emotional responses may come to generate intense anxiety, whereas others may become overdeveloped and rigid. For example, a child who is consistently ignored or neglected when crying or expressing sadness may come to associate those feelings with being weak or overly dependent, feelings that may come to generate intense anxiety and that as a result will be rigorously avoided. Another child, who is consistently given attention only when acting in a provocative or sexualized manner, may come to rely on taking a seductive stance when interacting with others. We have called these patterns of emotion and behavior, which form schematic representations of self–other interactions, "interpersonal" or "relational" schemas (Safran & Muran, 2000). Although these schemas are developed in the context of early attachments as a way of predicting and maintaining interactions with primary attachment figures, they can continue to influence interpersonal behavior throughout life.

The degree of flexibility and comfort with which an individual can interact with others varies a great deal. For some people, most, if not all, interpersonal encounters are relatively effortless and free from anxiety. For others the range of emotion they can comfortably express or respond to can become quite restricted, resulting in severe personality disorders. Most people, however, fall somewhere between these two extremes. Even those who, for the most part, are able to interact with others in a healthy and flexible fashion may have certain areas or types of interactions that are particularly problematic. For example, situations that evoke feelings of being disregarded, controlled, or threatened may activate a particularly rigid and maladaptive interpersonal schema.

Even circumscribed maladaptive relational schemas can have a powerful impact on a person's life, restricting the types of relationships they develop, situations they feel comfortable in, and work they do. This is one of the primary ways in which such schemas are self-reinforcing. Individuals may choose to avoid situations in which their problematic relational tendencies are evoked, thus depriving them of the opportunity to disconfirm their beliefs and expectancies. For instance, a patient who has difficulty relating to figures in authority may feel the need to avoid work opportunities that require supervision. Conversely, people tend to seek out others who are comfortable with their interpersonal style, although they may often be only partially aware that they are doing so. Although this behavior aids an individual in avoiding uncomfortable ways of relating, it also forces him or her to continue the problematic cycles that create the anxiety in the first place. For example, a man who has come to believe that others value him only if he is useful or strong may attract others who are needy and dependent. He may believe that expressing his own needs will threaten or even destroy his relationships. His experiences with those around him, who have sought him out because of his apparent strength and control, can serve to reinforce and reconfirm his belief. When he acts "in character," he may receive considerable gratification and positive reinforcement from those who have come to depend on his strength. Expressions of sorrow or neediness, however, may be met with confusion or distaste.

In addition to influencing the types of relationships that a person engages in, the patients' maladaptive relational schemas may cause them to act proactively to protect themselves from what they believe to be dangerous responses of others. For example, those who fear that others will reject, take advantage of, or act in a hostile or aggressive way toward them can become highly sensitized to any sign that this behavior *might* be forthcoming. Individuals whose learning history has led them to expect that relationships with others can be dangerous may become hypervigilant in their attempts to detect evidence or warning in time to protect themselves from the feared response. This may then lead them to behave in self-protective, albeit maladaptive, ways instead of taking the time needed to clarify others' intentions. For example, they may lash out or withdraw at even slight indications of misattunement or hostility.

Another way in which maladaptive cognitive–interpersonal cycles are self-reinforcing is that people often attempt to control or conceal emotions that they have come to believe are threatening to their relationships. Ironically, it is often the very attempts to protect relatedness by controlling unwanted or anxiety-provoking feelings that elicit the precise responses that they were designed to avoid. This can happen in several ways. First, the stance that the individual takes may end up pulling for the unwanted response. For example, the man who is afraid of appearing weak or dependent may attempt to act in a cool and controlled fashion, even when experiencing sadness or a desire for closeness. His attempts to manage what he believes to be unacceptable or dangerous feelings in a bid to gain or protect closeness may make him appear aloof or unapproachable to those who might be willing to get closer. Attempts by significant others to penetrate his protective style will likely only increase his anxiety, causing him to withdraw even further.

A second consequence of efforts to manage threatening affect is that such attempts are, more often than not, only partially successful. Feelings of anger or a need for contact, although denied and concealed, are often expressed in subtle, nonverbal ways without the patient's awareness. Despite the struggling individual's best attempts to ward off threatening feelings, he or she often ends up giving off paralinguistic and physical cues that communicate the very feelings that he or she is attempting to conceal. For example, a man trying to hide his anxiety may smile and joke, but a tightness around the mouth and eyes or a shift in vocal tone may give him away. Similarly, a woman attempting to conceal her anger may speak in a complementary way, but a slightly sarcastic tone may lead others to question her sincerity.

The expression of affect, whether overt or implicit, exerts a strong pull for a complementary or contrary response from others (Kiesler, 1988). For example, sadness can pull for sympathy, and expressions of hostility can evoke responses of aggression or submissiveness. When one is aware of what emotions are being communicated, it is, of course, possible to respond in a noncomplementary way. But as Safran and Segal (1996) point out, "when an individual exerts a very strong pull for complementary behavior . . . it is difficult not to respond accordingly" (p. 75). For example, a therapist confronted with an overtly hostile patient may find it impossible not to respond defensively to the patient's attacks.

When the affects expressed verbally and nonverbally are different, the result can often feel particularly confusing. The nonverbal cues can be so subtle that others can find themselves responding to the patient without having a clear understanding of what it is that they are reacting to. For example, a woman can speak sympathetically but convey disdain through minute shifts in vocal tone or facial expression, evoking feelings of anger or resentment. Similarly, a man may tell a story of great hardship and woe but also convey a sense of entitlement and resentment and therefore evoke anger rather than empathy from his listeners. This in turn frequently causes the listeners to respond in ways that confirm the patient's initial expectations, particularly if the listeners remain unaware of the nature or cause of their emotional responses.

WORKING WITH RUPTURES AND COGNITIVE INTERPERSONAL CYCLES

When maladaptive relational schemas are triggered in the therapeutic situation, the result is often a rupture in the alliance and a breakdown in the normal negotiating process. Such ruptures can take several forms. Patients who are acting in a preemptively defensive fashion can often lash out overtly, attacking or blaming the therapist, or else withdraw abruptly, becoming silent, changing the topic or even missing sessions. Because the patients are acting out of anxiety about what "might" happen, their responses may well be difficult to understand or may appear quite excessive given what has occurred in the session. If the patients' fears are not recognized and addressed, it is possible that they may drop out of treatment.

When patients attempt to ward off their own feelings rather than act out preemptively, the rupture can be harder to detect. As described, it may be extremely difficult for the therapist to identify exactly what is behind the breakdown in communication or even to realize that a breakdown has taken place. Because areas of rigidity in the patient's interpersonal schemas occur where the patient has trouble accessing and expressing particular feeling states or needs, it is difficult, if not impossible, for him or her to communicate those feelings or needs directly. The elusiveness of this process means that therapists will often become aware that they have been caught up in a particular interpersonal cycle only after some time has passed. It is only by keeping an eye on their own subjective experience and reactions that it is possible for therapists to begin to identify the cycle and start to disengage.

As mentioned, the traditional cognitive-behavioral approach to the alliance does much to implicitly promote ongoing negotiation with patients about the tasks and goals of therapy and to promote the alliance as an agent of positive change. At times at which the normal negotiating process breaks down, however, some of the traditional cognitive-behavioral therapy assumptions, such as the desire to overcome resistance and a focus on technique, can exacerbate rather than relieve ruptures. For example, a man who believes that relationships are contingent on his appearing competent and acquiescent comes into therapy for anxiety caused by problems at work. A therapist trained in cognitive-behavioral technique will certainly spend time at the beginning of treatment working to establish a strong working alliance and will continue to work collaboratively with the patient throughout treatment. The patient will try to do his best to be a "good patient" and comply with all therapeutic tasks, even when he does not understand or agree with them. Despite the anxiety that brought him into treatment, the patient may tend to minimize his difficulties or report that interventions have been effective even if he feels no relief. As he becomes frustrated or confused, the patient will do his best to ignore or at least hide these feelings from the therapist, believing them to be threatening or inappropriate. For her part, the therapist may begin to become aware that, despite the patient's superficial compliance and enthusiastic reassurances, little seems to be happening in the treatment. She may be confused and frustrated by the mixed signals that she gets from the patient, who may report his anxiety as being both quite severe and "not a real problem." The therapist's attempts to explore the patient's responses to the treatment and requests for feedback will be met with uniform expressions of enthusiasm and praise. As the therapist probes for the patient's response to treatment and signs of dissatisfaction, the patient may become more anxious as threatening feelings of frustration and anger are in danger of being exposed. He may react with annoyance at the therapist's continued inquiries, then quickly reassure the therapist that everything is all right. The therapist, trained to focus on technique and smooth over, rather than explore, difficulties in the alliance, will likely continue to ignore her own growing sense of discomfort and annoyance and, signaled by the patient's irritation, begin to avoid topics that the patient is implicitly warning her are "out of bounds." Despite the outward signs of compliance, the negotiating process that forms the basis of the working alliance has, in fact, broken down.

As the treatment continues, the therapist's belief that a warm and empathic stance is appropriate to all treatments and the lack of attention that cognitive-behavioral training places on the therapist's subjective experience may also hinder her ability to make sense of the interaction and may actually contribute to the cycle. Her attempts to maintain a professionally warm and empathic stance, in spite of her annoyance and confusion, will begin to sound more hollow, both to her and to the patient. The patient begins to feel that perhaps coming to therapy was a mistake. Cued by his own sense that the therapist is not being completely honest, he may believe that the therapist, despite her outwardly warm demeanor, is actually somewhat repelled by the weakness the patient displayed by admitting that he needed help—just as he had expected.

Although a patient like this may not drop out of therapy, outcome will certainly be negatively affected. The kind of process described here can be difficult to manage for any therapist, regardless of orientation, but altering the approach to the alliance and beginning to place more emphasis on exploring one's own subjective states can make it significantly easier for the therapist to recognize and work with ruptures.

To work with ruptures, it is first necessary for the therapist to recognize that he or she is involved in a maladaptive cycle and to begin the process of *disembedding* from the cycle rather than perpetuating it. To do this, the general technical principle we advocate is *metacommunication*, which, simply stated, is the practice of focusing on and communicating about the therapist–patient interaction *as it occurs* in session (see Safran & Muran, 2000, for a detailed description). To do this, therapists need to be aware of their own emotional states and reactions and be willing to make use of that awareness as they engage with their patients in a collaborative inquiry into what is going on in the therapeutic relationship. By exploring the patient's construal of events rather than continuing to react in a way that is consistent with the patient's beliefs and past experience, the therapist is able to begin to disconfirm those beliefs and offer the patient a new relational experience. This process of disembedding and disconfirmation through metacommunication is at the heart of working with ruptures. Some of the fundamental principles of the metacommunication process include focusing on the immediate details of experience and behavior, establishing a sense of collaboration or "we-ness" in the exploration, recognizing that the situation is constantly in flux, and being open to exploring and acknowledging one's own subjectivity and contribution to the interaction (Muran, 2002). For example, over the course of a session, the therapist might notice that her attempts to engage the patient were being subtly rejected, spurring her to try even harder. As she became aware of this interaction, she might comment on it directly to the patient: "I feel like I'm really pushing you to engage, but it still seems hard for you. I wonder if there is something that I'm doing that is making it difficult for you to open up."

A MODEL FOR RUPTURE RESOLUTION

As discussed, the purpose of focusing on and working with ruptures is not simply to repair them so that work can continue with a revitalized alliance. Rather, the goal is to help the patient to come to a fuller understanding of how he or she construes events, how that construal affects his or her interactions with others, and to provide him or her with a new experience of relating. Ideally, this will help the patient to develop more comfort with his or her own emotional states and needs and greater flexibility in expressing those feelings and needs with an improved expectation of maintaining relatedness with important others.

Although elsewhere (Safran & Muran, 2000) we have found it useful to distinguish withdrawal ruptures from confrontation ruptures and have described specific resolution models for each, it is possible to abstract a more general model consisting of five positions: (1) the relational matrix, (2) recognizing and disembedding from the matrix, (3) exploring the patient's construal, (4) exploring the avoidance of vulnerability/aggression, and (5) expressing the underlying wish or need. Each position describes a dyadic interaction between therapist and patient that is spelled out here.

Although for heuristic purposes, we present a consecutive series of separate and distinct positions, in practice it is often the case that work with ruptures moves back and forth through different stages, and it is necessary for the therapist to be aware of and respond to what is actually happening in the dyad in the moment rather than relying on the theoretical stepwise progression we describe here.

Position 1: The Relational Matrix and Rupture Markers

Ruptures typically begin when the patient perceives some action of the therapist as confirming his or her anxiety-provoking beliefs about relationships. For example, a patient who believes that expressing dissatisfaction is dangerous to his relationships might attempt to conceal his anger by being compliant or submissive. The therapist might well miss subtle signs that the patient is dissatisfied or concerned. Instead, the patient's overly submissive presentation may pull for the therapist to take a more active or controlling stance in the treatment, thus reinforcing the patient's beliefs that he or she needs to be accommodating and that attempts to be more assertive will be ignored or met with rejection or hostility. Another patient, who has a long history of relationships with disappointing and rejecting others, might be so prepared for the therapist to reject her that any of the therapist's inevitable shortcomings and minor failings could be seen as a sign of impending rejection and trigger an attack or precipitous withdrawal. The therapist's defensive or angry reaction to this apparently unprovoked hostility or retreat confirms the patient's expectations. It is important to note that, regardless of whether the patient's initial expectations are realistic or distorted, at this point the therapist and patient are *both* engaged in a cycle of reaction and counterreaction.

Position 2: Recognizing and Disembedding from the Relational Matrix

For the resolution process to begin, the therapist must first recognize that he or she has become embedded in a relational cycle with the patient. Some ruptures are easy to recognize. When a patient begins to openly criticize or blame the therapist or, somewhat more indirectly, to attack the technique, the setting, or the profession of psychology in general, there is little doubt that something has gone wrong with the ongoing negotiation process. Similarly, an abrupt withdrawal, such as a patient repeatedly missing visits, coming late, or constantly needing to change appointment times can be a clear indication that something is amiss. Even in these situations, however, patients may be unwilling or, as is more often the case, unable to describe what they are reacting to. As demonstrated earlier, other types of ruptures can be even more subtle and difficult to detect. When patients try to conceal their feelings of anger or dissatisfaction, it may be possible for the therapist to recognize that the negotiation process has been compromised only by noting changes in his or her own subjective experience. Feelings of annoyance, boredom, or wariness are among the cues that can allow a therapist to begin to question what is going on.

Because ruptures reflecting maladaptive interpersonal schemas can occur at any time in treatment, this ongoing attention to subjective states, which we have labeled mindfulness in action (Safran & Muran, 2000), needs to be an ongoing process. By maintaining a sense of awareness of their own emotional reactions, therapists can be alerted to strains in the relationship and begin to identify what patient behaviors are pulling for a particular complementary response (e.g., a brittle or sarcastic vocal quality, nervous shifting, sudden topic changes, an averted gaze, to name just a few). Additionally, although awareness of their own feelings is especially important for detecting subtle ruptures, it is essential that therapists be able to identify and use their own responses to all ruptures in order to facilitate the subsequent disembedding process.

Once the rupture has been detected and the therapist realizes that both he and the patient are caught in a cycle, he can begin the disembedding process in which both the therapist and the patient attempt to step back and communicate about what is going on. This process involves the therapist metacommunicating his observations about the cycle to the patient (actually communicating about the communication). For example, the therapist might draw the patient's attention to her sudden silence or acknowledge his own defensive response to the patient's criticism and invite the patient to explore the interaction. It is important here that the therapist recognize and is able to express his or her own contribution to the cycle. As described, a central feature of maladaptive interpersonal cycles is the complementary responses that are evoked in the therapist. Acknowledging the feelings that emerge in exchanges with the patient serves two important purposes. First it allows the therapist to regain his or her ability to talk about the rupture with the patient rather than continuing to respond reflexively. Second, just as patients are not completely able to conceal the emotions they believe will threaten the relationship, therapists cannot hide these feelings completely, either. Patients are well aware when the therapist's verbal and nonverbal messages do not match. Acknowledgment of these feelings by the therapist will allow the patient to make sense of his or her own emotional responses.

Metacommunication needs to be done with care. Therapists should not report every feeling that they are experiencing. But talking about the feelings that are central to the current dynamic gives patients important feedback about how they are affecting others and can serve as a model for the idea that expressing feelings, even dangerous ones, can lead to closeness rather than more hostility and can open up further exploration. For example, with a particularly hostile patient, a therapist might say, "I can't help feeling defensive when you yell at me, and it's difficult for me to respond to you right now." With a patient who is reluctant to try a new technique, the therapist might talk about the urge he or she feels to try to prove that it will work. A comment such as, "I feel like I'm trying to convince you that this will work, but I don't know that anything I say will persuade you" can open the way for a patient to talk about what is behind his or her reluctance.

Position 3: Exploring the Patient's Construal

The goal in this stage is to unpack and explore the patient's construal of events. Although doing this may allow the therapist to gain a clearer understanding of how the patient characteristically makes sense of interpersonal relationships, the focus here should remain on the interaction *in the moment.* The goal is not simply to provide the patient with greater understanding of the cycles that he or she can get caught in but to provide him or her with the experience of working his or her way out of those cycles with another person. To do this, the therapist needs to help patients to unpack their understanding of what happened to precipitate the rupture. The focus here is *not* on identifying or correcting cognitive distortions. Rather, the therapist and patient try to jointly come to a better understanding of the patient's response and what led to up to it. For example, if a patient angrily tells a therapist that his or her intervention was cold and unfeeling, the therapist might acknowledge the patient's feelings and ask what specifically had felt cold or hostile to the patient. It is critical that the therapist maintain a curious and empathic stance at this point and be open to any negative feelings the patient may express. Similarly, the therapist needs to be willing to recognize that he or she played a part in the rupture and, as that contribution becomes more clear, to acknowledge it. The goal here is not simply to fix the rupture and return to the application of technique or, to extend Raue and Goldfried's (1994) analogy, to put the patient back under so that surgery can continue. Rather, the aim is help the patient to understand his or her own experience better and to empathically validate the feelings that result from his or her construal. For example, if a patient is able to express anger or resentment because a therapist unexpectedly canceled a session, the therapist should not, at this stage, elicit alternative explanations or ask the patient how objectively likely his or her construal is. Rather, the therapist should focus on helping the patient explore and articulate his or her feelings of resentment, fear of abandonment or rejection, belief that he or she is not important to the therapist, and so on.

Position 4: Avoidance of Vulnerability/Aggression

Although exploration of the patient's experience of the rupture may in itself lead to a resolution, the exploration itself may cause significant anxiety and trigger avoidance of underlying feelings. Patients who use anger and aggression to mask or avoid the expression of feelings of vulnerability may experience considerable guilt and shift into a withdrawal state, attempting to smooth things over. Others may find that attempts to understand their feelings of vulnerability or anger create intense anxiety. These feelings may have been masked or avoided with great effort for years. It may be impossible for a patient to believe, despite the therapist's open and empathic stance, that his or her feelings will be accepted.

Just as therapists' ability to monitor subtle shifts in their own and their patients' emotional states is critical in detecting the initial rupture, it is crucial in being able to track the patient as they explore their construal of events. As the therapist becomes aware that the patient is becoming more anxious, the exploration needs to shift to the anxiety. For example, a patient who had become silent during the session began to explore his feelings that the therapist was not listening to him. As he spoke, however, the therapist noted that he began to talk about psychologists in general rather than the therapist herself. She noted the shift and wondered aloud if the patient had any concerns about how she might react if criticized. This allowed the patient to begin to talk about how he worried that she might not want to work with him any longer if he were not a "good patient." Another patient was very comfortable criticizing the therapist for his youth, inexperience, and general incompetence. The therapist acknowledged that he was young and relatively new to the profession compared with other therapists the patient had seen. The patient seemed to relax and started to talk about his fears that his problems were too much for any therapist to deal with. As he spoke, his tone shifted, once again becoming harder and more aggressive, and he again attacked the therapist, calling him weak and flimsy, wondering how he could possibly begin to tolerate or understand the patient's levels of pain. The therapist felt a strong urge to convince the patient that he could help and, in fact, had helped other patients. At the same time, he became aware of feeling both frustrated and helpless. He found that he did not believe he could say anything to this patient in the moment that would be experienced as helpful. Rather than give in to the temptation to prove his worth, the therapist tried to metacommunicate his feelings. "I really want to convince you that I can help, but I find that I don't believe I have the power to say anything to you that would satisfy you that that is true." Again, the patient was able to relax and express his belief that he was too damaged to ever feel better. The exploration continued to shift back and forth between the patient's feelings of vulnerability and pain and his attempts to blame the therapist's supposed incompetence. As the conversation progressed, the therapist was able to draw the patient's attention to these shifts and to begin to explore how dangerous it felt for the patient to reveal his own sense of despair and how much more comfortable it was to attack the therapist.

Typically, patients will move back and forth between expressing and avoiding their feelings, with the exploration of both the feelings and the avoidance helping them to better understand and more comfortably express a wider range of feeling states. Frequently, ruptures are partially resolved only to reappear in slightly different form as the underlying schema is reactivated by another encounter later in therapy, allowing for the process of exploration to continue.

Position 5: Expressing the Underlying Wish or Need

The preliminary expression of feelings in position 4 often continues to be associated with patients' beliefs that they are unacceptable or that needs will go unmet. As a result, a patient's initial expressions of a wish or need may be presented in a qualified or indirect way or in an apologetic, pleading, or insistent tone. As with any other stage in the process, the danger here is that if the therapist is not aware of his or her own feelings and responses, the complementary responses evoked by this qualified presentation can perpetuate a new enactment of the cycle. Providing the therapist can continue to be mindful of his or her own reactions, continued work can lead to the examination of the underlying wish or need. As the exploration continues, and the therapist continues to validate the patient's emotional responses, the patient gradually becomes more comfortable with his or her underlying feelings and needs and more capable of expressing them directly. Patients can begin to feel comfortable expressing a wider range of emotions and needs without feeling that doing so will endanger their ability to relate to others. They will also begin to understand that all of their wants and needs cannot be met and that the feelings of sadness and disappointment that result can be tolerated and accepted. At this stage, patients may be able to express disappointment that therapy cannot solve all of their problems, sadness at a recent loss, or anger at an abusive parent without feeling that the therapist has to make the feelings go away or fix the situation.

SUMMARY: SOME BASIC PRINCIPLES OF THERAPEUTIC METACOMMUNICATION

Metacommunication is an attempt to disembed from the relational matrix by focusing on the current interaction between the therapist and patient. The process involves engaging in collaborative exploration of and communication about what is going on within the dyad. Elsewhere we have elaborated a number of specific principles for therapists to follow (Safran & Muran, 2000). Here, we have attempted to show how some of the core ideas can be used to work with ruptures in a cognitive-behavioral treatment. In particular, we have focused on:

1. *Awareness:* The therapist needs to be open to exploring and acknowledging his or her own subjective experience, as well as that of the patient.
2. *A collaborative focus:* Like cognitive-behavioral therapy, our approach emphasizes the collaborative nature of the exploration of ruptures, with a particular focus on the therapist's recognition of his or her contribution to the relational matrix in which he or she has become embedded with the patient.
3. *A present, specific focus:* Focus needs to be on what is going on in the moment between the therapist and patient, with special attention paid to the details of emotional experience and behavior and with an awareness that the process is in a state of constant flux.
4. *An emphasis on understanding rather than change:* The goal of the exploration is to understand the patient's construal of events and to

accept and validate the patient's emotional responses and needs. It is the experience of having the therapist react in a different way than had been expected, while simultaneously recognizing and validating the patient's experience that leads to growth.

CONCLUSION

The approach to working with ruptures that we describe here is not fundamentally incompatible with basic cognitive-behavioral therapy technique. An awareness of and willingness to work in the relationship does not preclude or take precedence over the use of technique. As described, the traditional cognitive-behavioral therapy stance already does a lot to facilitate the use of the alliance as an agent of change under many circumstances. In situations in which the usual negotiating process breaks down, however, the ability to understand and work within the relationship can provide cognitive-behavioral therapists with a unique opportunity to explore and expand the patient's characteristic way of construing relationships. To do this, though, a number of important shifts need to take place.

1. The alliance needs to be viewed as an ongoing negotiation rather than a static construct.
2. Ruptures in the alliance cannot be seen as random events but must be recognized as windows into the patient's core interpersonal belief system. As such they should be seen as opportunities for learning and growth rather than simply obstacles to the smooth application of technique.
3. Therapists need to develop an ongoing appreciation of their own subjective feelings and responses as a source of information about what is going on with the patient.
4. Therapists need to be willing to explore the patients' construal of events and to take that construal seriously, including being willing to acknowledge their own contribution to rupture events.
5. Most importantly perhaps therapists need to be aware that any intervention is going to take on specific meaning within the interpersonal context in which it is applied and they need to be willing to explore that meaning-in-context with their patients.

Moments of rupture with patients can be very anxiety provoking. They can challenge a therapist's sense of competence and efficacy. It is extremely tempting in these moments to fall back on familiar technique and the implicit authority of the therapist role for support. Being willing to recognize and acknowledge feelings of anger, boredom, or inadequacy can be very difficult. Nevertheless, adopting the self-awareness and relational focus we are advocating here can provide therapists with additional tools to cope with and benefit from ruptures in the alliance and provide even greater flexibility for working with a wider range of patients.

REFERENCES

Beck, A. T., Rush, J., Shaw, B., & Emery, G. (1979). *Cognitive therapy of depression.* New York: Guilford Press.

Beck, J. S. (1995). *Cognitive therapy: Basics and beyond.* New York: Guilford Press.

Bordin, E. (1979). The generalizability of the psychoanalytic concept of the working alliance. *Psychotherapy: Theory, Research and Practice, 16*(3), 252–260.

Bordin, E. (1980). A psychodynamic view of counseling psychology. *Counseling Psychologist, 9*(1), 62–70.

Bordin, E. S. (1994). Theory and research on the therapeutic working alliance: New directions. In A. O. Horvath & L. S. Greenberg (Eds.), *The working alliance: Theory, research and practice* (pp. 13–37). New York: Wiley.

Bowlby, J. (1969). *Attachment and loss: Vol. 1. Attachment.* New York: Basic Books.

Bowlby, J. (1973). *Attachment and loss: Vol. 2. Separation, anxiety and anger.* New York: Basic Books.

Bowlby, J. (1980). *Attachment and loss: Vol. 3. Loss: Sadness and depression.* New York: Basic Books.

Burns, D. D. (1989). Agenda setting: How to make therapy productive when you and your patient feel stuck. In *The feeling good handbook* (pp. 523–543). New York: Plume.

Castonguay, L. G., Goldfried, M. R., Wiser, S., Raue, P. J., & Hays, A. M. (1996). Predicting the effect of cognitive therapy for depression: A study of unique and common factors. *Journal of Consulting and Clinical Psychology, 64*, 497–504.

Ellis, A. (1983). Rational-emotive therapy (RET) approaches to overcoming resistance: I. Common forms of resistance. *British Journal of Cognitive Psychology, 1*(1), 28–38.

Ellis, A. (1985). *Overcoming resistance: Rational-emotive therapy with difficult clients.* New York: Springer.

Ford, J. D. (1978). Therapeutic relationship in behavior therapy: An empirical analysis. *Journal of Consulting and Clinical Psychology, 46*, 1302–1314.

Forman, S. A., & Marmar, C. R. (1985). Therapist actions that address initially poor therapeutic alliances in psychotherapy. *American Journal of Psychiatry, 142*(8), 922–926.

Goldfried, M. R. (1982). Resistance and clinical behavior therapy. In P. L. Wachtel (Ed.), *Resistance: Psychodynamic and behavioral approaches* (pp. 95–114). New York: Plenum Press.

Horvath, A. O., & Symonds, D. (1991). Relation between working alliance and outcome in psychotherapy: A meta-analysis. *Journal of Counseling Psychology, 38*(2), 139–149.

Kiesler, D. J. (1988). *Therapeutic metacommunication: Therapist impact disclosure as feedback in psychotherapy.* Palo Alto, CA: Consulting Psychologists Press.

Leahy, R. (2001). *Overcoming resistance in cognitive therapy.* New York: Guilford Press.

Martin, D., Garske, J., & Davis, K. (2000). Relation of the therapeutic alliance with outcome and other variables: A meta-analytic review [Electronic version]. *Journal of Consulting and Clinical Psychology, 68*(3), 438–450.

Mitchell, S. A. (1988). *Relational concepts in psychoanalysis.* Cambridge, MA: Harvard University Press.

Muran, J. C. (2001). Meditations on "both/and." In J. C. Muran (Ed.), *Self-relations in psychotherapy process* (pp. 3–35). Washington, DC: American Psychological Association.

Muran, J. C. (2002). A relational approach to understanding change: Plurality and contextualism in a psychotherapy research program. *Psychotherapy Research, 12,* 113–138.

Raue, P. J., & Goldfried, M. R. (1994). The therapeutic alliance in cognitive behavioral therapy. In A. O. Horvath (Ed.), *The working alliance: Theory, research, and practice* (pp. 131–152). New York: Wiley.

Safran, J. D. (1998). *Widening the scope of cognitive therapy.* Northvale, NJ: Aronson.

Safran, J. D., & Muran, J. C. (1996). The resolution of ruptures in the therapeutic alliance. *Journal of Consulting and Clinical Psychology, 64,* 447–458.

Safran, J. D., & Muran, J. C. (1998). *The therapeutic alliance in brief psychotherapy.* Washington, DC: American Psychological Association.

Safran, J. D., & Muran, J. C. (2000). *Negotiating the therapeutic alliance: A relational treatment guide.* New York: Guilford Press.

Safran, J. D., Muran, J. C., Samstag, L. W., & Stevens, C. (2002). Repairing alliance ruptures. In J. C. Norcross (Ed.), *Psychotherapy relationships that work* (pp. 235–254). New York: Oxford University Press.

Safran, J. D., & Segal, Z. V. (1996). *Interpersonal process in cognitive therapy* (2nd ed.). Northvale, NJ: Aronson.

Shick-Tyron, G., & Kane, A. (1990). The helping alliance and premature termination. *Counseling Psychology Quarterly, 3,* 233–238.

Shick-Tyron, G., & Kane, A. (1993). Relationship of working alliance to mutual and unilateral termination. *Journal of Counseling Psychology, 40,* 33–36.

Shick-Tyron, G., & Kane, A. (1995). Client involvement, working alliance, and type of therapy termination. *Psychotherapy Research, 5,* 189–198.

Stern, D. B. (1985). *The interpersonal world of the infant.* New York: Basic Books.

Sullivan, H. S. (1953). *The interpersonal theory of psychiatry.* New York: Norton.

Sullivan, H. S. (1956). *Clinical studies in psychiatry.* New York: Norton.

Wachtel, P. L. (1993). *Therapeutic communication: Knowing what to say when.* New York: Guilford Press.

Yeomans, F., Gutfreund, J., Selzer, M., Clarkin, J., Hull, J., & Smith, T. (1994). Factors related to drop-outs by borderline patients; Treatment contract and therapeutic alliance. *Journal of Psychotherapy Practice and Research, 3,* 16–24.

Zetzel, E. (1956). Current concepts of transference. *International Journal of Psychoanalysis, 37,* 369–375.

Zetzel, E. (1965). The theory of therapy in relation to a developmental model of psychic apparatus. *International Journal of Psychoanalysis, 46,* 39–52.

15

Angry Patients: Strategies for Beginning Treatment

Raymond Chip Tafrate
Howard Kassinove

We have worked with hundreds of angry adults in various national and international research projects. Many of our participants arrived with a keen awareness of how their anger disrupted family and vocational relationships and resulted in losses that contributed to other negative emotions, such as anxiety and depression. In addition, these research participants have been quite willing to engage in a variety of program interventions. Some of these might be considered to be easy (e.g., problem discussion and rehearsal of coping statements in the office), whereas others might be seen as more threatening or requiring greater effort (e.g., listening to verbal insults or *in vivo* exposure to anger triggers). Participants are typically recruited through newspaper advertisements that propose free treatment for anger. Adults who believe they are experiencing problematic anger reactions are invited to participate in a screening process that involves completing a series of questionnaires, including the Trait Anger scale of the State–Trait Anger Expression Inventory (Spielberger, 1988, 1999). If they score above the 75th percentile, they are considered to have a level of anger that is problematic and are retained for the study. This selection method identifies adults who possess some level of awareness of their own problems with anger and its associated consequences and who are disposed to engage in treatment. We encounter little resistance from these adults and most show clear treatment gains.

We have been less pleasantly surprised to find that the same interventions that were successful in research programs are not easily implemented with psychotherapy outpatients in clinics and private practices who score in the same range on the Trait Anger scale. Even more challenging has been the task of trying to translate empirically supported anger interventions for use in criminal justice settings, such as prisons and alternative-to-incarceration centers. One reason for this implementation difficulty is that the existing treatment outcome literature for anger disorders is predominantly based on volunteer research participants (Tafrate, 1995). These participants do not fully represent the clinical cases seen by practitioners, who are likely to work with angry adults who have been coerced into treatment by courts, employers, or spouses. Research findings thus lack some degree of external validity in that the motivational level of volunteers is different from that of many patients who appear in a practitioner's office. Thus, in the area of anger, research findings may not easily translate into effective clinical practice techniques.

Although the treatment outcome literature on anger is relatively small and restricted to a few therapeutic approaches, dysfunctional anger does appear to respond to intervention. To date, four meta-analytic reviews have appeared (Beck & Fernandez, 1998; DiGiuseppe & Tafrate, 2003; Edmondson & Conger, 1996; Tafrate, 1995). In the vast majority of studies, treated research participants showed a moderate to large magnitude of improvement when compared with untreated controls across a variety of anger-related outcomes. Several forms of cognitive restructuring are among the interventions that received empirical support. Most studies using cognitive treatments focused on a self-instructional training model (Meichenbaum, 1985; Novaco, 1975). In addition, several investigations have shown support for both Ellis's (1962, 1973) rational–emotive behavior therapy model and the cognitive therapy model as originally formulated by Beck (1964), suggesting optimism about these approaches (Deffenbacher, Dahlen, Lynch, Morris, & Gowensmith, 2000; Tafrate & Kassinove, 1998). However, as noted, translating such research findings into acceptable and effective interventions for use in diverse clinical settings poses a number of challenges.

In this chapter we identify the typical roadblocks presented by angry patients seen in nonresearch settings, and we provide a series of steps for overcoming them. We note that no studies, as of yet, have examined the effect of including a motivational component prior to active cognitive and behavioral interventions. This element is critical because research participants seem to arrive with sufficient motivation, whereas patients in clinical settings often do not. Because anger interventions appear to work well with motivated research participants, overcoming motivational roadblocks in real-world mental health environments is an obvious next step in anger treatment outcome research.

Although we expect our research participants to score above the 75th percentile in trait anger, clinical practitioners do not deal much with traits.

Rather, their patients arrive with reports of angry *states*, and they have to help patients resolve problems and prevent the recurrence of those anger states. The more often that angry states can be prevented or reduced in intensity or duration, the more likely it is that the angry trait will be reduced. Thus, in *Anger Management: The Complete Treatment Guidebook for Practitioners* (Kassinove & Tafrate, 2002), we developed a five-stage anger episode model to provide for a clear analysis of individual anger events (see Figure 15.1).

Anger begins with a *triggering event* that is *appraised cognitively* in some way. Specific "hot cognitions" (Beck, 1976; Ellis, 1973; Safran & Greenberg, 1982) will lead to strong *anger experiences* (i.e., private events such as images, fantasies, and additional cognitions that may involve rumination about the triggers and the appraisals). The appraisals and private events lead to patterns of *anger expression*, such as shouting, use of profanity, sarcasm, bodily gestures, and so forth. (As an aside, we note that if the expressive patterns are motoric, e.g., hitting or punching, they represent aggression rather than anger.) Finally, every anger episode leads to *outcomes*. These outcomes may be negative, neutral, or even positive, such as when the anger leads to motivation for problem resolution. Some outcomes appear immediately, as in the case of a verbal argument that leads to avoidance of interactions by the parties, whereas outcomes such as heart disease

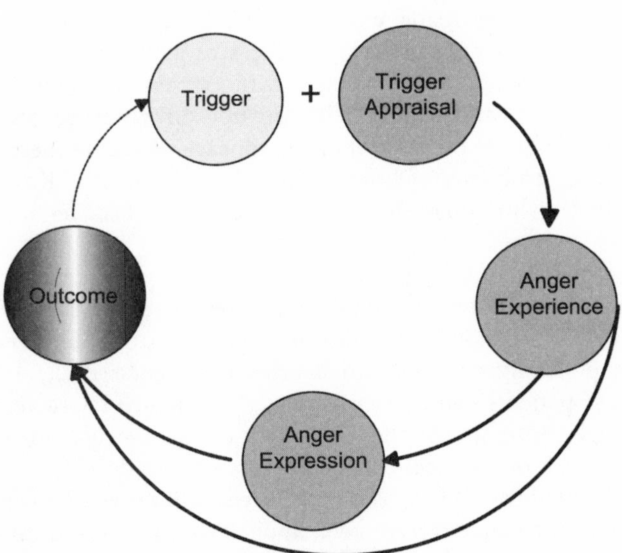

FIGURE 15.1. Anger episode model. Adapted from Kassinove and Tafrate (2002). Copyright 2002 by Howard Kassinove and Raymond Chip Tafrate. Permission granted by Impact Publishers, Inc., PO Box 6016, Atascadero, CA 93423.

or stroke may not appear for many years. In addition, negative outcomes associated with anger episodes may set the stage for increases in additional anger triggers. We believe that strategies for change are best targeted to the individual elements of this episode model. For example, triggers can be avoided; appraisals can be changed, leading to a more accepting philosophy; new and more appropriate assertive behaviors can be practiced, leading to changes in outcomes of anger episodes; and so forth. As an outgrowth of this model, we conceptualize anger interventions as falling into four distinct phases: *preparation*, *change*, *acceptance*, and *relapse prevention* (Kassinove & Tafrate, 2002). Preparation sets the stage for change and acceptance interventions, and relapse prevention strategies solidify treatment gains.

As noted previously, the most noticeable difference between research participants and outpatients seems to be in their willingness to participate eagerly in intervention programs. Thus the preparation phase of treatment is the focus of this chapter. We view strategies for building patients' awareness of their anger and increasing their motivation for change as prerequisites for using the change and acceptance methods of cognitive-behavioral therapy effectively.

ROADBLOCKS FACED WHEN WORKING WITH ANGRY ADULTS

The obstacles presented by angry patients are certainly not unique. Comparisons can easily be made with other traditionally defined "difficult" groups, such as substance abusers, compulsive gamblers, adults with impulse control disorders, and patients with certain personality disorders (e.g., paranoid and antisocial). It is also not surprising to discover that adults who are high on the trait of anger appear to have frequent comorbid substance use problems (Deffenbacher, 1993; Tafrate, Kassinove, & Dundin, 2002). Thus there are likely to be many obstacles to successful treatment.

Basic principles of cognitive and behavioral therapies, such as collaborative empiricism, an active–directive therapeutic style, Socratic questioning, and between-session homework assignments, grew out of early work done with primarily anxious and depressed patients (Beck, 1976; Ellis, 1962). These patients came to practitioners with such characteristics as a desire for help, insight that the anxiety or depression was their personal problem to work on, and others. The practice styles developed were quite useful for such adults. During the past 40 years, however, both Beck's and Ellis's models of treatment have been applied to a wider and ever-growing range of problems. Modifications, in terms of emphasis, would certainly be required to adequately address the unique characteristics of adults with other problems, such as anger disorders. However, few such modifications have been made, and the models of practice in the cognitive and behavioral therapies have remained rather uniform. We think the roadblocks presented by angry adults in clinical settings are sometimes exacerbated by the uniform, traditional approach taken by cognitive therapists. For example, rational–emotive behavior therapy practitioners, and certainly Ellis himself, are known for moving rapidly to intervene. Quick intervention may be useful at a generic level, as many patients remain in psychotherapy for only one to five sessions and as quick interventions may give practitioners the best opportunity to be helpful. At the same time, if angry adults appear in practitioner's offices because they have been coerced, then modifications in terms of the pace of treatment and the typical active–directive style may be required.

Roadblock 1: Lack of Motivation for Change

As noted previously, it seems certain that a subset of angry adults does exist who voluntarily seek treatment and who possess a high level of motivation to actively engage in change strategies. Thus we do not wish to portray all angry adults as unmotivated. Nonetheless, adolescents and adults with anger problems in outpatient settings and offenders in correctional settings have the reputation of being ambivalent about, or outright resistant to, treatment.

It is wise for practitioners to carefully consider the manner in which the patient was connected to treatment, the patient's rationale for seeking change, and the extent to which others applied overt and subtle coercion. Despite the observable nature and seriousness of many of the negative consequences associated with anger (Kassinove & Tafrate, 2002), it is common for angry adults to show less motivation for change than patients experiencing problems with anxiety or depression. Angry adults often lack awareness of the long-term costs associated with their anger episodes and have difficulty distinguishing between normal or common and disturbed anger experiences. Thus they do not see their anger as a serious problem, and they frequently reject making anger the focus of intervention. Rather than attempting to engage such patients in anger reduction, the therapist may target the first few sessions at increasing awareness of the costs associated with individual anger episodes.

Roadblock 2: Difficulties in Establishing a Therapeutic Alliance

It is certainly true that people profit from reading self-help books, listening to lectures, and so forth. Nevertheless, much therapeutic change occurs within the confines of an interpersonal practitioner–patient relationship. For such a relationship to be beneficial, it is important that an alliance be formed between the two parties. Although there are differences among alliance conceptualizations, most posit that a strong relationship has three key elements. These include agreement on (1) the goals of treatment and (2) the methods to be used to achieve the goals. In addition, (3) the presence of a positive bond between practitioner and patient is often considered to be essential (Bordin, 1979; Gaston, 1990; Horvath & Symonds, 1991; Saunders, Howard, & Orlinsky, 1989). In terms of developing the three areas of the alliance, there are differences among depressed, anxious, and angry patients.

Agreeing on a shared goal of treatment is the most difficult treatment roadblock to overcome. Angry adults frequently come for psychotherapy:

1. Seeking advice about how to change *others*, or
2. Wanting to *vent* about being the target of unfair behavior at the hands of others, or
3. Wanting *verification* that others are, indeed, evil or malicious, and
4. Typically wanting some kind of *revenge*.

On the other hand, practitioners often want to change their patient's anger by teaching self-control or acceptance. This, of course, does not mean that the practitioner agrees with the actions of the anger instigator or is promoting "forgetting" about the problem. Rather, practitioners act in accordance with the Yerkes–Dodson law (1908), which suggests that intense emotionality such as strong anger or fury is associated with poorer performance. Thus they seek minimization of anger through self-change, so that problems can be resolved, if possible. Patients, in contrast, want to blame and seek to punish others. For this reason, agreement on the goals of treatment is typically more difficult to achieve with angry patients than with persons suffering from anxiety or depression.

Once patients gain the insight that their anger is not working for them and the goal of anger reduction is established, the second component of the alliance is easier to achieve. Angry patients are often quite willing to engage in a variety of methods or therapeutic tasks to achieve their goals. We have rarely found resistance in this area of alliance development. Of course, it is useful to carefully explain the rationale for engaging in the chosen treatment activities, such as thought monitoring or exposure practice, and to ensure that what is expected is fully understood before proceeding.

The willingness of angry patients to quickly embrace active change strategies differs in some respects from that of depressed and anxious patients. For example, adults with anger problems (not comorbid with depression) generally possess a greater overall level of energy than do depressed adults. They are rarely helpless or mired in nonaction. Rather, they desire and are willing to take active steps to deal with problems and may become frustrated (or angry) with psychotherapists who take too long to prescribe a concrete plan of action. In comparison with patients with anxiety disorders, angry patients show a greater willingness to engage in exposure activities, in imagery, in simulations, and in real-life practice. The tendency to avoid the emotionally charged stimulus that often makes cognitive-behavioral treatments for anxiety slow is not typically problematic for angry patients. They jump right in. Additional discussions related to the use of exposure-based techniques for angry patients can be found in Brondolo, DiGiuseppe, and Tafrate (1997), Grodnitzky and Tafrate (2000), Tafrate and Kassinove (1998) and Kassinove and Tafrate (2002).

In terms of the relationship bond, angry patients who have agreed on the goal of treatment often do establish a positive connection and a productive working relationship with the practitioner. In clinic or private-practice settings, this bond is enhanced on the basis of the trust developed by openly discussing and agreeing on the goals and methods of intervention, the frequency and time of sessions, and so forth. Respect for and understanding of the patient's initial resistance to self-change is also very helpful in developing the bond. Nevertheless, issues related to external coercion and characteristics of the treatment setting require careful attention. Certain environments—such as in high schools in which an adolescent may be mandated for treatment as a condition of remaining in school, or in correctional institutions—pose serious alliance-related challenges. Because custody and security are the main missions of prisons, treatment issues are often considered to be low priorities. Inmate/patients are likely to be distrustful of anyone who is viewed as part of the institutional staff. Even when a positive relationship and bond are established, custody issues may interfere with treatment. For example, sessions may be interrupted or canceled due to security concerns (e.g., head counts may be mandatory and unannounced). Or inmate/patients may be moved from one institution to another with little notice or consideration given to their relationship with a given practitioner. Thus the relationship will be influenced to some degree by the setting in which the treatment is delivered.

Roadblock 3: Challenges to Anger-Related Beliefs Are Viewed by Patients as Invalidating

A third obstacle facing cognitive therapists is that anger is associated with a number of highly charged beliefs that differ from those that are common in anxious and depressed patients. Anger is an emotion that occurs most frequently in an interpersonal context and that most commonly involves people who are well known or liked (Averill, 1983; Kassinove, Sukhodolsky, Tsytsarev, & Solovyova, 1997; Tafrate et al., 2002). The perception that one has been transgressed upon by another person or group of people is a central focus of angry adults. This stands in contrast to depressed and anxious patients, who have beliefs related to a range of areas involving the self, other people, the future, and the external world. Anxious patients tend to overestimate danger from a variety of sources (e.g., internal sensations, loss of control, specific stimuli such as dirt, bugs, one's own unpleasant thoughts, evaluative situations, etc.), and depressed patients focus on self-denigration, helplessness, and pessimism regarding the future. Angry patients, in contrast, tend to focus on the unwanted behavior of others.

Because angry patients are prone to engage in demanding and distorted thinking concerning interpersonal relationships (e.g., "My husband should be more attentive" or "My wife just doesn't care about us at all"), it is reasonable to assume that these beliefs can easily become activated in the therapeutic relationship. Thus efforts to identify and especially to challenge anger-related thinking may be perceived as invalidating and met with resistance. Therapists are often viewed as taking the side of the offending person in the conflict. Thus, without careful preparation, cognitive interventions can prompt resistant responses and, at times, anger directed at the practitioner.

Specific cognitions associated with anger have emerged from descriptive research and clinical experience. They involve misinterpretations of the motivations of others, distortions, rigidly held views about the perceived triggers, and the belief that one is unable to deal effectively with aversive people and situations that "should" be different than they are.

Misinterpretations and Distortions

Aspects of anger-engendering triggers are often distorted, seen in an unrealistic manner, or exaggerated. The tendency to make negative attributions, for example, has been well documented in angry and aggressive children and adolescents who typically show deficits in interpreting the intentions of others (Dodge & Coie, 1987) and who often misinterpret ambiguous or benign interactions as hostile (Dodge, Price, Bachorowski, & Newman, 1990). Anger-prone adults seem to possess a similar negative bias when they interpret ambiguous and potentially provocative situations. Adults who are high on the trait of anger report more distortions and exaggerations in their own thinking during anger episodes than do less angry adults (Tafrate et al., 2002). Thus patients with anger problems may be predisposed to misinterpret verbal statements made by practitioners. Cognitive therapists are especially prone to become the targets of distorted thinking and patient anger when the accuracy of a patient's thinking is challenged. The following brief exchange illustrates this process. John is a graduate student in mathematics.

THERAPIST: John, where is the evidence that your professor, Dr. Patterson, is "out to get you"?

JOHN: Well, he wouldn't let me make up the exam that I missed and he gave me a zero. Now I'm going to fail the course.

THERAPIST: So, your evidence is based on this one example?

JOHN: You're not there, so you have no idea how he treats me. He talks down to me all the time. I don't think he likes me.

THERAPIST: Let's examine the specific things that he does that lead you to think that he doesn't like you and is out to get you.

JOHN: You make it sound like I am making this stuff up. I'm telling you he doesn't like me and you are acting like you don't believe me!

In this example, the therapist did not clearly and affirmatively acknowledge John's perception of a transgression. Attempts to challenge his view of the situation are thus met with resistance statements, and the therapist's persistence resulted in a shift of focus away from the original anger trigger to the therapist's behavior. It may be necessary to spend more time with angry clients validating their perceptions by using reflective statements early in the treatment process.

Rigidly Held, Demand-Based Assumptions

The most common anger-related belief is that persons who are viewed as the source of anger "should" or "ought to" have acted differently, as they could have if they "really wanted to" (Tafrate et al., 2002). Thus the trigger is conceived to be a person who could have controlled his or her behavior but simply did not. Patients engaged in demand-based thinking elevate their personal wishes to dictates or rigid rules that are then imposed on others and the world. Helping them replace demanding and inflexible beliefs (e.g., "My husband ought to be more appreciative of what I do") with a more preference-based view (e.g., "I would like my husband to be more appreciative of what I do") is a treatment goal emphasized in the rational–emotive behavior therapy approach.

Demand-based assumptions frequently have a moral tone, and there is sometimes some kind of associated belief about discrimination (e.g., "Short people shouldn't be discriminated against. That's why I didn't get the job. This company should be more fair to job applicants"). Thus angry patients typically see themselves as having been treated unfairly. And therapists' efforts to challenge their demand-based assumptions are sometimes seen as confusing. For example:

THERAPIST: Why must your boss treat you with respect?

CAROL: Because that's the way you are supposed to treat people.

THERAPIST: I agree, it would be "nice" and even "preferred." But why "must" people always treat others with respect?

CAROL: So, you are saying it is OK for my boss to treat me like crap?

In this example, the therapist's efforts to challenge the abstract assumption that people must always treat others with respect is quickly seen by the patient as the therapist taking the wrong side of a moral argument. Such straightforward challenging will often backfire with angry patients.

"Awfulizing" and Low Frustration Tolerance

Angry patients have a tendency to exaggerate the level of hardship associated with aversive life events and thus define them as "awful" and "terrible," even when they are best objectively defined as persistent irritants. Also, in spite of their bluster, many patients who experience frequent and intense anger have a poor view of their own ability to handle difficult or challenging situations. Negative events, instead of being viewed as a normal part of life or a challenge to be solved, are, instead, viewed as situations that the patient cannot "stand," "take," or "tolerate." They may continually complain in session about how they cannot tolerate a bad or unfair situation, which diverts time and effort away from productive problem solving. If not handled delicately, efforts to reduce the complaining and to de-"awfulize" or decatastrophize can be viewed as unsupportive. Although it is often unpleasant for therapists to listen to such complaining, angry clients seem more willing to engage in active problem solving once they believe they have been thoroughly understood.

Negative Ratings of Others or the Self

When angered, an individual tends to view the offending person in extreme terms, usually with complete condemnation. Not only are angry patients likely to be harsh when thinking about others, they may be equally prone to self-criticism and are thus vulnerable to experience other negative emotions following anger episodes (Tafrate et al., 2002). Because angry patients are frequently vocal about the negative behaviors of others, practitioners may forget to inquire as to how they view themselves. The tendency to view the behaviors of others in black-and-white terms (i.e., "great" or "evil") can also easily extend to the patient's view of the therapist. Therapist mistakes are often costly when they lead to the patient adopting a sweeping negative view of the practitioner.

Core Beliefs

There has been relatively little theorizing about core beliefs in angry patients. However, Beck (1999) has recently proposed that people who react impulsively, with anger and aggression, have a tendency to view themselves as vulnerable and to see others as hostile. Negative core beliefs are hypothesized to underlie distorted automatic thoughts. For example, if a client deep down believes "others are hostile," then it will follow that "others should not be trusted." Such an assumption sets the stage for distortions of reality (e.g., "I'm being treated poorly"), especially in ambiguous or stressful situations, leading to more frequent anger. For a more detailed discussion of conceptualizing various levels of client cognition, we refer the reader to Beck (1995).

DEVELOPING AN ALLIANCE AND INCREASING MOTIVATION

Before formal intervention begins, it is important to build the alliance and increase motivation to change. The first step is to develop *awareness*; that is, to assist patients in understanding that their anger episodes are not working for them in terms of achieving important life goals and that they are associated with significant costs. Practitioners can identify and make explicit numerous negative anger-related consequences when beginning treatment (Kassinove & Tafrate, 2002). These include interpersonal conflicts with family members, coworkers, or strangers; medical problems such as cardiovascular disease, stroke, and cancer; negative evaluations by others (being disliked); lowered self-evaluation due to recognizing the negative anger outcomes; erratic and aggressive driving; occupational dissatisfaction and maladjustment; inappropriate risk taking, such as making needless risky choices that are less likely to pay off in the long run and may be quite self-defeating; verbal conflicts; physical aggression; interactions with the criminal justice system; and the use of alcohol and other drugs.

Unfortunately, just pointing out these negative costs rarely wins over angry patients who are not motivated to change. Indirect, patient-centered methods have long been thought to be more effective (Rogers, 1957). We recommend refraining from the traditional active–directive presentation style of the cognitive and behavioral therapies in favor of a motivational interviewing format as outlined by Miller and Rollnick (1991). The goal in this approach is to subtly increase awareness of the negative costs of anger without increasing patient resistance. As noted earlier, once a commitment to change exists, then an active–directive style, as well as a variety of change strategies, will usually be acceptable to angry patients.

Using motivational interviewing with angry patients involves the same principles as originally developed and applied to patients with substance abuse problems (Miller & Rollnick, 1991). The beginning stage of treatment involves using *reflective statements* to highlight potential areas of patient ambivalence toward change. This is done in a nonjudgmental way, allowing the therapist to empathize with the patient's perceptions of being mistreated. The therapist's role is simply to make the ambivalence more explicit and, where possible, to highlight the costs associated with anger episodes. Costs may be further amplified through the use of open-ended questions designed to elicit patient statements regarding problematic aspects of their anger experiences. Thus therapists should keep in mind the list of costs noted previously as a context from which to formulate reflective statements and questions in order to encourage patients to acknowledge the downside of anger. The list is not meant for didactic presentation. Once the patient expresses some concerns regarding the costs connected with anger, a plan of action is developed collaboratively, which may include targeting patient thinking patterns.

To illustrate this approach, portions of a case follow. This case involves a patient who was coerced into treatment, has little insight and motivation, and is hostile toward the therapist. It highlights the more difficult aspects of working with angry patients.

THERAPIST: Carl, tell me what you would like to focus on. [open question]

CARL: Well, I don't really want to be here. It was my company's idea. My supervisor has been a pain in the neck and there has been some friction between us.

THERAPIST: You're saying it's not really your idea to come to treatment. [reflection]

CARL: Yeah. I was told to see somebody. Of course the higher-ups take my supervisor's side. Nothing happens to her, even though she caused the problem. But I'm the one who has to come for counseling.

THERAPIST: It seems unfair to you that you were asked to come here and she wasn't. [reflection]

CARL: Damn right it's unfair! I don't have a problem with anger. But when someone treats me like crap I'm going stick up for myself.

THERAPIST: Sounds like sticking up for yourself is important. [reflection]

CARL: You bet.

THERAPIST: You're saying that anger was not part of this situation at all. So, it is definitely not an anger issue. [reflection, instead of questions]

CARL: No, I was pretty pissed off. Things got heated.

THERAPIST: Let me make sure I understand. You were feeling angry and getting heated and also sticking up for yourself. [reflection]

CARL: Yeah. That's right.

THERAPIST: What happened when things got heated? [open question asked only after a number of reflective statements that elicited agreement from the patient]

CARL: Well, I thought, "Ann shouldn't have changed my territory without discussing it with me first. I tried to talk to her about it, and she just told me that changes had to be made and that I could take it or leave it."

THERAPIST: You were feeling angry when you realized that she hadn't taken the time to talk with you about the changes. [reflection]

CARL: Yeah. I mean this is my life we're talking about. I worked on developing this territory for seven years and she just goes and changes it without a word.

THERAPIST: That sounds like a tough spot to be in. How did you react? [empathizing with patient; open question only after patient agreement with reflective statements]

CARL: Well, I told her that she can't just do this and I called her a bitch. Then I threw a chair across the room and walked out. I just lost it.

THERAPIST: It seems like you didn't like the way she treated you and you reacted pretty strongly. [reflection]

CARL: Yeah, I did. That's why I have to come here if I want to keep my job.

THERAPIST: You mentioned that you put in seven years into this job. Tell me why it is important to keep it. [open question; therapist has identified one area of potential "goal agreement" as trying to keep the job]

CARL: I make a decent salary, and I don't want to start all over somewhere else, and I have a family to support.

THERAPIST: So, this job sounds really important to you. [reflection]

CARL: Yeah.

THERAPIST: It seems important for you to keep the job and also unfair that in order to keep it you have to come for counseling [double-sided reflection—acknowledges both sides of the dilemma]

CARL: Right.

THERAPIST: So, where does that leave you? [open question putting the responsibility for change back on the patient]

CARL: I guess I need to come here.

THERAPIST: Sounds like you are making the choice to come here, even though you don't like the situation that brought you here. [reflection]

CARL: Yeah.

THERAPIST: Well, what would you like to get out of it? [again, not trying to convince the patient of a problem; also shifting responsibility to him]

CARL: I'm not sure. Maybe a way to patch things up at work and learn ways to not get so bent out of shape.

THERAPIST: If we could come up with some ways to help you keep your job and react with less anger to unfair situations that might come up in the future, would that be helpful to you?

CARL: Yeah. [We now have agreement on the goal. The focus was kept on the single situation that brought him into treatment. No attempt was made to label him an angry person or to suggest that he has an anger problem.]

A second strategy for increasing awareness and developing an alliance is to keep the focus of early sessions on monitoring individual episodes of anger. The emphasis is on understanding the anger sequence and the components of the experience—including cognitions—and on connecting anger episodes with short- and long-term consequences. In this approach, exploration, not change, is the main focus of the sessions.

As noted at the outset of this chapter, practitioners will find it useful to have a formal model of "typical" anger episodes, both to provide a framework for shared understanding and to help practitioners and patients jointly conceptualize anger episodes as they appear in the patient's life. Our model (Kassinove & Tafrate, 2002) helps the practitioner and patient:

- Understand the environmental and internal causes of anger.
- Focus on the current anger experience.
- Learn about the manner in which the anger is being displayed.
- Think of more desirable reactions to aversive life events.
- Recognize the many costs of anger.
- Develop interventions to achieve a less angry life.

In the larger sense, the model also helps practitioners and patients recognize the differences between typical, or normal, anger and exaggerated problematic anger reactions that require intervention.

We have translated our anger episode model into an Anger Episode Record (Figure 15.2) as a simple way to help patients understand the component parts of their anger reactions. By monitoring and reporting individual episodes of anger, both the patient and practitioner can specifically target key features of anger that are problematic. Thus treatment can be tailored to a patient's symptom patterns. Examining multiple episodes over time allows practitioners to better understand typical functioning.

Several features of this model make it useful for overcoming roadblocks to effective treatment. First, as noted previously, patients may not be aware that their anger is exaggerated, beyond the scope of "normal," and may be oblivious to the short- and long-term costs associated with their anger experiences. It is these costs that make their anger reactions problematic. The insight that anger is having a negative impact on functioning is a prerequisite to engaging in active cognitive and behavioral change strategies. Thus the model connects specific anger events to consequences. Second, because patients often initially possess a tendency to simply blame the external world for their anger reactions, the model highlights the *combination* of triggering events *and* patient thinking patterns as causative of anger. Thus, in early sessions, patients can be introduced to the role of thinking in a way that minimizes the likelihood of the therapist being viewed as invalidating the seriousness of the transgression for the patient. Third, patients may be more willing to "admit" to certain anger-related behaviors when they are diagrammed on paper as opposed to being questioned in an in-person discussion.

Of course, as is typical in cognitive-behavioral interventions, an ongoing self-monitoring strategy such as an Anger Episode Record can be used to provide an indicator of treatment progress. Patients can be instructed to complete one record for every anger episode they experience, and the number of episodes reported early in treatment can serve as a baseline from which improvement can be measured. Other dimensions of anger can also serve as indictors of progress, depending on areas that the practitioner wishes to target. These might include average intensity of anger episodes, duration, number of episodes containing aversive verbalizations or aggressive behaviors, and number of episodes containing negative consequences. We recommend that the first Anger Episode Record be completed with the patient so that the practitioner is available to answer questions. Patients can then be asked to complete the record as homework, and responses can be discussed in the following session. Sample dialogue, using the Anger Episode Record, follows.

THERAPIST: Carl, everyone feels anger at times. Anger can be difficult to understand because it is made up of a number of different components or parts that go into the reaction. People are complicated, and, in order for me to understand you better, I would like to get into some of the

ANGER EPISODE RECORD: Triggers + Appraisals → Experiences → Expressive Patterns → Outcomes

<u>Directions</u> Fill out one record completely for each episode of anger that you experience.

Triggers Describe the event(s)

This anger episode occurred on:
Monday Tuesday Wednesday
Thursday Friday Saturday Sunday

This anger episode occurred in the:
Morning Afternoon
Evening Late at night

This anger episode occurred:
At home At work
Other______________

The target of my anger was: ________________

The situation surrounding my anger was:
____

+

Appraisals Place a check next to each thought that you have/ had about the trigger.

___"Awfulizing" (e.g., I thought this was one of the worst things that could be happening)
___Low frustration tolerance (e.g., I thought I could not handle or deal with this situation)
___Demandingnes (e.g., I thought the other person should have acted differently)
___Other rating (e.g., I thought the other person was "bad," "worthless," or, an "asshole," "#@*%&," etc.)
___Self-rating (e.g., Deep down I thought I was less important or worthwhile)
___Distortion (e.g., My thinking became distorted I didn't see things clearly)
___Unfairness (e.g., I thought the other person acted unfairly)
___Revenge(e.g., I thought the other deserves to suffer or be punished)
___Other ________________________________
___Other ________________________________

Experiences

How *intense* was your anger in this situation? 0 | | | | | | | | | 100
none mild moderate strong extreme

How long did your anger last? ___ minutes ___ hours ___ days

What physical sensations did you experience? (Place a check next to each physical sensation you experienced.)

__ Muscle tension
__ Nausea
__ Diarrhea
__ Flushing
__ Fluttering in stomach
__ Indigestion
__ Upset stomach
__ Feelings of unreality
__ Sweating
__ Headache
__ Tingling sensations
__ Trembling
__ Fatigue
__ Rapid heart rate
__ Rapid breathing
__ Positive energy
__ Dizziness

Expressive Patterns

(Place a check next to each behavior you engaged in during this anger episode.)

___ ***Aversive verbalizations*** (e.g., yelling, screaming, arguing, threatening, making sarcastic, nasty, or abusive remarks)
___ ***Bodily expressions*** (e.g., rolling eyes, crossing arms, glaring, frowning, giving a stern look)
___ ***Physical aggression*** (e.g., fight, hit, kick, push, or shove someone; break, throw, slam, or destroy an object)
___ ***Passive retaliation*** (e.g., say something bad or do something secretly harmful to the person; deliberately not follow rules)
___ ***Hold anger in*** (e.g., keep things in and boil inside; harbor grudges and not tell anyone)
___ ***Avoidance*** (e.g., escape or withdraw from the situation; distract myself by reading, watching TV, or listening to music, etc.)
___ ***Try to resolve the situation*** (e.g., compromise, discuss, or come to some agreement with the person)
___ ***Substance use*** (e.g., drink beer or alcohol; take medications: aspirin, valium, etc.; take other drugs—marijuana, cocaine, etc.)
___ ***Other*** ___

Outcomes

How did you feel after the anger passed? *(Check all that apply.)*

__ Irritated/Annoyed	__ Relieved	__ Depressed
__ Satisfied	__ Disgusted	__ Happy
__ Sad	__ Triumphant	__ Concerned
__ Joyous	__ Guilty/Ashamed	__ Foolish
__ Anxious/Fearful		

What other feelings did you have after the anger passed?

___

How did this anger episode affect relationship(s) with others?

This episode had a *(check one)* ___negative ___ positive

impact on a:
__ Work/professional relationship
__ Social/friendship
__ Romantic relationship
__ Family relationship
__ Other ___

List the *positive short-term outcomes* of this anger episode:

___

___

List the *negative short-term outcomes* of this anger episode:

___

___

List the *positive long-term outcomes* of this anger episode:

___

___

List the *negative long-term outcomes* of this anger episode:

___

FIGURE 15.2. Anger Episode Record. Reprinted from Kassinove and Tafrate (2002). Copyright 2002 by Howard Kassinove and Raymond Chip Tafrate. Permission granted by Impact Publishers, Inc., PO Box 6016, Atascadero, CA 93423.

specific elements that make up your anger. I would like to go through the situation that happened with your supervisor, Ann.

CARL: I already told you what happened.

THERAPIST: You did. But, in order for me to help you in the future, it would be useful to get more of an idea of the specific chain of events as you experienced them.

CARL: OK.

THERAPIST: This is called an Anger Episode Record, and I'm going to ask you to fill in information for each of the boxes. Even though we have already discussed much of the information in the first box, I would like you to put in the details. *(Carl writes in the date, time, and situation.)* Moving to the second box, what was going through your mind when you threw the chair and called Anne a bitch? Look at the statements and see if any are similar to what you might have been thinking. *(A list of common angry thoughts is provided and Carl indicates which ones were present during his anger experience.)* [Patients typically need help in this area in terms of monitoring their anger episodes.]

CARL: I was thinking that she shouldn't be treating me like this.

THERAPIST: Does that seem similar to the first type of thought presented?

CARL: Yes.

THERAPIST: How about any others?

CARL: Well, I definitely thought that she was acting like a real bitch. So, "other rating" seems on target. Also, I think that my thoughts were pretty exaggerated at that moment. I would not act so strongly now that I have stepped back from it a bit. [Carl is already making the connection between his thoughts and his angry reactions.]

THERAPIST: So, three of the thoughts that seem most on target for you in this situation are demandingness, other rating, and distortion.

CARL: Yes.

THERAPIST: In terms of the experience itself, how would you rate the strength of your reaction? Use the 0–100 scale.

CARL: Pretty strong. I would say about a 95. *(Carl completes the remainder of the experiences box. He reports the physical sensations of fluttering in stomach, trembling, and headache and thinks that his anger lasted, at its peak, for about 20 minutes then started to diminish.)*

THERAPIST: In terms of how you acted at the moment, what items seem most on target? (*Again, from the checklist of typical anger-related behaviors, Carl acknowledges engaging in aversive angry verbalizations, bodily expressions, physical aggression in that he threw a chair, and then avoidance following the incident.*) There are a number of different outcomes that people can experience related to their anger. How did you feel after the situation ended and your anger passed somewhat? Again, look at the list of feelings and select those most on target.

CARL: I felt depressed, guilty and ashamed, and foolish. [Negative feelings after the incident are a potential negative consequence for this particular episode.]

THERAPIST: OK. Moving to the next box, how do you think this episode affected your relationships with others?

CARL: Well, it obviously affected my work relationships. They sent me here, and if I have another outburst I will lose my job.

THERAPIST: How else did this episode affect your work relationships?

CARL: I think other people lost respect for me.

THERAPIST: In what way did that occur? [The therapist deviates from the form to explore the negative consequence in more depth. Following a brief discussion of how his colleagues lost respect for him, the focus then shifts to his wife.]

CARL: It also affected my relationship with my wife. She was upset that my temper got me in trouble.

THERAPIST: Has she been concerned about your temper?

CARL: Yeah.

THERAPIST: What did she say about the situation? [Again, exploring the negative consequence further in terms of his marital relationship. Next, both positive and negative long- and short-term consequences are explored.]

THERAPIST: What short-term positive outcomes were related to your anger?

CARL: Well, I was able to tell her [supervisor, Ann] exactly how I felt about the situation.

THERAPIST: How was that positive for you?

CARL: I didn't just want to go along with my territory being changed. I needed to stick up for myself.

THERAPIST: So, sticking up for yourself was positive in some ways. Were there any immediate or short-term negative consequences connected with your anger?

CARL: Yeah. I left the office and was afraid to come back. My colleagues lost respect for me. And my supervisor wanted me fired. My wife was upset that I might lose my job. [At this point the therapist could choose to explore in more detail those negative consequences that were not already reviewed. In this manner the therapist could emphasize the negative outcomes related to the anger that the patient notes. Thus it is the patient who is identifying the problematic aspects of his anger and not the therapist. This is likely to diminish resistance.]

THERAPIST: What about the long term? What are the positive and negative outcomes for you?

CARL: I don't see any positive long-term outcomes.

THERAPIST: How about negative long-term outcomes?

CARL: Well, I have to come for counseling. That will take a while. And for a long time people will be scrutinizing my every move. And I may not get a raise this year.

THERAPIST: Sounds like there are a number of negative long-term effects.

CARL: Yeah.

THERAPIST: Tell me about each one of those. [Again, exploring the negative aspects of anger in more detail. Once this episode is completed, the patient is asked to use the record in between sessions to better understand additional anger experiences.] Carl, now that you understand how to do it, I would like you to take several of these records with you and fill them out the next time you feel angry. This will allow us to see how you are handling things and also help us find areas to work on that might be useful to you. Do you have any questions about the records?

CARL: No.

We have used more comprehensive instruments based on this anger episode model with patients and clients in various clinical settings and in descriptive self-report research studies as a guide to help participants better understand and communicate symptoms related to their anger. Our samples have included "normal" nonangry college students and adults, adults from the community with high trait anger, and samples of adults from other countries, such as Russia, India, and Israel. The simplicity of the model has made it possible for patients to form a conception of the emergence of their anger and for us to collect information efficiently from individuals from a wide variety of backgrounds.

INTRODUCING COGNITIVE INTERVENTIONS

As noted, a self-monitoring form introduces the idea that a *combination* of outside events and thoughts create anger experiences. Thus the role of thinking in anger can be introduced easily, as is shown in the following:

THERAPIST: On the four records that you completed this week, it looks like you clearly experienced some difficult situations. Also, you often noted that your thinking was exaggerated.

CARL: Yeah.

THERAPIST: Could you give me an example of how your thinking might have been exaggerated? [Therapist is moving the focus of the session to cognitions.]

Self-monitoring makes the negative costs associated with anger more explicit, assists clients in understanding of the role of thinking in the anger sequence, and sets up a foundation on which to engage in cognitive therapy.

CONCLUSION

As opposed to research participants who volunteer for treatment, patients with anger problems who are seen in clinical settings are less inclined to see anger reduction as a worthwhile treatment goal. Thus it is wise very early in treatment to address roadblocks such as a lack of awareness of the costs of anger, difficulties establishing aspects of the therapeutic alliance, and seeing attempts to challenge thinking as invalidating. The first step proposed in this chapter emphasizes the intentional use of empathy and motivational interviewing tactics in the first few meetings. The focus is then changed to an exploration of individual episodes of anger, using the anger episode model and Anger Episode Record, to emphasize the negative consequences and the role of thinking in the anger sequence. Finally, once thinking patterns are introduced as a focus of treatment, active interventions such as rational–emotive behavior therapy or cognitive therapy can be implemented.

REFERENCES

Averill, J. R. (1983). Studies on anger and aggression: Implications for theories of emotion. *American Psychologist, 38,* 1145–1160.

Beck, A. T. (1964). Thinking and depression: Theory and therapy. *Archives of General Psychiatry, 10,* 561–571.

Beck, A. T. (1976). *Cognitive therapy and the emotional disorders.* New York: International Universities Press.

Beck, A. T. (1999). *Prisoners of hate: The cognitive basis of anger, hostility, and violence.* New York: HarperCollins.

Beck, J. S. (1995). *Cognitive therapy: Basics and beyond.* New York: Guilford Press.

Beck, R., & Fernandez, E. (1998). Cognitive-behavioral therapy in the treatment of anger: A meta-analysis. *Cognitive Therapy and Research, 22,* 63–74.

Bordin, E. S. (1979). The generalizability of the psychoanalytic concept of the working alliance. *Psychotherapy: Theory, Research and Practice, 16,* 252–260.

Brondolo, E., DiGiuseppe, R., & Tafrate, R. C. (1997). Exposure-based treatment for anger problems: Focus on the feeling. *Cognitive and Behavioral Practice, 4,* 75–98.

Deffenbacher, J. L. (1993). General anger: Characteristics and clinical implications. *Psicologia Conductual, 1,* 49–67.

Deffenbacher, J. L., Dahlen, E. R., Lynch, R. S., Morris, C. D., & Gowensmith, W. N. (2000). Application of Beck's cognitive therapy to general anger reduction. *Cognitive Therapy and Research, 24,* 689–697.

DiGiuseppe, R., & Tafrate, R. (2003). Anger treatment for adults: A meta-analytic review. *Clinical Psychology: Science and Practice, 10,* 70–84.

Dodge, K. A., & Coie, J. D. (1987). Social-information-processing factors in reactive and proactive aggression in children's peer groups. *Journal of Personality and Social Psychology, 53,* 1146–1158.

Dodge, K. A., Price, J. M., Bachorowski, J., & Newman, J. P. (1990). Hostile attributional biases in severely aggressive adolescents. *Journal of Abnormal Psychology, 99,* 385–392.

Edmondson, C. B., & Conger, J. C. (1996). A review of treatment efficacy for individuals with anger problems: Conceptual, assessment, and methodological issues. *Clinical Psychology Review, 16,* 251–275.

Ellis, A. E. (1962). *Reason and emotion in psychotherapy.* New York: Lyle Stuart.

Ellis, A. E. (1973). *Humanistic psychotherapy.* New York: McGraw-Hill.

Gaston, L. (1990). The concept of the alliance and its role in psychotherapy: Theoretical and empirical considerations. *Psychotherapy, 27,* 143–153.

Grodnitzky, G. R., & Tafrate, R. C. (2000). Imaginal exposure for anger reduction in adult outpatients: A pilot study. *Journal of Behavior Therapy and Experimental Psychiatry, 31,* 259–279.

Horvath, A. O., & Symonds, B. D. (1991). Relation between working alliance and outcome in psychotherapy: A meta-analysis. *Journal of Counseling Psychology, 38,* 139–149.

Kassinove, H., Sukhodolsky, D. G., Tsytsarev, S. V., & Solovyova, S. (1997). Self-reported constructions of anger episodes in Russia and America. *Journal of Social Behavior and Personality, 12,* 301–324.

Kassinove, H., & Tafrate, R. C. (2002). *Anger management: The complete treatment guidebook for practitioners.* Atascadero, CA: Impact.

Meichenbaum, D. H. (1985). *Stress inoculation training.* New York: Pergamon.

Miller, S., & Rollnick, W. R. (1991). *Motivational interviewing: Preparing people for change.* New York: Guilford Press.

Novaco, R. (1975). *Anger control: The development and evaluation of an experimental treatment.* Lexington, MA: Lexington Books.

Rogers, C. R. (1957). The necessary and sufficient conditions of therapeutic personality change. *Journal of Consulting Psychology, 21,* 95–103.

Safran, J. D., & Greenberg, L. S. (1982). Eliciting "hot cognitions" in cognitive behaviour therapy: Rationale and procedural guidelines. *Canadian Psychology, 23,* 83–87.

Saunders, S. M., Howard, K. I., & Orlinsky, D. E. (1989). The Therapeutic Bond Scales: Psychometric characteristics and relationship to treatment effectiveness. *Psychological Assessment, 1,* 323–330.

Spielberger, C. D. (1988). *Professional Manual for the State–Trait Anger Expression Inventory.* Odessa, FL: Psychological Assessment Resources.

Spielberger, C. D. (1999). *Manual for the State–Trait Anger Expression Inventory—2.* Odessa, FL: Psychological Assessment Resources.

Tafrate, R. (1995). Evaluation of treatment strategies for adult anger disorders. In H. Kassinove (Ed.), *Anger disorders: Definition, diagnosis, and treatment.* Washington, DC: Taylor & Francis.

Tafrate, R., & Kassinove, H. (1998). Anger control in men: Barb exposure with rational, irrational, and irrelevant self-statements. *Journal of Cognitive Psychotherapy, 12,* 187–211.

Tafrate, R., Kassinove, H., & Dundin, L. (2002). Anger episodes in high and low trait anger community adults. *Journal of Clinical Psychology, 58,* 1573–1590.

Yerkes, R. M., & Dodson, J. D. (1908). The relation of strength of stimulus to rapidity of habit-formation. *Journal of Comparative and Neurological Psychology, 18,* 459–482.

16

Medication Compliance with Difficult Patients

Lynn Marcinko

"I was mortified. I walked into a store and the woman behind the counter asked me how my dog was, knew my brother-in-law's name, and asked how I was doing on my medications. I had never met her before in my life."

Jennifer, a 28-year-old, attractive and intelligent woman started cataloguing the effects of her most recent manic episode. She had refused to take any mood stabilizers for fear they would make her gain weight. She had been manic for some time before agreeing to start on lithium. In the process of trying several mood stabilizers with her psychiatrist, she had become less manic and developed partial insight into her illness. Unfortunately, her preoccupation with her illness had itself become a symptom, and she had been speaking to anyone who would listen about her condition, including the woman behind the counter. She sat in my office with a stack of e-mails from friends that stated that they no longer wanted to speak to her. Her initial medication refusal had cost her dearly.

Jennifer's case illustrates the importance of addressing medication compliance in therapy. As cognitive therapy expands into the treatment of the severely and persistently mentally ill, medication compliance is being recognized as an increasingly important factor in therapy. Researchers (e.g., Hale, 1995) estimate that up to 70% of patients with recurrent depression are noncompliant with medications and that approximately 50% of patients with schizophrenia do not comply with prescribed medications. This high rate is one of the primary causes of readmission to the hospital (Weiden & Olfson, 1995). As effective as medication can be in controlling symptoms, their real-world efficacy is nonexistent if the patient refuses treatment.

Cognitive-behavioral therapy appears to be particularly well suited to dealing with the problem of medication compliance in general due to its active, solution-focused approach to problems. Recent studies have shown the modality's effectiveness in decreasing the frequency and severity of psychotic symptoms, as well as in decreasing the frequency and severity of manic episodes (e.g., Seckinger & Amador, 2001; Barrowclough et al., 2001). However, with some notable exceptions (e.g., Beck, 2001; Newman, Leahy, Beck, Reilly-Harrington, & Gyulai, 2002), the literature on the mechanics of applying cognitive therapy and the specific adaptations to the cognitive model for medication compliance in the severely and persistently mentally ill has been sparse.

Medication noncompliance may be a function of practical issues, psychological issues, or a combination of the two (Beck, 2001). For instance, practical issues contributing to medication noncompliance include a lack of access to the medications, problems with side effects, or a poor understanding of a complicated medication regimen. Psychological issues may include the patient's fears about the reaction from peers toward his or her taking medication, an unwillingness to accept the diagnosis, or beliefs that they should be able to handle the illness on their own. Most medication compliance issues are often a combination of practical and psychological issues. For example, a patient believes that taking the medication is a sign of their ultimate weakness and an acceptance of a psychiatric diagnosis. This belief then decreases the patient's motivation to engage in active problem solving in order to address issues related to accessing the medication.

Previous psychotherapy programs aimed at increasing medication compliance have met with limited success (e.g., Colom, Vieta, Martinez, Jorquera, & Gasto, 1998; Valenstein, Barry, Blow, Copeland, & Ullman, 1998). This result may be due in part to an attempt to improve compliance through a lateral extension of methods from the medical model. In this model, patients are presumed to be rational, willing participants in their treatment. Patients are provided education about their disorder, the regimen is explained to them, and they are expected to comply. As Fenton, Blyler, and Heinssen (1997) suggest, even the term "compliance" is laden with paternalistic connotations and may alienate patients who are already highly marginalized and stigmatized. Severely and persistently mentally ill patients are already compromised with respect to their decision making and problem solving abilities due to the cognitive effects of their illnesses. If they experience their therapists as pejorative, it may have a negative effect on compliance.

A treatment approach designed to target both the practical and psychological issues associated with noncompliance appears to be in order.

That is, the approach should possess the flexibility to accept the patient's perspective and concerns about taking the medications as well as to address issues pertaining to access to medication and understanding of medication regimens. Recently Beck (2001) and Newman and colleagues (2002) suggested straightforward cognitive-behavioral methods for dealing with medication compliance problems for a host of psychiatric disorders. Other studies have shown that cognitive-behavioral therapy is instrumental in increasing medication compliance (e.g., Lecompte & Pelc, 1996; Lam et al., 2000; Cochran, 1984) . Several empirical studies indicate that the use of cognitive therapy increase medication compliance (e.g., Cochran, 1984; Klingberg, Buchkremer, Holle, Moenking, & Hornung, 1999).

Despite the compelling case for the use of cognitive therapy to address medication compliance in the severely and persistently mentally ill, dealing effectively with reasons for noncompliance in this population may violate some basic principles of cognitive-behavioral therapy. Many patients with severe and persistent mental illnesses may not benefit from the psychoeducational aspect of cognitive-behavioral therapy (e.g., Amador & Johanson, 2000), as they do not agree that they have a problem. Specifically, educating the patient about a diagnosis of schizophrenia can prove to be a frustrating experience for patient and clinician.

Patients with psychosis and bipolar disorder may underreport or deny symptoms or adherence problems. Because their illnesses are severe, persistent, and debilitating, patients are often reliant on their families to care for them. With severe, persistently ill, and impaired patients, effective treatment requires an emphasis on assessment, adopting a long-term approach to treatment, increasing the involvement of the treating physician and the patient's family, and balancing active problem solving and cognitive restructuring approaches with acceptance of the patient's ambivalence.

In the current chapter I seek to integrate principles from cognitive-behavioral therapy, dialectical behavior therapy (Linehan, 1993), and Amador's LEAP program (Amador & Johanson, 2000) with an aim to increasing medication compliance in patients with bipolar and psychotic disorders. Linehan's dialectical behavior therapy is a cognitive-behavioral treatment developed for patients with borderline personality disorder, many of whom are reluctant to adhere to treatment protocols. Dialectical behavior therapy places a heavy emphasis on acceptance and environmental interventions and focuses on the therapeutic relationship as a catalyst for change.

Amador's LEAP program (Amador & Johanson, 2000) is designed for family members of patients with psychosis and bipolar disorder. Amador suggests that families learn how to balance acceptance and change strategies for dealing with their affected loved one. Specifically,

Amador outlines skills for Listening, Empathy, Accepting, and Participating (LEAP).

In this chapter I discuss seven principles for improving medication compliance in patients with severe and persistent mental illness utilizing cognitive and behavioral techniques. The chapter is organized in the order in which the principles tend to present themselves over the course of treatment. The principles are as follows:

- Thoroughly assess.
- Be mindful of the level of insight while providing psychoeducation.
- Develop and utilize the therapeutic alliance.
- Adopt a long-term approach to medication compliance.
- Increase communication and cooperation from collateral sources.
- Practice acceptance.
- Practice change strategies, problem solving, and cognitive restructuring.

THOROUGHLY ASSESS

The spirit of change implied in cognitive-behavioral therapy may place the therapist and the patient on opposite ends of a power struggle if a change in beliefs is advocated before the problem is adequately assessed. When a patient has a long-standing bipolar disorder or psychosis, the patient often comes into the office prepared to ignore, attack, or otherwise do battle with the therapist regarding medications. Simply mirroring the patient's beliefs about medications accurately and acknowledging the wisdom in his or her current approach (Linehan, 1993) can result in change.

The therapist is also encouraged to assess comorbid medical illnesses; current medication usage, including the use of benzodiazipines; side effects of the medications, especially the cognitive effects; and substance use, as all have been shown to affect adherence (Fenton et al., 1997). For instance, patients may discontinue their medication in favor of drinking because their physician has informed them not to drink while taking the medications.

The therapist's own thoughts regarding the use of medication can become a roadblock to successful treatment as well. As Beck (1995) and others suggest, assessing one's own thoughts about the treatment, in this case, regarding medication, can help elucidate thoughts that are interfering with the therapist's optimal handling of medication issues. Chances are, when working with long-standing noncompliance, the therapist's thoughts do not differ significantly from the thoughts of the family members or physician (i.e., "Can't they see how much easier their life would be if they took the medications?"). Patients maybe impervious to such attempts to sway their behavior. Completing thought records on one's own thoughts, completing a case conceptualization form for the patient, and conducting functional analyses of the behavior can all serve to increase the therapist's understanding of the problem at hand and improve empathy for the patient's plight.

Case Conceptualization

A case conceptualization is useful in assessing the thoughts, assumptions, and beliefs that mediate medication compliance (Persons, 1989; Beck, 1995). Beck's (1995) Cognitive Conceptualization Diagram can be used to categorize automatic thoughts, as well as core beliefs, that serve to influence the patient's medication-taking behavior. A case conceptualization is a structural approach to dealing with the thoughts associated with the noncompliance (i.e., core belief → assumption → compensatory strategy → situation → automatic thought → emotion → behavior). The conceptualization can then be used to inform strategies for intervening at different levels of thought, including examining and challenging distorted or unhelpful beliefs. Figure 16.1 illustrates the Cognitive Conceptualization Diagram for Jennifer.

Jennifer had a core belief—"I am not good enough." Her intermediate belief with respect to medication was, "I must never be sick because that proves that I am defective and not good enough." Her compensatory strategy was to deny her illness to others for fear that she would never find a mate if people knew she was sick. The resulting behavior was refusal to take her medications. In this case, developing the case conceptualization collaboratively was a good opportunity for the patient to see how her behavior made sense in light of her core beliefs.

Linehan (1993) and others (e.g., Krumboltz & Thoresen, 1969), advocate taking the stance of a "naive observer" when one is conducting a behavioral analysis of a problem behavior (or in this case, developing a case conceptualization). This means that the clinician must not assume that he or she knows why a behavior or thought is occurring, what the pertinent links in the behavioral chain are, or which thoughts, feelings, or behaviors get the patient from one link to the next. Essentially, it is important for the clinician not to assume that he or she knows why the patient is not complying. The following exchange illustrates this point:

JENNIFER: I don't think I need meds anyway. I mean I am not even sure I have bipolar disorder anyway. Look at how many times you guys change the rules about the diagnosis. Nobody knows anything. Why should I take it if you guys aren't even sure what I have?

Patient's Name: Jennifer **Date:** 09/01/02
Diagnosis: Bipolar affective disorder type I **Axis II:** Borderline personality disorder traits

Relevant Childhood/Developmental Data		
Mother constantly worried about her own weight and the weight of patient. "You'll never get a man if you're fat." Father invalidates patient's emotional experience. Unfavorably compared with sister.		
Core Beliefs		
"I am unlovable." "I am helpless." "I am not good enough." "I am not worth it."		
Conditional Assumptions/Beliefs/Rules		
"It is horrible to have anything wrong with you. You cannot be sick and loved." "I must never be sick. Otherwise, that proves that I am defective and not good enough."		
Compensatory Strategy(ies)		
Deny illness to others and self. Actively attempt to get others to take care of her.		
Situation 1 Told she needs medication by physician.	**Situation 2** Medication change	**Situation 3** Problems with boyfriend
Automatic Thought "That would mean I am sick . . . no way."	**Automatic Thought** "The medications have to be perfect or I will never get better."	**Automatic Thought** "If I am on the right dose of the right medications I should have no side effects and all of my personal problems will be over. I am not responsible for my behavior. It's not my fault."
Meaning of the AT "I am not good enough."	**Meaning of the AT** "I am helpless."	**Meaning of the AT** "I am helpless."
Emotion Anger, sadness	**Emotion** Sadness	**Emotion** Sadness, anger at physician
Behavior Refuse medications	**Behavior** Inaction	**Behavior** Refusal to work on interpersonal skills or problem solving

FIGURE 16.1. Cognitive Conceptualization Diagram for Jennifer. Diagram adapted with permission of Judith S. Beck, PhD. Copyright 1995.

THERAPIST: So you're saying a couple of things . . . you don't think you need the meds, you're not sure you have bipolar disorder, and since you don't feel confident in the ability of the professionals to diagnose, you don't trust that the treatment prescribed is worth doing. Did I get that right?

JENNIFER: Yeah, it's like everyone is so convinced that this medication is going to do great things for me, and all I know is that I am nauseous, I can't read or write well, and I am tired all the time. And I have taken it before . . . it didn't do anything except make me gain weight.

THERAPIST: The side effects are a problem too. And since you haven't seen a positive outcome yet symptom-wise, you don't see how it's worth it. I can see how you got there; your treating clinicians, including myself, were unclear about your diagnosis, and the criteria have changed since you first got sick. I can imagine that's totally frustrating. Is there more about that?

JENNIFER: I know *(rolling her eyes)* that everyone wants me to take this medication, but I just don't. I guess even part of me knows I should be taking the medication and I don't. I am not good at doing things I am supposed to.

THERAPIST: So even though you can see how medication could help you, you are finding it hard to follow through with taking it.

JENNIFER: Yeah, it's that knowing and doing thing.

THERAPIST: I think that's a tough one for a lot of people. I know when I have trouble following through with something like going to the gym, it's in part because I have trouble holding on to the long-term benefits when the short-term ones of sitting on the couch and eating potato chips seem so much more appealing.

JENNIFER: Yeah, you get it. Besides, I don't ever get to really see how the meds help me anyway. All I see are the side effects.

THERAPIST: Sounds like what you're saying is that although you see some benefits, you don't take it in part because you believe you aren't good at doing good things for yourself.

JENNIFER: Yeah.

THERAPIST: And the reason you don't do good things for yourself is. . . .

JENNIFER: Oh, I do some good things for myself. Like I can buy myself nice things.

THERAPIST: Right, I am talking here about the difference between self-indulgence and self-care. The reason I have a hard time caring for myself is. . . .

JENNIFER: I am not worth it.

THERAPIST: So you are walking around with the belief that you are not worth it. Okay, that makes sense. So help me figure this out, if you don't believe you are worth it, how does that get you to not taking your medication?

JENNIFER: Well, if I am not worth it, then doing something good for myself is kind of a moot point. You don't do good things for someone who's worthless, right? And ultimately, even though I hate them, there is part of me that knows that taking the meds is good for me. I am not worth it, therefore I don't take my meds.

THERAPIST: So you would have to really work against a core belief in order to take your medication regularly. I can see how hard that might be. You are also saying that the side effects are a problem. That is one of the biggest reasons that people don't take their meds, so let's look at that. . . .

Here, the therapist is not focused yet on challenging or working to modify the beliefs of the patient. Rather, she is attempting to build rapport, validate the patient's struggle, and solicit information regarding problems associated with noncompliance. Strategic self-disclosure on the part of the therapist can be beneficial, if the therapist has struggled with something similar. The therapist was effective in soliciting the information from the patient regarding medications in part because the patient did not experience the therapist as assuming that she knew how the patient moved from one level to the next.

Consider Functional Assessments of Behavior

Despite the utility of the case conceptualization, our patients' behaviors do not occur in a vacuum. Environmental contingencies shape all of our behaviors. Therefore, it is also useful to assess the *function* of the beliefs and behaviors associated with noncompliance, that is, the consequences the patient is soliciting by having the thought, by engaging in the behavior, or by experiencing or expressing the emotion. For instance, the function of not complying with medication may be to reduce the demands of the environment, to reinforce the patient's sense of autonomy, or to increase the likelihood of hospitalization, if that is reinforcing. The therapist may wish to assess not only the *actual* function of the noncompliance for the individual but also the *hoped for* and interpersonal functions of the noncompliance in the patient's environment. In a way this is similar to doing a cost–benefit analysis with an emphasis on the consequences of the behavior in the patient's environment.

The therapist should be curious about who or what is reinforcing the noncompliance. For example, a patient who historically receives little nurturance from her husband has his full attention when she decompensates. This is not meant to imply that the patient deliberately engages in noncompliance as a way to receive nurturing from her husband, but it does suggest that she has been subtly reinforced for decompensating nonetheless. Conversely, what could the patient imagine would be sufficient reinforcement for complying? What would have to change in her environment? Behavioral chain analyses are helpful here. For instance, avoidance of the side effects of weight gain or motor and concentration difficulties that accompany antipsychotic and mood-stabilizing medication reduces adherence (Fenton et al., 1997). The patient may fear that her family and others will reject her if she is fat or exhibiting odd motor movements in public. Accordingly, it is advisable to involve the patient's social network in treatment when possible, particularly when the functional analysis reveals contingencies related to the patient's significant others. The following exchange illustrates the use of assessing the "hoped for" function of noncompliance.

THERAPIST: So when you think about the fact that you aren't taking the medication that everyone else wants you to take, what do you think is the function of that behavior?

JENNIFER: I don't know. I just don't take the meds. I forget.

THERAPIST: That may be. You may forget, and at the same time, what is your secret wish? If I forget to take my meds then I can . . .

JENNIFER: Be normal. Party with my friends. Not have to think about it.

THERAPIST: Those are all compelling reasons not to take your medication. So "being normal" is an important part of it.

JENNIFER: It's like those guys on TV who get into those high-speed chases. They know they're going down eventually. I don't think any of them really expect that they are going to get away, but they keep going because as long as they are running, they are still free.

THERAPIST: So in some ways, the function of the noncompliance is to increase a sense of freedom in your life, a sense of normalcy. What are you hoping that other people will do when you don't comply with your meds?

JENNIFER: I am not hoping for anything from them. I am not doing it for them.

THERAPIST: At the same time, your not taking the meds has an impact on the people around you, right? They have a lot of opinions and behaviors that go with your not taking your meds. What are you hoping they might do . . . if I don't take my meds, then maybe they will. . . .

JENNIFER: Leave me alone. Let me do my thing and solve my own problems.

THERAPIST: So one of the hopes is that by not complying with the meds, people will recognize your independence. Am I getting that right?

JENNIFER: Yeah, now that you say that though. . . . I don't know. It sounds strange.

THERAPIST: Well, I can see how insisting on doing things your way is a way to let everyone else know you are your own person. I can imagine that feels a little empowering. So, what actually happens?

JENNIFER: I get harassed and hospitalized.

THERAPIST: So . . . ummm. . . .

JENNIFER: (*Laughs.*) Yeah, doesn't look good, does it?

THERAPIST: At the same time, I can see how it would get them to leave you alone . . . if you don't comply often enough. . . .

JENNIFER: Yeah, they will eventually get disgusted with me and give up or something. Ewww . . . that's not how I want to do it though.

THERAPIST: Right, you'd rather have integrity about it. It's important to recognize how the approach you are taking now still kinda works though.

JENNIFER: Yeah, but who wants that?

Again, the therapist here is not emphasizing challenging the thoughts yet. The questioning is mild and focused on mirroring, empathizing, and validating the patient. There is some guided discovery here, but the conclusions about the functions and the consequences of the strategy are left to the patient.

BE MINDFUL OF THE LEVEL OF INSIGHT WHILE PROVIDING PSYCHOEDUCATION

Denial of illness can be a significant roadblock to medication compliance at any time, and it is especially significant during the acute phase of illness (Cuffel, Alford, Fischer, & Owen, 1996). Collaborative empiricism, a central tenet of cognitive therapy, involves treating patients as informed consumers and providing them with information about their illness. The challenge arises when the patient does not want to hear the information provided or frankly disagrees with the diagnosis and treatment plan.

In the therapist's attempt to provide psychoeducation, merely assessing the symptoms may be incredibly painful for the patient, and providing psychoeducation about the disorder can be overwhelming and experienced as "flooding" by the patient. Thus, in the process of providing psychoeducation, the therapist should be mindful of the patient's shifts in affect and subtle and not-so-subtle objections. The therapist should ask the patient to rephrase or summarize what is being said and to identify any obstacles or misunderstandings that might ensue. The therapist can ask the patient to describe the symptoms of schizophrenia, automatic thoughts about those symptoms, what it would mean if they were diagnosed, and what the worst-case, best-case, and most likely scenarios would be if they accepted the diagnosis and took medication.

Unilateral attempts to insist on the treatment protocol are rarely effective. Statements such as, "You'll be on these medications for the rest of your life," "There is no cure for your illness, you are just going to have to manage it," or "You must not want to get better, because everyone knows that people with your problem need these meds," all exemplify the unrealistic expectation that clinicians can rely on the status of their position and expertise to ensure patient compliance. Amador and Johanson (2000) point out that whether we like it or not, the patient is the boss. If patients do not want to take their medications, they will not.

Alternative forms of psychoeducation in the face of denial include honoring the patient's ambivalence, agreeing on the life problems that the patient is having, but also agreeing to address presumed causes in the future. This is a good opportunity to reframe the patient's conviction about the need for medication as a set of beliefs that may or may not be true and that therefore can be experimentally tested. Additionally, the therapist can acknowledge that medication compliance is a problem in the eyes of the therapist, family, and so forth, not of the patient. However, if the patient wants the therapist to work on other goals with him or her or to help him or her pursue his or her values, the therapist would be more motivated to do so if the patient agreed to work on medications as well.

DEVELOP AND UTILIZE THE THERAPEUTIC ALLIANCE

The better the therapeutic alliance, the better the treatment adherence (e.g., Cohen, Parikh, & Kennedy, 2000). Several studies suggest that if the therapeutic alliance is secure, patients will be compliant with medications, even if they do not believe they are sick (Fenton et al., 1997). Increasingly, however, patients with schizophrenia and bipolar disorder receive care from a physician for medications and from a nonphysician psychotherapist for therapy. Little systematic research has been done on nonphysician therapists, medication compliance, and cognitive-behavioral therapy.

Several studies suggest that a primary reason that patients report medication nonadherence is complication from side effects (Valenstein et al., 1998). Compounding this problem, physicians are often remiss in their duty to assess side effects and therefore miss opportunities to reassess the medication profile and to optimize compliance on their end (Fenton et al., 1997). Fletcher (1989) frames this type of low adherence as a relationship problem. For instance, underreporting of nonadherence or side effects is framed as a strategy by the patient to preserve the relationship with the physician and avoid confrontation. Ultimately, a way to increase adherence is for the therapist and patient to collaborate with the physician to reduce the side-effect profile.

Studies assessing medication compliance for schizophrenia agree that the relationship that the patient has with his or her physician has a significant impact on medication compliance, whether or not the patient believes that he or she has an illness that requires medications (Fenton et al., 1997).

The therapist should attempt to improve the patient's interpersonal and assertiveness skills to ensure that the patient is receiving adequate care and attention from the treating physician. The clinician can model effective communication with the physician through role plays in session and can examine the patient's automatic thoughts and assumptions in communicating with the physician. Patients may have maladaptive thoughts regarding their relationship with their physicians that can be addressed through straightforward cognitive therapy techniques. We can examine some of the cognitive distortions associated with the relationship that patient's have with their treating physician and propose rational responses (see Table 16.1).

ADOPT A LONG-TERM APPROACH TO MEDICATION COMPLIANCE

One physician generally begins his sessions with recently diagnosed patients with bipolar disorder by saying gently but firmly, "You can look forward to three or four hospitalizations before you really understand the gravity of your illness and the importance of remaining compliant with your meds. Most of your hospitalizations will be a direct result of problems with compliance to your medications. Right now you probably don't believe that. I wouldn't either if I were you. My job is to work with you so you don't seriously harm yourself or others while you are learning this lesson." Because many antipsychotic and mood-stabilizing medications have a long half life, the patient may not see the relationship between medication

TABLE 16.1. Sample Distortions about the Physician–Patient Relationship

Cognitive distortion	Example	Rational response example
All-or-nothing thinking	"My doctor is no good. He doesn't listen to what I want at all."	"It may be true that I have had trouble getting the doctor to listen to my objections. I can either learn to be more effective in my communication, get another doctor, or accept that he may never be willing to take me off of medications completely."
Overgeneralization	"My doctor once gave me medications that had a lot of side effects. She doesn't know what she's doing."	"Side effects are unpleasant. At the same time, neither of us knew that I would develop side effects from that medication. She has prescribed me other things that have worked well."
Mind reading	"My doctor doesn't like me."	"Maybe and then again maybe not. There isn't a lot of evidence to suggest he doesn't. Let's say it's true though. What would I need to do to improve my relationship with him?"
Personalization and blame	"It's my doctor's fault that I am not getting better."	"Although I put my trust in a doctor's care, it is ultimately my illness, and I need to take responsibility for it and do my part to deal with my illness."
Catastrophizing	"I am never going to get better, this is awful! My life is over!"	"I have better days and worse days. Everyone has some limitations, I can choose to focus on those or I can work with what I have got."
Emotional reasoning	"I don't feel like dealing with my doctor."	"Is that going to move me closer or further away from health?"

(continued)

Cognitive distortion	Example	Rational response example
"Should" statements	"I shouldn't have to be the one to talk to my doctor. He's the doctor; he should know what to do!"	"That would be nice, and yet, the reality that I am in means that if I want to take care of my health, I can't expect my doctor to read my mind."

noncompliance and hospitalization. The therapist should indicate the necessity of continuous medication compliance to ensure proper blood levels. However, if the patient does not believe that he or she has a problem that necessitates medication, then indicating that proper blood levels are needed for the medication to be effective is a moot point.

Thus it may not be possible to use traditional cognitive strategies immediately. The therapist may have to "ride out" a lack of compliance and even entertain having the patient committed if he or she poses a credible threat to him- or herself or others or if his or her self-care skills (food, clothing, and shelter) are seriously compromised. In the case of patients who refuse to take medication and drop out of therapy, the therapist is reminded to adopt a long-term approach. Creating a safe enough place for the patient to return after refusing medications is key. Patients are often ashamed that they did not listen and sheepish about returning. Furthermore, if they continue to have diminished insight despite an acute episode and if the therapist is associated with a perceived misdiagnosis, the likelihood that patients will return for help is low.

Motivational interviewing (Miller & Rollnick, 1991) and dialectical behavior therapy for substance abuse (Dimeff, Rizvi, Brown, & Linehan, 2000) may be helpful in framing the dialectic between aiming for compliance and, at the same time, acknowledging and accepting that there will be slips. Adopting a long-term approach to medication compliance implies recognizing that it is likely in psychotic disorders, acute manic phases, and major depressive episodes that patients may insist that they no longer need the medication and discontinue it. For instance, a profoundly depressed patient may have the thought, "nothing will make a difference anyway, I might as well stop taking my medication." If the patient insists on discontinuing medication, as a last resort the physician, therapist, and patient can frame this decision as an opportunity to collect data. The therapist can ask the patient what would be compelling enough evidence to suggest that the patient needed medication and how that data would be collected. The therapist may also wish to point out that the short-term consequences of not taking medications (i.e., cessation of sedation, decreased appetite) are in fact reinforcing and valid. These consequences should not be dismissed.

INCREASE COMMUNICATION AND COOPERATION FROM COLLATERAL SOURCES

Including the family increases the likelihood of medication compliance and reduces the likelihood of relapse (e.g., Craighead, Miklowitz, Frank, & Vajk, 2002). Patients whose families refuse to be part of treatment have lower compliance rates (Mari & Streiner, 1996). However, family members may be unwilling to participate in the patient's treatment because the patient burned bridges between them over the long course of his or her illness. If family members are involved, the interactions can be so strained that they actually increase the likelihood of rehospitalization (Rosenfarb, Miklowitz, Goldstein, Harmon, Nuechterlein, & Rea, 2001). Providing services for family members, including psychoeducation, emotional support, problem-solving skills, and access to emergency resources during crises, have been shown to reduce hospitalization rates and to facilitate recovery in patients with bipolar disorder (Dixon et al., 2001).

Familial and cultural beliefs about the role of medication in the treatment of mental illness can also complicate compliance. For instance, we have found at our clinic that in some Latino families, the possibility of mental illness and the need for medication are viewed as a significant weakness that should be turned over to God. The prospect of having a psychiatric problem that requires medication can be viewed as bringing shame upon the family. Trips to the pharmacist can be discouraged for fear that a neighbor might see the patient picking up medications. The therapist can help the patient conduct a cost–benefit analysis that identifies values in the patient's culture that *are* consistent with taking medication, such as taking care of one's health and contributing to the community. Through Socratic questioning, the clinician can help the patient see that taking the medications may help him or her to be even more assimilated into their culture. For instance, if praying is important to the patient, then the therapist can explain that taking medication that reduces extraneous voices and beliefs actually facilitates a communion with God.

The choice not to take medication may be a valid way for the patient to deal with a difficult family situation. Families may hide the medication from the patient, throw the medications away, lock the patient in her room when she is supposed to come for sessions, and otherwise interfere with compliance. For some patients it is a choice between taking medications and losing connection with their families, often their only source of financial and social support.

Although these examples are extreme, practitioners in private practice may face milder versions of the same relationship patterns. A disapproving look from a spouse or comments to the effect of, "How long do you have to take those things?" can undermine the progress that the therapist and patient have made in session. For instance, spouses are often upset about the sexual side effects of some medications and may encourage their spouse to discontinue them.

In contrast, many families are desperate for ways to improve the patient's medication compliance. In such cases, getting the patient's permission to include his or her family in medication compliance sessions, getting commitments from the patient to practice interpersonal skills with his or her family and physician, and engaging the family in problem solving increases the chances of compliance. For instance, if the assessment reveals that the patient is forgetting to take the medications, family members can assist by putting the medications next to the patient's plate at dinnertime, by connecting them with resources such as the National Alliance for the Mentally Ill (*www.nami.org*), or by having them read literature such as *I Am Not Sick, I Don't Need Help!* by Amador and Johanson (2000) or *Surviving Schizophrenia* by E. Fuller Torrey (1995).

Family members often contact the therapist to inform him or her about compliance problems, as patients may underreport. In this case, listening to the family member vent, redirecting their questions to the patient, and letting him or her know that you will be including the patient in all the information conveyed are all ways to gently remind the family member that your patient is the identified patient and naturally your first priority. At the same time, gathering this information can be useful in the case of a patient who underreports symptoms and adherence problems. Dealing effectively with family members may also increase the chances that the treatment plan you have developed with the patient generalizes to the patient's natural environment.

PRACTICE ACCEPTANCE

Many theorists and practitioners highlight the importance of balancing acceptance strategies with change strategies (e.g., Linehan, 1993; Hayes, Strosahl, & Wilson, 1999). However, the role of acceptance in medication compliance has only recently been described (Newman et al., 2002). It is easy to see how acceptance could be applicable to the problem of medication compliance: If patients were able to accept the need for medications, the limitations of the medications in treating psychiatric disorders, and the discomfort that accompanies taking them, then it is likely that medication compliance problems would diminish.

There are several areas of acceptance for patients to entertain—acceptance of the illness itself, acceptance of the change in their lives associated with the illness, acceptance of the symptoms, and acceptance of what the medications can and cannot do. All of these issues can potentially bring about a sense of loss and shame for the patient. Acceptance, however, is difficult to teach to patients because it is difficult to define as a behavior. It is often demonstrated by inaction (Dougher, 1994). "Enduring," "tolerating," and "allowing to be" are offered as alternative descriptions. Hayes et al. (1999) and others (e.g., Dougher, 1994) speak of *nonacceptance* in terms of the Western approach to problem solving. According to a "Western" ideal about a "good life," one should not have problems to begin with. However, if one does have a problem, one identifies the cause of the problem, one eradicates the cause of the problem, and the problem is supposed to go away. Therefore, if one does not accept something or insists that it not be there, it should magically go away. One can see, however, that trying to eradicate thoughts and feelings (which are often viewed as the cause of the problem) or even the need for partially effective medications can cause more problems. Accordingly, lower levels of acceptance of the diagnosis of bipolar disorder and high levels of denial undermine medication adherence (Greenhouse, Meyer, & Johnson, 2000). Similar findings have been reported with schizophrenia (e.g., Amador & Johanson, 2000). However, many patients with bipolar disorder and schizophrenia understand that they have the illness but still wish to discontinue their medications when their symptoms remit.

Acceptance involves a choice of pursuing one set of behavioral contingencies versus another. In order to accept, one has to have some awareness of the competing contingencies. The therapist may help the patient identify the costs and benefits of each of these approaches to solving their problems. Medications can make patients gain weight, decrease their sex drive, decrease their concentration, and make them tremble in public. The perceived benefits are often low, and these side effects can lead the patient, even if he or she understands the illness, to reject the medications. Often patients show unrealistic expectations and all-or-nothing thinking that a medication should exist that has no side effects. Acceptance of the medications implies that one may indeed gain weight, but that one still has to take them to stay out the hospital. Additionally, accepting "what is" does not imply that the patient must like the circumstances or judge them to be "good" (Linehan, 1993).

One patient told her therapist that if she accepted the need for medication, then she should no longer feel angry, sad, resentful, and so forth. The therapist was able to point out that the goal of acceptance was not only to fully accept the circumstances of her life (i.e., her diagnosis and need for medication) but also to accept that there would be a predictable set of private events (thoughts, feelings, sensations, and memories) that would accompany the acceptance. Their presence was to be accepted as well. Beck referred to this as "distancing" (Beck, Rush, Shaw, & Emery, 1979). Once the patient no longer insisted that her feelings and thoughts not be there, she was then in a better position to challenge her thoughts and make a less reactive decision about how to handle her emotions. Adopting a "yes/and" approach with the patient can also help foster acceptance. For instance, wanting to reject the medications makes sense, and at the same time, continually rejecting medications keeps the patient far away from his or her life goals. The therapist must also recognize that, in using acceptance as a tool with patients, goals and values are implied. One simply cannot accept all possible contingencies because they are inherently at odds.

There are situations that the therapist must accept as well. Trying to solve every problem is also a form of nonacceptance because it insists that a set of contingencies should not exist. Some patients will resist any attempt to make them compliant with their medication regimens. Therapists cannot and should not be so invested in their own wish to be effective that they do not accept the situation before them.

PRACTICE CHANGE STRATEGIES, PROBLEM SOLVING, AND COGNITIVE RESTRUCTURING

Acceptance of the problem allows both the patient and the therapist to approach problem solving more effectively. Following are practical suggestions for dealing with medication compliance problems gathered from therapists and patients alike.

- *Don't reinvent the wheel.* Get the patient's idea about what might increase compliance
- *Increase contact.* Start seeing the patient more often and assess medication compliance at every session.
- *Simplify.* Have patient encourage physician to make dosing one time a day, preferably at night, so that many of the side effects occur while patient is sleeping.
- *Alerts.* There are several programs now for PDAs (personal digital assistants) with alerts. One may also set alarms on digital watches or utilize machines that dispense the pills at certain times.
- *Pill dispensers.* Sometimes the answer is as simple as giving the patient a "days of the week" pill dispenser and showing them how to use it.
- *Consider injectables.* The best solution for many patients who do not manage their medications reliably is to use injectable medications, such as Prolixin Dacanoate, which needs to be given only every three or four weeks. Some patients prefer this solution so that

they do not have to think of mental illness and medications so often.

Cognitive Restructuring

The goal of cognitive restructuring in this case is to reduce the distress that the patient has about taking medication by examining distorted beliefs about medications and their effects, by helping the patient categorize the types of thoughts and their impact on the patient's behavior, and finally by helping the patient to evaluate and change negative, incorrect or dysfunctional beliefs about medication.

Table 16.2 includes suggestions for aiding the patient in challenging dysfunctional thoughts and behaviors associated with medication compliance. Although a few are standard for cognitive therapy (i.e., examining the evidence), a few are more experiential and draw on Gestalt and other techniques. The goal here is to balance the cognitive restructuring techniques with the acceptance and validation strategies explained previously.

TABLE 16.2. Cognitive Strategies for Increasing Medication Compliance

Desired outcome	Ask the patient what his or her desired outcome is with respect to refusing medications. What does the patient think is going to happen if he or she keeps refusing medications?
Examining personal rewards	What would be enough of an incentive for the patient to take the medications? What changes would the patient have to see in his or her life in order to make the medications worth it?
Examining interpersonal rewards	What rewards would the patient receive from the environment if he or she is compliant with medications? How would the patient like others to respond if he or she complied? How could the patient make that happen?
Shades of gray	If the medications were to reduce the patient's symptoms by 20%, would that make it worth the side effects and inconvenience? 30%? 40%?
Validating the valid, invalidating the invalid	For instance, "Makes sense that you would want to stop taking the medications when your symptoms are gone, and if you do it will make a relapse more likely."
Examining the evidence	What is the patient's evidence that the medications are ineffective?

(continued)

Examining the quality of the evidence	Where is the evidence coming from? Friends? The Internet? How does the patient evaluate whether the information is credible? Would it stand up in court?
Experiential techniques	Have the patient make verbal commitments to the costs and benefits of taking the medications. For instance, "Even though I know that I will be dizzy and gain some weight, I am willing to take the medications because I get to keep my children if I do."
Attentional focus	Identify medication-deterrent thoughts. Have patient treat them as if they are slightly unwelcome guests at a swank party. Make room for them, but don't pay them much attention.
Experimental techniques	Have the patient come up with several criterion variables and agree that these variables, if they appear, are signs that the patient needs to be taking medication.
Bibliotherapy	*An Unquiet Mind*, *A Beautiful Mind*, and other books and films that illustrate the struggle with accepting a mental illness and taking medications may help the patient.
Identifying with others	Although the Internet may not be the best resource for information about medications and its effects, patients often take comfort in online support groups, lists of famous people who have suffered from disorders such as theirs, and the like. Providing disclaimers and psychoeducation about the nature of information on the Internet is worthwhile. Patients with bipolar disorder are often heartened by the number of famous people who have spoken publicly about their illness.
Thinking about it on continuum	It may be true that the medication isn't wholly effective to control the patient's symptoms and that the side effects may, in fact, be significant. Work with the patient to think about it in terms of diminishing returns. Are the medications doing enough to warrant continuing them? Help the patient avoid thinking, "Oh, forget it! I already missed a dose, I might as well go off them altogether."
Looking at the patient's contribution to the problem	What behaviors has the patient engaged in that are bringing about the opinion that he or she should take medications? What would his or her mother, doctor, etc., say he or she has done that has upset them or made them suggest this? Is it possible for the patient to control these behaviors so that people will reduce their demands about taking the medications?
Predictions	Have the patient predict the severity of side effects and chart them over time.

(continued)

TABLE 16.2. *(continued)*

All or nothing	Challenge beliefs that medications should remove all of the patient's interpersonal and life problems or, conversely, that medications have no positive effects.
Designing the perfect medication	Have the patient create a wish list of medication effects on his or her life. See how many you can address using problem solving and consultation with the physician. Practice acceptance with the rest.
Examining permissive thoughts	"It will be okay if I skip this dose. Nothing bad will happen." Get detailed history of previous skips. Examine evidence that nothing bad happens. In the short term, this may be true, but generally this behavior is linked to noncompliance and hospitalization in the long run.
Future perspective	Have patient imagine him- or herself after 10 years of noncompliance with medications. What does his or her life look like?
Challenging magical thinking	"If I ignore it, it will just go away." How often has that worked?
Visualizing coping	Have patient visualize time in the future when he or she does not want to take medications and have him or her acknowledge why he or she doesn't want to take it but imagine doing it anyway.
Alternative interpretations	How many of the problems he or she is facing does he or she feel are symptoms and how many are things he or she can control without medication? Set up experiments to change behavior and thoughts associated with the illness
Reducing emotional reasoning	"I am feeling worse, therefore I should take more," or, "I am feeling better, therefore I don't need meds at all." Examine the evidence the patient has for how medications are supposed to be taken. Acknowledge that this is a reasonable approach to something like food, clothes, or even other medications, but not reasonable for mood stabilizers, antidepressants, etc.

CONCLUSION

I have attempted to outline some factors to consider when handling medication compliance with patients presenting with severe and persistent mental illnesses. The crux of the chapter is to encourage the therapist to accept the patient where the patient is and to cultivate a willing stance for dealing with the issues at hand. By fostering a sound therapeutic alliance and remembering that one can only go as fast as the slowest person in the room, the therapist may be able to improve the lives of patients even when they possess limited insight into their illness.

REFERENCES

Amador, X., & Johanson, A. (2000). *I am not sick, I don't need help!: Helping the seriously mentally ill accept treatment.* Peconic, NY: Vida Press.

Barrowclough, C., Haddock, G., Tarrier, N., Lewis, S. W., Moring, J., O'Brien, R., et al. (2001). Randomized controlled trial of motivational interviewing, cognitive behavior therapy, and family intervention for patients with comorbid schizophrenia and substance use disorders. *American Journal of Psychiatry, 158*(10), 1706–1713.

Beck, A. T., Rush, A. J., Shaw, B. F., & Emery, G. (1979) *Cognitive therapy of depression.* New York: Guilford Press

Beck, J. S. (1995). *Cognitive therapy: Basics and beyond.* New York: Guilford Press.

Beck, J. S. (2001). A cognitive therapy approach to medication compliance. In J. Kay (Ed.), *Review of psychiatry: Vol. 20. Integrated treatment of psychiatric disorders.* Washington, DC: American Psychiatric Press.

Cochran, S. D. (1984). Preventing medical noncompliance in the outpatient treatment of bipolar affective disorders. *Journal of Consulting and Clinical Psychology, 52*(5), 873–878.

Cohen, N. L., Parikh, S. V., & Kennedy, S. H. (2000). Medication compliance in mood disorders: Relevance of the Health Belief Model and other determinants. *Primary Care Psychiatry, 6*(3), 101–110.

Colom, F., Vieta, E., Martinez, A., Jorquera, A., & Gasto, C. (1998). What is the role of psychotherapy in the treatment of bipolar disorder? *Psychotherapy and Psychosomatics, 67*(1), 3–9.

Craighead, W. E., Miklowitz, D. J., Frank, E., & Vajk, F. C. (2002). Psychosocial treatments for bipolar disorder. In P. E. Nathan & J. M. Gorman (Eds.), *A guide to treatments that work* (2nd ed.). New York: Oxford University Press.

Cuffel, B. J., Alford, J., Fischer, E. P., & Owen, R. R. (1996). Awareness of illness in schizophrenia and outpatient treatment adherence. *Journal of Nervous and Mental Disease, 184*(11), 653–659.

Dimeff, L., Rizvi, S. L., Brown, M., & Linehan, M. M. (2000). Dialectical behavior therapy for substance abuse: A pilot application to methamphetamine-dependent women with borderline personality disorder. *Cognitive and Behavioral Practice, 7*(4), 457–468.

Dixon, L., McFarlane, W. R., Lefley, H., Lucksted, A., Cohen, M., Falloon, I., et al. (2001). Evidence-based practices for services to families of people with psychiatric disabilities. *Psychiatric Services, 52*(7), 903–910.

Dougher, M. J. (1994). The act of acceptance. In S. C. Hayes, N. S. Jacobson, V. M. Follette, & M. J. Dougher (Eds.), *Acceptance and change: Content and context in psychotherapy* (pp. 46–53). Reno, NV: Context Press.

Fenton, W. S., Blyler, C. R., & Heinssen, R. K. (1997). Determinants of medication compliance in schizophrenia: Empirical and clinical findings. *Schizophrenia Bulletin, 23*(4), 637–651.

Fletcher, R. H. (1989). Patient compliance with therapeutic advice: A modern view. *Mount Sinai Journal of Medicine, 56*(6), 453–458.

Greenhouse, W. J., Meyer, B., & Johnson, S. L. (2000). Coping and medication adherence in bipolar disorder. *Journal of Affective Disorders, 59*(3), 237–241.

Hale, A. S. (1995). Atypical antipsychotic and compliance in schizophrenia. *Nordic Journal of Psychiatry, 49*(Suppl. 35), 31–39.

Hayes, S. C., Strosahl, K. D., & Wilson, K. G. (1999). *Acceptance and commitment therapy: An experiential approach to behavior change.* New York: Guilford Press.

Klingberg, S., Buchkremer, G., Holle, R., Moenking, H. S., & Hornung, W. P. (1999). Differential therapy effects of psychoeducational psychotherapy for schizophrenic patients: Results of a 2-year follow-up. *European Archives of Psychiatry and Clinical Neuroscience, 249*(2), 66–72.

Lam, D. H., Bright, J., Jones, S., Hayward, P., Schuck, N., Chisholm, D., et al. (2000). Cognitive therapy for bipolar illness: A pilot study of relapse prevention. *Cognitive Therapy and Research, 24*(5), 503–520.

Lecompte, D., & Pelc, I. (1996). A cognitive-behavioral program to improve compliance with medication in patients with schizophrenia. *International Journal of Mental Health, 25*(1), 51–56.

Linehan, M. M. (1993). *Cognitive-behavioral treatment of borderline personality disorder.* New York: Guilford Press.

Mari, J. J., & Streiner, D. (1996). The effects of family intervention for those with schizophrenia. *Cochrane Database of Systematic Reviews,* Issue 3.

Miller, W. R., & Rollnick, S. (1991). *Motivational interviewing: Preparing people to change addictive behavior.* New York: Guilford Press.

Newman, C. F., Leahy, R. L., Beck, A. T., Reilly-Harrington, N. A., & Gyulai, L. (2002). *Bipolar disorder: A cognitive therapy approach.* Washington, DC: American Psychological Association.

Persons, J. B. (1989). *Cognitive therapy in practice: A case formulation approach.* New York: Norton.

Rosenfarb, I. S., Miklowitz, D. J., Goldstein, M. J., Harmon, L., Nuechterlein, K. H., & Rea, M. M. (2001). Family transactions and relapse in bipolar disorder. *Family Process, 40*(1), 5–14.

Seckinger, R. A., & Amador, X. F. (2001). Cognitive-behavioral therapy in schizophrenia. *Journal of Psychiatric Practice, 7*(3), 173–184.

Torrey, E. F. (1995). *Surviving schizophrenia: A manual for families, consumers, and providers* (3rd ed.). New York: HarperPerennial.

Valenstein, M., Barry, K. L., Blow, F. C., Copeland, L., & Ullman, E. (1998). Agreement between seriously mentally ill veterans and their clinicians about medication compliance. *Psychiatric Services, 49*(8), 1043–1048.

Weiden, P. J., & Olfson, M. (1995). Cost of relapse in schizophrenia. *Schizophrenia Bulletin, 21*(3), 419–429.

17

Conclusions

Robert L. Leahy

Therapists who see patients on an ongoing basis understand that the typical treatment module or treatment plan approach, advocated by those who wish to employ "empirically based treatments," is not always effective. Patients come to therapy with a set of expectations, strategies, environmental and familial problems, or developmental, emotional, and schematic issues that make straightforward, technique-driven therapy problematic. Some therapists may comfort themselves by labeling the patient as "not ready for therapy" and may self-righteously dismiss the patient as a "help rejecter." This attitude is unhelpful, to say the least. The question arises, "How can the therapist adapt the therapy to the idiosyncratic needs of the patient?" If the standard treatment is not working, then what changes need to be made?

Clinicians from different orientations will provide different answers to this question. One response may be consideration of differential diagnosis. After all, if the patient is demonstrating volatility of mood, the therapist may consider that the diagnosis should be changed from borderline personality disorder to rapid cycling bipolar disorder. Differential diagnosis may be an essential first response to roadblocks, as this may represent modification of pharmacological treatment. Thus the therapist may consider a different class of antidepressant (for unipolar disorder) or the use of mood stabilizers, anticonvulsants, or atypical antipsychotic medication (for bipolar disorder). Another response to roadblocks, indicated in a number of the chapters in this volume, is to examine familial and environmental factors that may impede treatment. For example, some patients are reluctant to mention their financial hardships when seeking treatment; others are experiencing pressure from family and friends who tell them treatment is unnecessary; and still others view psychotherapy, from a sociocultural perspective, as a stigma.

Another fundamental issue involved in roadblocks is inadequate socialization to the therapy model. Utilizing bibliotherapy may help offset this problem, but it may also be useful to spend considerable time explaining the disorder to the patient. Some clinicians fear labeling a patient with a "mental illness," as if mental illness is a stigma. This covert shaming of the patient only feeds into the sense that the patient may have that his or her problems are too shameful to be discussed openly. My preference is to "medicalize" the disorder by directly going to the diagnostic system and explaining the differential diagnosis, the pharmacological treatments available, and the relevance of cognitive-behavioral treatments. However, this diagnostic approach at intake may be off-putting to some patients, who view their illness as a weakness or a moral failure. Comparisons to other illnesses—such as pneumonia, diabetes, or hypertension—may remove the pejorative label. Examining the family history of mental illness—history of depression, anxiety, and substance abuse among other family members—may help the patient recognize the genetic link, thereby reducing the personalization and moral stigma of the illness.

Another fundamental roadblock is the patient's lack of belief that the therapy will be helpful. Many patients that we see come with a long history of both mental illness and ineffective treatment. Why should this patient believe that this therapy will be any different? While avoiding making promises to perform, the therapist may examine how the current treatment will be different from past treatments and may invite the patient to take an "experimental" approach: "Let's try some new medications and new interventions and evaluate how they are working." For example, a patient who has been depressed for the past four years and who has been on an SSRI medication may justifiably have feelings of hopelessness. The patient may say, "I have been in psychodynamic therapy and have taken medication but nothing has changed." Here differential diagnosis may be important. A medical workup might reveal a thyroid condition that is untreated. The patient might examine whether a variety of other classes of medications, higher doses of the current medication, or combinations of medications have been tried. Perhaps there is a persisting environmental or social relationship that contributes to the depression—such as persisting marital conflict—that can be addressed. Perhaps the focus should now be on behavioral activation, isolation, or passivity and rumination. The question should be, "Now that we know what has been tried, let's examine what has not been tried."

Both Schaffer (Chapter 10) and Marcinko (Chapter 16) provide specific recommendations for using motivational interviewing strategies to enhance therapeutic cooperation. These are valuable recommendations, as many patients come to therapy with mixed feelings, long histories of frustration in treatment, doubts about the very nature of the current treatment, and some investment in their current problem. Motivation for change may be an outcome of effective treatment, rather than a precursor.

Beyond these fundamental questions—which are often revolutionary in individual treatment—there are a number of ways in which roadblocks can be addressed. In this overview and conclusion I have focused on the use of case conceptualization, metacognitive and emotional issues, severity of illness, and the interpersonal nature of these roadblocks.

ROADBLOCKS AND CASE CONCEPTUALIZATION

One size does not fit all. Simple technique-driven therapy may fall short of its goals when the patient's approach to therapy is not consistent with the therapist's approach. In my earlier book *Overcoming Resistance in Cognitive Therapy* (Leahy, 2001), I indicated that the cognitive-behavioral model stresses the importance of structure, direct questioning of current thinking, empirical evaluation of the patient's cognitive schemas, self-help, and here-and-now issues. The therapist presumably involves the patient in "collaborative empiricism," identifying with the patient the thoughts to be tested and the goals to be pursued (Beck, Rush, Shaw, & Emery, 1979). It sounds wonderful—but many patients come to therapy with precisely the opposite ideas about therapy. They may view the therapeutic interventions as invalidating, risky, threatening to their personal schemas, and undermining their strategies of self-limitation (Leahy, 2001; Safran, 1998). Ignoring these issues will result in therapeutic impasses, passivity, withdrawal, premature termination, and other notable failures in the therapeutic process.

Why does this patient find it difficult to benefit from the manual-based, traditional cognitive-behavioral therapy? Some pharmacologists may respond that the patient's biochemical imbalance makes cognitive therapy useless—although there is no empirical evidence that pharmacological treatments are any more effective than cognitive-behavioral therapy for unipolar depression or the entire range of anxiety disorders and phobias. Psychodynamic therapists may propose that the patient is not "ready" for change, although readiness for change may be the equivalent to the hopelessness and helplessness intrinsic to major depression. The cognitive-behavioral approach suggests that the patient can change even if he or she is not "ready." Just as we might exercise when we are not motivated, we can also change our behavior even if we do not like to.

Three questions are posed in this volume:

1. What are the signs of therapeutic roadblocks?
2. What kind of conceptualization is useful in understanding these problems?
3. What strategies are helpful in reversing these problems?

The intention here is not to label the patient as simply "resistant" or "noncompliant" (although these labels may be accurate), but rather to move beyond the mere description of this phenomenon to how the resistance can be useful in deepening the therapy and making more significant changes.

In this volume, experienced cognitive-behavioral therapists have identified numerous dimensions of resistance to change or noncompliance. What may be especially helpful to the reader is to recognize that roadblocks in therapy may be evaluated from many different clinically valuable perspectives. The chapters in this book provide a rather comprehensive approach to many of the impasses that therapists will encounter.

Freeman (Chapter 2) provides an opening overview to the general nature of impasses in therapy, indicating that the therapist needs to evaluate issues such as familial, environmental, skill deficits, psychoeducation, and other "generic" issues. Needleman (Chapter 1) recommends that each patient's presenting complaints be contextualized by the case conceptualization. I have found that many novice cognitive therapists forego developing a case conceptualization and seem to mechanically throw techniques at the patient. This process results in the patient's perception that the therapist is naïve and does not understand the unique nature of the patient, thereby undermining therapy. Indeed, I have noticed in our clinic that when the therapist takes the time and effort to develop the case conceptualization, premature dropouts are avoided.

Why this resistance to using case conceptualization? Some therapists may incorrectly believe that it is too difficult or that we do not have enough data on the patient to develop a conceptualization. Or they may believe that only experienced therapists, with years of accumulated artistry and wisdom, are capable and worthy of developing these conceptualizations. I believe that these assumptions are incorrect. Therapists may benefit from reading Judith Beck's (1995) excellent *Cognitive Therapy: Basics and Beyond,* Jacqueline Persons's (1989) seminal book *Cognitive Therapy in Practice: A Case Formulation Approach,* or Needleman's (1999) own excellent book *Cognitive Case Conceptualization: A Guidebook for Practitioners* to see that case conceptualization is an attainable skill for the therapist. Just as the patient has homework to do, so also does the therapist.

Case conceptualization is immensely helpful in overcoming roadblocks. Indeed, many of the chapters throughout this book employ various kinds of case formulations or case conceptualizations, whether in dealing with emotions, therapeutic relationships, couples, families, or medication compliance. The value of case conceptualization is to help the therapist and patient understand the rationale for the resistance, noncompliance, or roadblocks in therapy. For example, the patient who believes that separation from her spouse is a sign of her failure and that her obligation is to protect the feelings of those who depend on her may find simple cost–benefit analyses and problem-solving strategies for separation to be cold, overly rational, and personally meaningless exercises. Simply identifying and challenging her negative fortune telling, catastrophizing, and personalizing will not be enough. It is more helpful for her to understand how her caregiver role, with reverse parenting in her family of origin—in which she took care of her parents and "protected" them from each other through her mediation of their conflicts—established a role for her in all intimate relationships. This case conceptualization allowed her to understand that because she was so busy protecting the needs of everyone else, her own needs were not identified or met. Indeed, she felt guilty about having needs, equating them with both defectiveness and anxiety. Similarly, she believed that no one could ever understand her needs, a belief reinforced by her narcissistic father and narcissistic husband. Moreover, her intolerance of her anxiety and her inability to identify and label her needs contributed to her reliance on binge eating, drinking, and dissociation. Developing this case conceptualization with her allowed her to develop the emotional and cognitive capability to separate from her husband and pursue more meaningful interpersonal goals. Therapeutic progress would not have been possible if the therapist had simply gone through a list of techniques, concluded that this would not work, and farmed her off to a pharmacologist to medicate her depression. Her reality would not have changed.

Perhaps the most compelling reason for utilizing a case formulation is to *anticipate* roadblocks and noncompliance, as Tompkins (Chapter 3) indicates. What does self-help homework mean to the patient? For the dependent patient, self-help may suggest that the therapist will not help and that the patient is being abandoned: "I came here for you to help me." Self-help may become an occasion for self-criticism and humiliation in some patients or control and subjugation in others. Still other patients may view self-help as further invalidation, suggesting that they do not have "real reasons" for feeling depressed. Perhaps because cognitive therapy is so action oriented and interactive, there are even more opportunities for roadblocks to arise. In nondirective therapies in which self-help homework would not be utilized, many of these issues would never arise. Ironically, cognitive therapy may elicit *more* resistance or noncompliance precisely because more is expected of both patient and therapist.

EMOTION AND ROADBLOCKS

Part II of this book, on metacognition and emotion, could not have been written 10 years ago. The foremost spokesperson for the area of metacognition, Adrian Wells (Chapter 4), provides an insightful and clinically useful guide to understanding why anxious individuals might resist change. Indeed, the belief that worry protects and prepares an individual implies that decreasing worry may imprudently expose one to harm. And the beliefs that worry can never be controlled but also always needs to be controlled place the unfortunate worrier in a catch-22 situation—trying to control the uncontrollable. Identifying and eliminating the "safety behaviors"—the superstitious behaviors that the patient engages in to neutralize the worry or to feel less vulnerable—are essential in modifying roadblocks in cognitive therapy.

Accessing emotions in order to activate the hot cognitions that may be core for the patient is a key focus in Holland's chapter (Chapter 6). Ironically, some people seek cognitive therapy because they wish to avoid more troubling memories and emotions. For example, a rather "matter-of-fact," "problem-solving" man, complaining of worry, wanted to acquire some tools for dealing with his anxiety. His view of therapy was that it would be a "skill-acquisition" experience, with a focus on self-statements and relaxation. Although the therapy did include these techniques, the therapist noticed that he was reluctant to talk about his family. Closer inquiry into this issue revealed that earlier memories of emotional deprivation and threats of abandonment by his mother were so emotionally evocative that he believed that he needed to avoid these feelings. This discovery then led to a discussion of his thoughts about his feelings—or what I would call his "emotional schemas." His belief was that he should always be rational, logical, and in control and that if he allowed himself to have strong feelings, then they would overwhelm him. Much of his anxiety was compounded by his fear of his anxiety and his belief that no one would understand him.

Evoking these deeper feelings by utilizing emotion-focused techniques described by Greenberg (2002) allowed him to overcome a roadblock in therapy. Ironically, the roadblock appeared to be his belief that he should always be rational and in control of his feelings—a set of "skills" he thought he would obtain in cognitive therapy. Attracted by the apparent "rational" basis of the therapy, he was surprised to learn that the therapy could help him access his emotions, make sense of his memories, identify the dysfunctional thoughts encapsulated in his emotional schemas, and test his belief that his emotions could not be tolerated. Indeed, this is a form of emotional exposure or emotional processing that allows access and resolution of more fundamental problems.

Emotional focus and emotional processing, coupled with empathy and validation, have proven to be effective in connecting patients to the therapy. With borderline, dependent, and avoidant patients—as well as patients with binge-eating disorder—I have found it immensely useful to begin the initial evaluation by focusing attention on how the individual conceptualizes his or her own emotions. For example, a female patient with borderline disorder, rapid cycling bipolar disorder, and a history of substance abuse was helped in her initial contact with the therapist by focusing on how she attempted to but failed in regulating her intense emotional state. Focusing on her thoughts and feelings about intense emotion—such as, "I can't stand these feelings" and "No one can understand how bad it feels"—allowed the patient to recognize that the therapy would be especially attuned to her emotional dysregulation and her chronic sense of emptiness, loneliness, and invalidation. These were the emotional issues of specific importance to her—and these would be a focus of the therapy. This led to a strong commitment to the therapeutic modality, something that she was seldom able to make in her prior treatments.

Thus the value of emotional focus in cognitive therapy is that the therapy becomes ecologically valid—it is part of the patient's "real" phenomenal world. This does not imply that the traditional cognitive and behavioral techniques—such as activity scheduling, relaxation, identifying and challenging automatic thoughts, and examining schemas—would not be utilized. Indeed, these techniques would prove useful in emotional regulation and emotional processing. The important difference, however, is that the patient's emotional experience would be the core focus. The therapy would continue to return to questions about her internal and interpersonal dialogues concerning her emotions: "How does this make you feel?" "How do you feel about telling me about your feelings?" and "What are the thoughts that you have about your emotions?"

SEVERITY OF ILLNESS AND COMPLIANCE

There are now effective adjunctive cognitive therapy interventions for patients with severe mental illnesses, such as psychosis or bipolar illness (Haddock et al., 1998; Lam et al., 2000; Newman, Leahy, Beck, Harrington, & Gyulai, 2001; Turkington & Kingdon, 2000). In dealing with individuals with severe chronic mental illness, the therapist often finds that the nature and severity of the illness impedes treatment. Thus, as Haddock and Siddle (Chapter 7) indicate, the paranoid delusions of the psychotic patient may make it difficult for the patient to accept the vulnerability of placing any trust in the therapist. Similarly, for the manic patient who believes that his mania is enjoyable and realistic, therapy may appear to deprive him of his opportunity to get as much out of life as he can. Negotiating precommitment strategies with patients—for example, to wait 48 hours before making important decisions—may be a useful strategy to utilize when the bipolar patient is in the euthymic phase. As with all chronically and severely mentally ill patients, there is the consideration of medication. As Marcinko (Chapter 16) illustrates, the patient's delusional beliefs may make medication problematic. Developing a motivational strategy of interviewing—presenting medication as an alternative with pros and cons to be evaluated by empirical testing—may be helpful. However, many patients paradoxically believe that because they are feeling fine when they are on medication, they therefore do not need medication; but when they are psychotic, they may view the medication as a persecution. Marcinko identifies how the use of case conceptualization and cognitive therapy techniques can assist the patient in modifying his distorted beliefs about medication. Because medication compliance is essential in the treatment of individuals with psychoses and bipolar disorder, it is essential for the therapist to be able to address the roadblock of noncompliance. Indeed, some might argue that this is one of the most important factors that may contribute to the added benefit of using cognitive-behavioral therapy with patients with bipolar disorder (see Lam et al., 2000; Newman, Leahy, Beck, Reilly-Harrington, & Gyulai, 2002).

Perhaps there is no more obvious situation in which resistance to change can occur than couple therapy. Any therapist who has experience working with couples knows that the two parties in the relationship seldom share the same motivation for working on the relationship. Not only do they differ in the motivation to change, but many patients in couples therapy also harbor beliefs that therapy will make matters worse or that therapy should be an opportunity to assign guilt. Hidden agendas may be examined in the course of treatment. My experience has been that these agendas arise when utilizing traditional cognitive-behavioral techniques. For example, a husband may be reluctant to engage in active listening—rephrasing, empathizing, and validating. His belief is that this active listening will only encourage his wife to complain more and that he will be overwhelmed with her complaints. Thus the husband withdraws or attempts to minimize his wife's expression. This further contributes to her belief that he has no interest in her feelings and that her only course of action is to escalate her complaints. (Needless to say, this role pattern can be reversed, with the husband acting as complainer.)

Identifying the underlying assumptions and thoughts that inhibit the members of the couple from utilizing active listening, rewarding, edited communication, or sensate focus can often be far more important than the actual "exercises" themselves. For example, the husband's belief that "I will change after my wife changes" will lead him to sabotage any homework assignments. Examining the consequences of this belief—and how it reinforces his wife's belief that he does not care about the relationship—may allow the patient to experiment with acting against this resistance. An experiment can be set up whereby he engages in active listening and pleasure days (i.e., engaging in positive behavior toward his wife) while predicting what he believes the outcome will be.

As with resistance in individual therapy, resistance in couple therapy often illustrates core impasses for the couple that may be the source of the couple's persistent problems outside of therapy. When the therapist encounters resistance from one or both members of the couple, this resistance can become a focus of inquiry—often revealing core assumptions and schemas that have contributed to the ongoing conflict. For example, when the therapist asked the husband to engage in positive tracking and rewarding behavior, the husband's noncompliance revealed his entitlement assumptions in the marriage—"My wife should change before I change" and "I shouldn't have to reward her for things she is supposed to do." His reliance on passivity and entitlement led his wife to withdraw attention from him and focus primarily on the children, thereby reinforcing his belief that he was not important to her. Thus his resistance to doing homework in therapy uncovered an ongoing problem in their relationship that could be more directly addressed.

Similarly, as Dattilio (Chapter 12) discusses, understanding how the consumer of therapy perceives the therapist and the process of change can be an essential factor in overcoming impediments to treatment. Therapists are not neutral stimuli for patients—especially in family therapy. Cultural differences perceived between therapist and patient may lead the patient to react to the therapist with envy, disdain, distrust, or fear. Psychoanalysts have referred to this as the "transference"—a term that implies a generalization from earlier family-of-origin roles (Menninger & Holzman, 1973). It may not be necessary to refer the patient's reactions to family-of-origin issues; the patient's beliefs may be currently quite transparent. One question that is important to ask in couple or family therapy is, "How does each patient view this process? How do they view the therapist?" Cognitive-behavioral therapy often appears technique driven, with clear-cut interventions offered to patients to utilize. However, if one family member in the session views the therapist as undermining his authority in the family, then that patient will undermine the authority of the therapist.

THE INTERPERSONAL NATURE OF ROADBLOCKS

The therapist can be direct about doubts that individuals have. Questions such as, "Do you think I am being fair with each of you?" or "Do you have any doubts about what we are doing?" can open the dialogue. Even identifying common perceptions can facilitate discussion of ambivalence. For example, I often tell couples that a common complaint about therapy is that the exercises seem artificial and lacking in spontaneity. This almost always elicits some agreement and discussion. Often, underlying assumptions about relationships are identified: "We should always be spontaneous"; "She should want to do these things—I shouldn't have to tell her"; "If we need this kind of instruction, then our relationship is hopeless." These critical thoughts may be tested by asking the patient to examine other important relationships in which one has to be artificial and nonspontaneous at times and the costs and benefits of practicing these skills, setting up predictions of how one will feel after these exercises are conducted and examining the possibility that practicing any new skill at first always feels artificial until it later becomes "natural."

Therapists who work with patients with borderline personality disorder can appreciate the many kinds of "treatment-interfering behaviors" (TIB) described by Foertsch and colleagues (Chapter 13). Not to anticipate roadblocks with these patients is always a mistake. Noncompliance with scheduling, parasuicidal behavior, and other TIBs are the highest priorities; the therapy cannot proceed without resolving these important problems. I have found that examining the patient's rationale for noncompliance can assist these patients. For example, the patient who relies on too many doctors for treatment may, on inquiry, reveal her belief that she is afraid of being abandoned by one doctor, so she diversifies her help providers. Thus, if she loses one doctor, she will have another to fall back on. Given her history of troubling therapeutic relationships, this belief makes sense to her. Similarly, the patient who relies on cutting herself may reveal that this has proven to be the most effective way of managing intense moods or that this is the only way she knows of to communicate her emotional pain to her distant father. Identifying the functionality of these behaviors, as Foertsch and colleagues suggest, is an essential step in developing alternative coping strategies for the patient. Simply telling the patient to stop doing these things without helping the patient understand the purpose and the alternatives will contribute to more therapeutic impasses.

Stevens, Muran, and Safran (Chapter 14) indicate that therapeutic ruptures may serve as opportunities to explore the patient's interpersonal belief system—that is, how the patient typically experiences ruptures and problems in relationships. The emphasis in their approach is primarily on increasing awareness as a means of change. Interestingly, the dyadic nature of therapy—patient and therapist—and the importance of the therapist's own experience of the relationship are highlighted by Stevens and colleagues in evaluating therapeutic ruptures, by Foertsch and colleagues in the use of dialectical behavior therapy, and by Dattilio in examining the therapist's underlying assumptions. In my own work, I have suggested that the "countertransference," understood primarily in cognitive-therapy terms, can be a useful window into the interpersonal history and current relationships that the patient experiences (Leahy, 2001). These interpersonal, or social-cognitive, approaches to roadblocks allow us to consider the reciprocal nature of the roadblocks. Some patients work better with certain therapists—not simply because of the therapist's skills but at times because of the therapist's own role behavior. Indeed, it is quite possible that the same patient may exhibit different roadblocks with different therapists.

Although the countertransferential nature of therapy has not been a focus for the chapters in this book, I have found this to be an important component in addressing roadblocks. For example, I will identify my own automatic thoughts, assumptions, and schemas that seem to be activated by certain patients. I then attempt to examine how my personality and my needs might begin to interfere with this therapy. Having evaluated how these human and neurotic tendencies may play themselves out, I then evaluate how this insight might tell me something about the patient's effects on others. If I am feeling frustrated and helpless, then how does this patient make others feel? If she is making others feel helpless and frustrated, then what schemas are activated in the patient? For example, if a patient with borderline personality disorder makes the therapist feel helpless, then this situation might activate the patient's hopelessness—or, concurrently, it may allow the patient the comfort of maintaining boundaries against the risk of merging or becoming too identified with the therapist.

FINAL THOUGHTS

Impasses are like pain or physical symptoms—they tell us to look further for what lies beneath. It is ironic that therapists often focus on their frustration in not being able to pursue their agenda of challenging thoughts, assigning behavior, and decreasing emotional discomfort. The question should be, "How can this frustration tell me more about this person?" "How does the patient's apparent resistance make sense to him?" Impasses may be viewed as a far richer source of information than compliance is. They may tell us something about why certain problems persist, as the rejection of help may imply that the help is viewed as more problematic than the depression or anxiety.

Just the other day a patient wanted to refer a friend to me for fear of flying. I thought, "I have so few openings in my schedule that I would rather refer this simple problem to someone else." I am sure that for this individual the fear of flying is very problematic. The problem for me was that there was not enough resistance, enough complexity, and enough of a problem to make it seem interesting. I preferred getting a new referral that was a more complicated, more chronic, or more difficult problem to solve. Perhaps it is this sense of challenge, curiosity, and even the willingness to sacrifice a bit of one's own discomfort that can make these "challenging" individuals far more interesting and intrinsically rewarding to work with. It is important to avoid taking the resistance personally and more important to be personally interested in the resistance.

I remember in high school the satisfaction of proving a geometry problem. At the end of puzzling through the challenge, one could write "Q.E.D"—in Latin, *quod erat demonstrandum*—"which was to be proved." It was the satisfaction of solving the puzzle. The bonus in solving these complex puzzles of resistance is that another human being can feel that life has more hope—a challenge worth pursuing. QED.

REFERENCES

Beck, A. T., Rush, A. J., Shaw, B. F., & Emery, G. (1979). *Cognitive therapy of depression.* New York: Guilford Press.

Beck, J. S. (1995). *Cognitive therapy: Basics and beyond.* New York: Guilford Press.

Greenberg, L. S. (2002). Integrating an emotion-focused approach to treatment into psychotherapy integration. *Journal of Psychotherapy Integration, 12*(2), 154–189.

Haddock, G., Tarrier, N., Spaulding, W., Yusupoff, L., Kinney, C., & McCarthy, E. (1998). Individual cognitive-behavior therapy in the treatment of hallucinations and delusions: A review. *Clinical Psychology Review, 18*(7), 821–838.

Lam, D. H., Bright, J., Jones, S., Hayward, P., Schuck, N., Chisholm, D., et al. (2000). Cognitive therapy for bipolar illness: A pilot study of relapse prevention. *Cognitive Therapy and Research, 24,* 503–520.

Leahy, R. L. (2001). *Overcoming resistance in cognitive therapy.* New York: Guilford Press.

Menninger, K. A., & Holzman, P. S. (1973). *Theory of psychoanalytic technique* (2nd ed.). New York: Basic Books.

Needleman, L. D. (1999). *Cognitive case conceptualization: A guidebook for practitioners.* Mahwah, NJ: Erlbaum.

Newman, C. F., Leahy, R. L., Beck, A. T., Harrington, N. R., & Gyulai, L. (2001). *Bipolar disorder: A cognitive therapy approach.* Washington, DC: American Psychological Association.

Persons, J. B. (1989). *Cognitive therapy in practice: A case formulation approach.* New York: Norton.

Safran, J. D. (1998). *Widening the scope of cognitive therapy: The therapeutic relationship, emotion and the process of change.* Northvale, NJ: Jason Aronson.

Turkington, D., & Kingdon, D. (2000). Cognitive-behavioural techniques for general psychiatrists in the management of patients with psychoses. *British Journal of Psychiatry, 177,* 101–106.

Index

"f" indicates a figure; "*t*" indicates a table

B

D

E

H

I

L